BACH FLOWER REMEDIES

FORM AND FUNCTION

By the same author:

Victorian Ceramic Tiles
   Studio Vista 1972
The Decorative Tradition
   Architectural Press 1973
A Guide to the Bach Flower Remedies
   C.W. Daniel 1979
Song of the Reeds
   Anne Jope 1980
Patterns of Life Force
   Bach Educational Programme 1987
Collected Writings of Edward Bach (editor)
   Bach Educational Programme 1987
The Healing Herbs of Edward Bach (with Martine Barnard)
   Bach Educational Programme 1988

BACH FLOWER REMEDIES
FORM & FUNCTION

JULIAN BARNARD

FLOWER REMEDY PROGRAMME 2002

First published in Great Britain 2002
by Flower Remedy Programme
PO Box 65, Hereford HR2 0UW

British Library Cataloguing in Publication Data
A catalogue record for this book
is available from the British Library

ISBN 0 9506610 7 4

Designed & typeset in Garamond
by Glenn Storhaug at Five Seasons Press, Hereford
Jacket printed by The Senecio Press, Charlbury, Oxford
Printed and bound in Great Britian by MPG Books Ltd, Bodmin, Cornwall

Contents

Acknowledgements

A big thank you to all who have helped with the ideas, writing,
editing, design and production of this book.
Graham Challifour: for listening, for advice and help
with illustrations.
Geoffrey Meadon: for the index.
Frank Page: for editing and corrections.
Tamsin Smith: for research.
Glenn Storhaug: for design and production.
The staff of Healing Herbs: who worked on with dedication
when I was away.
Those who have attended talks and workshops and shared
their experience and understanding.

The illustrations are by the author.
Most are original line drawings, others taken from photographs and
modified, while a few are redrawn from old illustrations. The picture
of Dr Bach on page 18 is from an original drawing by Julian Franks;
that on page 282 from an original drawing by Jean Addison—with
thanks to them both.

This book is dedicated to my two children

Alex and Taraka Barnard

Author's Preface

Writing the introduction for *The Healing Herbs of Edward Bach* in 1988, I suggested that book represented a departure rather than any kind of arrival. It has taken fourteen years to come to this point—a long time to be developing an idea. But the central proposition remains the same: the gesture of the plant and the gesture of the person are equivalent. The great strength and stature of the Oak is a reflection of the emotional condition of a person in the Oak state; the refinement and aloofness of the Water Violet type is paralleled by the delicacy and grace of the plant. What Bach discovered about the properties of those flowers he used as remedies can still be discovered today. We have only to look at them closely to make the same observation.

Observing a plant's gesture is helpful for those learning about the Bach remedies. It informs the emotional states. A description based upon the flower is as valuable as a description based upon the person. Both are needed. But the implications of this material, which portrays the form and function of Bach's flowers, could be carried beyond immediate application in diagnosis and therapy. If the remedies really work—and I, like many others, have experienced their working—there is real meaning in the way that a plant grows. The idea which instructs form cannot be based upon chance. There is, as Bach would say, a Grand Design behind the physical world of living beings. A grand design and a grand designer. This book is an attempt to represent aspects of that design at work.

Julian Barnard
Walterstone, Hereford
May 2002

Introduction

THE PHRASE 'BACH FLOWER REMEDIES' means different things to different people. Seven British judges have given the opinion that 'Bach flower remedies' is both an apt and accurate way to describe the discoveries of Dr Edward Bach. They said it is the only way to avoid the circumlocution 'a flower remedy prepared according to the original directions of Dr Edward Bach'. They said 'Bach flower remedy' is the generic—the type, the kind of remedy—just like 'herbal remedies' or 'homœopathic remedies'. And 'Bach' never should, never could, be used to identify the goods of one particular manufacturer. In other words 'Bach' could not be a valid trademark. That is what the judges said: one in the High Court, three in the Court of Appeal and three in this country's highest court, the House of Lords. It helps define what Bach flower remedies are.[1] You may think this a strange way to begin a book. But undue emphasis has been placed upon this phrase by those wishing to develop it as a brand name for commercial purposes. It only becomes necessary to define words after misuse. A part of the plan here is to suggest a redefinition of Dr Bach's work and his discovery of the flower remedies.

Many books have been written about Bach remedies, and most have focused on the therapeutic effects of taking essences. Fine: it is a valuable sharing of experience. But the time has come for a new assessment. It is now seventy-five years since Dr Bach found Impatiens growing by the banks of the River Usk, near the Welsh border town of Crickhowell. Over the years attention has always been focused upon either the remedies or the name Bach. Little has been done to place his work in a wider context. Nobody has properly considered how Dr Bach made these discoveries, why the remedies are prepared as they are, or why they have particular qualities. It is as if it has been forgotten why Bach flower remedies are made from flowers. Nor have the philosophical implications of his work been fully explored. There has been a tendency to use the remedies and forget the philosophy—often the way. But it misses the point.

In a lecture given shortly before his death,[2] Dr Bach stated that the real purpose of the remedies he had found was to 'bring us nearer to the

Divinity within'. It is this 'Divinity within which heals us'. All the philosophy, for him, pointed in this direction: it is the 'one Truth [which] has
mostly been forgotten'. Throughout his work Bach was trying to show
how health and disease are intimately linked to the way in which a person
lives and the need to make changes in that way of living. He did not
separate the person from the disease (his was a holistic view) believing
that what happened to the physical body was related directly to a patient's
mentality, their spiritual and emotional circumstances. He pointed to
the value of learning to take individual responsibility for health. Bach
remedies help with this and support the process of change. But to take a
remedy without understanding the source of healing is to miss the context
of learning offered.

The context for Bach's work can be understood from his writings.[3] For
him, medicine failed because it dealt with physical results and not real
causes. Even an apparently successful treatment was 'nothing more than
temporary relief unless the real cause has been removed'.[4] The real cause,
like the real cure, did not originate at the physical level. Disease was the
result of conflict between 'soul and mind'. These are terms which Bach
did little to define, but he pointed to a conflict between man's personality
and higher self, which he linked to a spiritual dimension from which
healing came. If plants help to heal it is because they too are linked to
this spiritual dimension. They are an expression of divine forces at work
in nature, part of a sacred world.[5] Scientific medicine is responsible for the
view that a human body is no more than a machine for living in. Bach saw
it rather as a temple for the spirit. His ideas were the principal obstacle
to acceptance of his remedies—the reason Bach has remained outside the
canon of medicine which places human action at the centre of operations,
rather than 'Divine Spark'.[6]

This is uncompromising material with which to work. Read what Bach
said and you will see that he did not pull his punches. The wording could
be modified according to the audience but the message remained the same.
Eradicating the symptoms of disease is temporary respite if the cause of
disease is not recognized and dealt with; and this does not take place at the
physical level alone. Yet some synthesis must be made: between religion
and science, between medical treatment and self-healing through the
spirit, between accepting help and taking individual responsibility. Bach
can be placed in the general stream of alternative and complementary
therapies without compromising the integrity of his message.

Millions of people use flower remedies and believe they work, although it may be difficult to explain why and how. There is a gulf between practice and theory. The problem lies with inadequacies of language and a lack of framework for explanation. There is no structure in physical sciences to explain the non-physical. And few will give a fair hearing to evidence, unless that evidence is obtained by conventional studies. This is the classic dilemma: how to prove scientifically something which does not fit into the framework of scientific belief. Attempts have been made but evidence can be both ignored and misinterpreted.[7] If there is reality in Dr Bach's discoveries then there must inevitably be a change in the perspective from which we view our world and what life is. Practical experience must modify scientific theory. The relationship between people and plants needs to be reconsidered.

Plants are sentient life forms, they are responsive to their environment; they can feel, react and move. They have consciousness. Research work at the Bose Institute, Calcutta, in the 1920s, showed that plants have a nervous system.[8] Sir Jagadis Chunder Bose (1858-1937) designed sensitive equipment which recorded plant reactions to a stimulus. Experiments in the USA, using a polygraph (lie detector), showed that plants reacted to human thought.[9] Bach discovered that particular plants are able to alleviate or counteract human emotional problems: Impatiens helps someone to release pain and irritation, Mimulus to overcome fear, Scleranthus to resolve vacillation and indecision. This is not based upon the physical chemistry of leaves and flowers but on the properties of some subtle energy within the plant—a kind of plant spirit or consciousness, which we have forgotten or lost contact with.

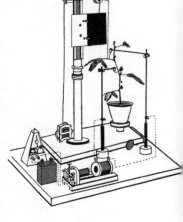

Recording plant responses

Theories on evolution, developed by Charles Darwin, concern only the physical form of species. He proposed that there would be adaptation to environmental influences through the survival of those best able to adapt.[10] Consciousness forms no part of that story. Yet it is logical to suppose, just as physical form has adapted and evolved, so too consciousness. Suppose that consciousness is integral to life and in some limited form was present from the beginning. As life forms evolved and grew in complexity, so too consciousness. As all physical forms relate through a common ancestry, so too all forms of consciousness. The discoveries of the human genome project show that humans share ninety-eight per cent of their

DNA with chimpanzees, fifty per cent with bananas, thirty-eight per cent with a daffodil.[11] There are grounds for the hypothesis that chimpanzees, bananas and daffodils share something of human consciousness.

This idea comes hard for Westerners because of the cultural atmosphere in which we have breathed for so long. We are taught that *Homo sapiens* has evolved as the dominant species on earth by virtue of intelligence, cunning and moral superiority. The problem began with the *Book of Genesis* and the Garden of Eden. On the sixth day God told Adam that he had dominion over all the creatures and could do what he liked with the plants (*Genesis* 1, 28-30). Then he was given the task of naming the animals and birds (*Genesis* 2, 19). Here began the idea that humans were both separate and superior to the rest of creation. In theological terms it gave rise to the notion that only mankind had a soul and that other life forms were subservient, other lives meaningless. The naming of species was a first step towards separating ourselves from the rest of nature.

Science developed through the naming of parts—its focus was the physical world. Adam was the first scientist. The narrowness of this science has become apparent, so full of fact and empty of meaning. But it is difficult to find an alternative which is more than hope and speculation. Wishful thinking may not lead to reality; one person's experience may not be shared by all. What if Dr Bach saw ghosts, lights, and patterns of energy, thought forms? Was it just imagination? What if he felt things not the result of physical forces? The chances are that you, the reader, will be in sympathy with that. But I do ask you not to accept what is written here in an uncritical way because of that sympathy. Please try to apply some science to the proposals made in this book. Only if something can be shown to be consistently true to any observer is it scientifically proven. So see if an idea can be validated, see if it meets objective criteria of observation. And then, if it does, the process of redefining our science and perception of reality can begin.

What exactly am I asking for? It is this. An essence prepared from one of Bach's flowers modifies a particular emotion. If the way that plant grows illustrates objective information about the emotion, a reconsideration of science is called for. Linnaeus devised a system of taxonomy based upon the reproductive structure of the flower. A further system could be based upon the quality of the plant's gesture: its root, its stem, leaf, flower, seed and way of growing. Observations could be used to agree a new language of evaluation to describe emotional states (fear, anger, doubt, resentment) in terms accurately and consistently reflected in the gesture of the plant.

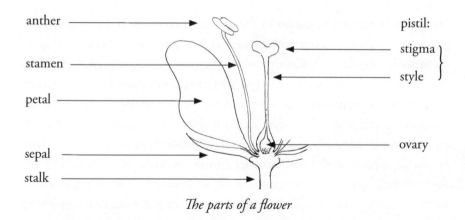

anther

pistil:

stamen

stigma

style

petal

sepal

ovary

stalk

The parts of a flower

A flower essence made from Gorse acts upon a person in a particular state of mind (hopeless and in despair) as a spur to renewal and a spring to new life. The spur and the spring are graphically represented in the gesture of the plant. Similarly, thorns on the stem of Wild Rose illustrate the need for stimulus to overcome apathy in that remedy state. The fact that Water Violet grows floating in water, without a root anchor, shows the detachment of this type of person. The explosive temperament of the Impatiens type is reflected in the exploding seedpods of the plant. At its simplest this means that yellow flowers hold in common certain ideas. Plants with hairy leaves have common attributes. The structure of a shrub or tree indicates the idea constructed within the physical and vibratory body of a species. This forms part of the identity of the plant.

It might be argued such observations are too subjective to be of value. But then I would ask you this: will you try an experiment? Gather a group of people and begin to make observations about a plant or tree. See what they say. Look at Aspen, Impatiens, Gorse, or any of Bach's remedy plants, then, after a while, read what has been written here about that flower. See if there is common ground. See if an objective language begins to form: a language of root, stem, leaf, flower and seed. I have done this with many groups of people and found that the observations are always consistent and directly relevant to the description of the emotional state which Bach wrote for the remedy. And, interestingly, on every occasion someone finds something new to say, a new observation about the plant.

Each of the Thirty-eight Bach remedies holds information of this kind—the gesture of the plant illustrates the emotional state of the person who needs that remedy. Form and function, therefore, extend beyond the confines of conventional botany to include a further level of study. First there is information based upon the physical attributes of the plant, then information about its gesture, the idea that it expresses. This second level includes the first but looks at a wider picture. The thorns of Wild Rose make this point. A functional view would suggest roses have thorns for protection. Alternatively, the thorns serve some evolutionary purpose by supporting the stems. Darwin observed that climbing plants use thorns to catch on to their neighbours, as other climbers use tendrils.[12] But the symbolic aspect of the rose and its thorns opens a new possibility for understanding, one not bounded by physical science. Develop this and it becomes evident that in plant study there can be a science of metaphysics and inner meaning. Bach's discovery of the flower remedies provides a key to understanding this meaning.

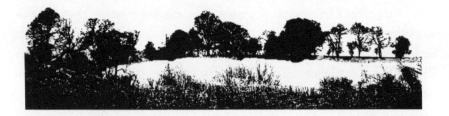

1 · A Growing Sensitivity

ANY ACCOUNT OF THE BACH FLOWER REMEDIES must start with the man who discovered them: Dr Edward Bach. The essential facts of his story are given by Nora Weeks in *The Medical Discoveries of Edward Bach*, first published in 1940, four years after his death. While we might like to know more about the personal drama of Dr Bach's life and may read her account as more hagiography than incisive biographical research, it does relate the basic events. This material has been repeated by most writers on the subject ever since. Research has been done which at least calls into question some of the gloss put on his life, but until now it has not been published. If Bach were here today it would be instructive to ask questions on those subjects where Weeks is strangely quiet—what of the family, your two wives, your daughter?—but there is the suspicion that such an interview would not get very far. Perhaps the private life of Bach was just that.

Yet a part of Bach's story is essential to our understanding of the Thirty-eight flower remedies he found. Events which led up to his decision, in 1930, to leave London and search for new herbal remedies tell much about the man and the process of discovery. This in turn tells us about the flower remedies. Edward Bach completed his basic training in medicine in 1912, at the age of twenty-six. In the following year he worked in casualty handling the blood and guts of medicine. He was beginning on the most physical level where, however brilliant the surgeon, the needle and knife are the instruments of emergency and last resort. Cutting open the physical body remains the coarsest form of medical intervention. Bach moved on quickly to more subtle forms of treatment and began work as a bacteriologist using the microscope in a laboratory. There he studied the different types of bacteria which inhabit the human gut. The presence of these bacteria is perfectly natural in a healthy person but in those who are chronically ill, hugely-increased populations can become an indication of the body's imbalance and may poison the system. This study went under the title of *intestinal toxaemia* and his researches led to the development of vaccines, the popular new form of medical treatment at the time.

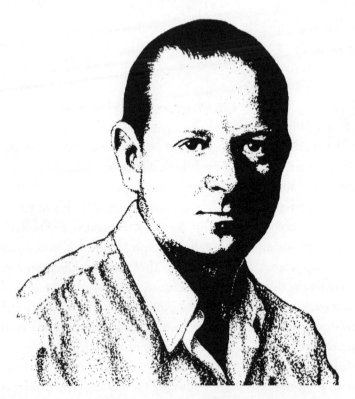

Bach was born in 1886, soon after Pasteur's development of a rabies vaccine. By the end of the nineteenth century, immunology and vaccine therapy were at the forefront of medical research. In the same way that the pharmaceutical industry of the late twentieth century was taken up with genetic engineering and biotechnology, the laboratory pioneers of a hundred years ago were convinced that vaccines and immunology held the key to world health and the future of medicine.

We learn from Nora Weeks that Edward Bach, while still a boy, was determined to be a doctor. What could inspire him more than the work of Pasteur, Koch (whose pupil Petri gave his name to the petri dish) and their colleagues? This was a time which seemed to be a turning moment in history, with brilliant reputations being made by the men in medicine who revealed the secrets of disease. The German bacteriologist, Robert Koch, had isolated the agent causing anthrax in 1876 and the tubercle bacillus in 1882; he went on to research cholera, rinderpest and malaria. The major contagious diseases like typhoid, diphtheria and polio were suddenly open for study and treatment in a new way. Science was rolling back the frontiers of knowledge and with the proven benefits of Lister's antiseptics it appeared that microbes were the enemy of health and of mankind. The battleground was the cell, which had both friends and foes—stalwart armies of phagocytes and the threatening germs of infection.

Pasteur's work had established what came to be known in the 1880s as the 'germ theory': the idea that disease is a result of germs invading the body. These germs, though microscopic, were hugely powerful. They were the unseen killers, the invisible enemy. Germs were the simple agent which defeated the all-conquering Martian armies in H. G. Wells' science fiction story of 1898, *The War of the Worlds*. Aware of contemporary science, Wells allowed his readers to sigh with relief as the planet was saved from science fantasy by science fact. The Martian invasion force carried strange and powerful heat rays, weapons of mass-destruction; mankind was helpless. Ironically it was the germs, the very organisms which appeared to threaten us most acutely, which ended up saving the day for humanity: the Martians were slain by the disease bacteria against which their body systems were helpless and unprepared.

Without going into the detail of the issues raised by these advances in medicine, it is helpful to have some idea of what is involved. Behind immunology there is a pleasing simplicity: the body has an integral defence (the immune system) which will fight off invaders. It is possible to isolate the potential invader, bacterium or virus, which causes the problem. Once isolated the bacterium can be grown in a culture, made inactive and then delivered into the blood stream of an animal or human being. The immune system reads the 'vaccine' as the real thing and initiates the production of antibodies to defend itself. But once antibodies are present, should an active invader of that type subsequently come on board, the body is ready with antitoxins to neutralize the infection. That is the simple outline—the subject is complex and there are many variants on the basic theme of antigen-antibody reaction.

Vaccines of this kind were produced, then as now, using cows and horses as hosts to generate antibodies which are then transferred to humans. This was the process begun by Jenner with his use of the cowpox (*vaccinia*) virus to inoculate or vaccinate against smallpox (1796). By the 1900s it had become an industry. Researchers were needed both to isolate the pathogens which characterized individual diseases and to develop vaccines which might be used to counter them. Research might be directed at a specific illness or it might be more general, seeking information about the way the immune system works. Entering the field as a young medical graduate, Dr Bach must have consulted with his colleagues and professors to see where an opening lay. There was the attractive prospect of discovering a new vaccine or form of treatment which might bear your name. This was indeed to be the case for Bach: he discovered the Bach nosodes.*

Dr Bach began researching into what had hitherto been considered an unimportant class of *bacilli* associated with chronic disease. Since they did not directly cause any specific illness they had been ignored. Yet their presence 'in such a large percentage of cases when no other abnormal or pathogenic organism could be isolated'[1] offered a new line of investigation. By taking a sample of the patient's stool, it was possible to grow a culture of the bacteria present in the faeces. These could then be identified under a microscope. The predominant bacteria were then used to make a vaccine which was re-administered to the patient. The effect of the vaccine was to stimulate a response which changed both the bacterial population and the general health of the patient.

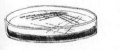
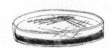

Bacteria grown in petri dishes

By 1919 Bach had taken up a post at the London Homœopathic Hospital. He was working in bacteriology still as a pathologist, not as a homœopath. But contact with the writings of Hahnemann and with the homœopathic doctors at the hospital nudged his research in a new direction. Previously he had prepared a vaccine from the bacteria of an individual patient and administered it in a liquid form with a hypodermic syringe. Now he began to use homœopathic methods to prepare vaccines in tablet form, taken by mouth. Again, we see that Bach was moving towards more sensitive and subtler forms of treatment, less damaging to the person. He avoided the needle of the hypodermic syringe because it punctured the skin and invaded the body.

In a paper delivered in 1920 he proposed that vaccine therapy was closer to homœopathic than allopathic medicine:

> *The resemblance of vaccine therapy to homœopathy is very close, so close that it is more a question: are they not identical?*[2]

In the case of his own vaccines, Bach presented evidence that their preparation, dosage and therapeutic action were distinctly homœopathic. Thinking, no doubt, that what he was discovering would be discovered by others in pursuit of the truth, he believed that all medicine would soon turn to homœopathy:

> *The attitude today of the medical profession in general is one of regard towards homœopathy; but when, as is shortly certain to happen, it is*

---

* Nosodes are homœopathic remedies prepared from the discharges of an illness.

generally recognized and appreciated that all modern research at the hands of the allopaths is rapidly proving and drifting in the direction of Hahnemann's laws, then will homœopathy be acknowledged to be the wonderful science that it is.[3]

It is extraordinary that Bach was so optimistic at that time. He saw allopathic medicine and homœopathy on a converging path of mutual respect and recognition; it was the path he thought that he was walking.

In 1918 the worst influenza epidemic in history had killed more than twenty million people worldwide and afflicted fifty times as many. In England and Wales 200,000 died. Vaccines appeared to offer the only real prospect for treatment or prevention. Nora Weeks says that Bach 'was allowed unofficially to inoculate the [British] troops in certain home camps with his vaccines, thereby saving many thousands of lives'.[4] Without evidence it is hard to know what to make of this assertion. However, it was demonstrable that an individual who suffered a mild form of infection could survive and remain immune—the epidemic illustrated the principle of vaccine therapy. At the same time it raised another point: what is it that makes a person susceptible? Why, if so many were infected, were some left untouched?

Bach must have asked himself such questions. Already his clinical experience had shown that a ward full of patients suffering the same disease had differing attitudes *emotionally* towards themselves and their condition. The emotional state of the patient influenced the prognosis. Fear was the great killer. So the fact that homœopathy gave a place to the mental state of the patient made it at once a beckoning prospect for Bach. Homœopathy offered a more complete picture of human health and disease.

During the 1920s Bach worked on with growing success. He had written a book—*Chronic Disease, a working hypothesis*—co-authored with Dr Charles E. Wheeler. The book deals with vaccine therapy and is notable for its advocacy of a raw food diet as a way of assisting the treatment of cancer; this in 1925.[5] Bach had come to the conclusion that diet was a vital factor in the equation since it influenced the *pH* (acidity) of the intestines and thereby the bacterial population in the colon. But reading his book illustrates only too graphically the work involved in a bacteriological study of the gastro-intestinal tract: faeces being the vehicle which carries the little fellows from the patient to the laboratory, so to speak. Bach was later to be attracted to flowers because of their healthy and healing qualities.

In contrast, he spent half his working life looking at faecal swabs and bacteria growing in a petri dish. He was later to speak of a desire to work not with the products of disease, but with the 'remedies of the meadow and of Nature'.[6]

As it happens, similar research on diet has been undertaken recently at Addenbrooke's Hospital in Cambridge, England. It appears to point to the same conclusions as Bach made more than seventy years ago. What Bach called 'errors in diet' cause manifold problems. If we eat the wrong food we end up deficient in the products necessary for health. We will also lack the substances which nurture those useful bacteria that keep the gut wholesome and provide a healthy lining to the bowel. Conversely, a wrong diet will encourage the proliferation of toxin-forming bacteria. These toxins can be absorbed into the body through the wall of the bowel. Furthermore, toxins produced from the wrong food, particularly those produced by cooked flesh, poison the system. Dr Bach thought the problem focused on the acid-alkaline balance of the faeces within the colon. He believed this should be acid.[7] An alkaline or neutral *pH* encourages the growth of bowel flora which are harmful. The problem is almost always chronic, resulting from poor dietary habits over many years, probably since childhood. Bach drew his conclusions from examination of patients suffering from long-term disease, people who were often terminally ill. However, the process is applicable to us all whatever our age, whatever our current health.

What then is a good diet, according to Bach? The essentials are plenty of raw food: fruit, nuts, cereals and vegetables. While a vegetarian diet may look to be preferable, it is no more beneficial than meat or fish diets if the vegetables are cooked. More important, perhaps, processed and preserved food should be avoided. Bach readily agreed that this would curtail the eating habits of modern western society. The purpose was to cultivate a pale-yellowish, odourless stool, indicative of a healthy colon! The problem, for most of us, he identified as a dark, foul-smelling stool from a bowel which is putrefying and toxic. These dietary problems are associated with clear symptoms which vary according to the type of bacteria involved. Bach wrote of headaches, lassitude, fatigue and anxiety. More generally, however, intestinal toxaemia is 'gradually and insidiously lowering the vitality of the individual and giving increased susceptibility to both acute and chronic disease'.[8]

Dr Bach had a successful medical practice and a team of laboratory technicians who, no doubt, did much of the routine work of examining the bacterial condition of the patients. He had developed seven bacterial vaccines or nosodes (the Bach nosodes) and these were used with success to treat a variety of illnesses. In the process, Bach observed that there were characteristic 'types' both physical and mental, who matched one or other of the seven vaccines. Indeed, he was often able to detect which of the seven bacteriological groups matched the patient simply by meeting and observing the person. In this respect he was already moving toward a way of working centred more upon the individual person and less on the pathological detail found in the laboratory tests.

As early as 1920 Bach was describing the characteristic behaviour which he associated with certain bacteria:

> Thus, individuals having unusual fears, such as dread of fire, heights, crowds, traffic, have almost invariably an organism of the paratyphoid group of bacilli.[9]

Or, as another example, the 'highly strung, nervy person with anxious expression' often has the Proteus group. The patient who appears to be in perfect health, yet has underlying chronic disease: Coli mutabile. People who bruise easily: Dysentery. Proteus, Coli mutabile and Dysentery are three of the seven bacterial types. At this stage he was describing observations from a notebook, not a fully formed hypothesis. But already the idea is emerging: the association between the personality and some physical factors which dispose towards disease.

In this Bach was following the homœopaths and their 'drug pictures' which drew a wider portrait of symptoms both physical and mental.*

---

* Hahnemann had been explicit about the way to observe a patient's demeanour:
'When the physician has finished noting down these statements he then notes what he himself perceives . . . Examples of the physician's observations:
1. How does the patient gesticulate during the visit?
2. Is he vexed, quarrelsome, hasty, inclined to weep, anxious, despairing or sad; or is he comforted, calm, etc.?
3. Is he drowsy or generally dull-witted?
4. Does he speak in a demanding manner, very faintly, inappropriately, or in any other way?
15. Does the patient lie with his head bent back? With his mouth half or open wide…?
16. With what exertion does the patient straighten himself up?
Organon of the Medical Art, Dr Samuel Hahnemann, edited by Wenda Brewster O'Reilly, transl. Steven Decker; Birdcage Books, Washington USA, 1996; pp. 134-135.

He was not content simply to make a diagnosis and name the disease, give some medication, then await results. He wished to understand the whole person, the varying influences upon health and, most of all, the cause of disease. 'Our object,' he says, 'is not to cure cancer, our aim is to prevent'.[10] Having treated people who were chronically ill, he saw that disease in the physical body was often the result of a long-acting process. Therefore he wished to look at the way we become ill, not merely fire a gun at the disease in the hope that this would destroy the pathogens. The process of distinction here is between the way mainstream medicine was going and the way Dr Bach was headed.

It was fundamental to his view of health that the body should not become a battleground for medicine. If the germ theory saw the patient as invaded by disease then some felt that the task of medicine was to counter-attack with pharmaceutical products which defeated the enemy: even today the military analogy comes first to hand when we talk of pain killers, the battle against Aids or a brave fight against cancer. Bach was inclined to a different view, but he too slipped into the language of warfare to explain why:

> The main reason for the failure of modern medical science is that it is dealing with results and not causes. For many centuries the real nature of disease has been marked by materialism, and thus disease itself has been given every opportunity of extending its ravages, since it has not been attacked at its origin. The situation is like an enemy strongly fortified in the hills, continually waging guerrilla warfare in the country around, while the people, ignoring the fortified garrison, content themselves with repairing the damaged houses and burying the dead, which are the results of the raids of the marauders. So, generally speaking, is the situation in medicine today; nothing more than patching up those attacked and the burying of those who are slain, without a thought being given to the real stronghold.[11]

So, treat the cause of disease; don't just tamper with the symptoms. But the cause will not be found by looking with the purely materialistic eye of modern science. Clearly he had been having some success with vaccines but a tension can be detected between the desire to effect a change for the patient and the knowledge that such a change could be symptomatic rather than fundamental.

Some of Bach's views on vaccine therapy may be deduced from his paper read to the Homœopathic Society in 1920. He begins with an outspoken criticism of the way vaccines are used: 'broadly speaking they are a hopeless failure compared with what they should be . . .'.[12] The reasons were first quality, and secondly, ignorance amongst practitioners as to the proper methodology. The quality question arose because 'large firms' were producing vaccines 'on an enormous scale'. To maximize the yield they grew and re-grew cultures so that they no longer carried the true imprint of the original organism. The practitioners, on their side, wanted straightforward remedies that were easy to prescribe while the manufacturers wanted remedies which could be mass-produced from an original without variation. In many respects we face similar problems today.

In his criticism, Bach is allying himself with the homœopaths and taking his lead from Hahnemann. Addressing the Homœopathic Society in 1929,[13] Bach gave an account of his work over the past decade and the development of the Bach nosodes, making a series of observations about Hahnemann and his *Organon of the Art of Healing* (published in Germany, 1810).[14] Hahnemann, apparently, used the products of disease to make homœopathic remedies: Bach did the same thing with his nosodes. Bach paralleled intestinal toxaemia with Hahnemann's psora. He quoted Hahnemann's principle that every epidemic and collective disease is different and will manifest different and individual symptoms in the patient. Bach stressed the need for proper administration of repeat doses, based upon the response of the patient: 'a law with which all homœopaths are familiar, but which will take a long time for allopaths to appreciate'.[15] What he referred to as the law of correct repetition of doses pointed a finger at the ignorance of general medical practitioners who were using homœopathy.

Continuing his list of concerns, Dr Bach suggested that for his nosode therapy a register of correctly trained practitioners might become necessary. His experience had shown him that the way the medicine was administered was every bit as important as the treatment itself. Yet there were two choices here: either Bach inclined to a more technical form of treatment requiring greater expertise and training, or he looked down a different road towards simplicity and self-administration. There was a signpost for his later proposal of a system of medicine in which 'everything may be done by the people themselves, even, if they like, to the finding of the plants and the making of the remedies'.[16] But this anticipates his discovery of the new remedies which were waiting in the wings. At this stage Bach was still taken up with homœopathy.

It is clear, then, from reading Bach's published writings and from reading Hahnemann's *Organon* that this treatise on homœopathy had a most profound influence upon his thinking. If Hahnemann was 'a giant in medicine whose equal has never existed',[17] what did Dr Bach learn from his reading? The early chapters of the *Organon* were an intense critique of medicine in the nineteenth century. What Hahnemann called 'the old school' was roundly condemned for what was essentially malpractice. Allopathic medicine, he said, works upon the suppression of symptoms, and while suppressive medicines are popular with patients they are deadly because the suppressed malady breaks out in worse form in a more critical place.

By contrast, Hahnemann spoke of bringing about a cure by stimulating the life force (*lebenskraft*) of the patient which activates in response to homœopathic medicine. This was what appeared so close to Dr Bach's vaccine therapy. He had been stimulating the patient's immune system by reintroducing the bowel bacteria. So his experience in medicine already made him open to the ideas of the *Organon*.

Hahnemann, in humorous tones perhaps, referred to the supposed recognition of a disease through pronouncing its name (preferably a Greek one) as if by knowing this name the allopath had known the disease for a long time and could deal with it as an old acquaintance. (The great endeavour of our contemporary diagnosis is similar: the patient goes to hospital for test after test until a name is finally given to the disease and the case declared hopeless.) Bach, by contrast, was to say 'it is the patient to be treated and not the disease'[18] or 'in true healing the nature and the name of the physical disease is of no consequence whatever',[19] or again, 'it does not matter what the disease is, the mood alone has to be treated'.[20] Hahnemann, too, wrote of the need to see each patient as an individual and emphasized the procedure for 'taking the case'—listening to the patients' accounts of how they feel and how the illness affects them individually. This became the basis for Bach's prescribing both his bowel nosodes and his flower remedies.

Hahnemann wrote of the need to test and prove the medicines and treatment upon oneself. These 'self-provings', as they are called in the language of homœopathy, involved the practitioner becoming acquainted with the physical and mental pattern of the illness through reaction to the physical substance which would become the medicine in its prepared homœopathic form. This proposition appeared halfway through the

Organon in paragraph 119 and it is, perhaps, the fulcrum of the whole book. To work with healing upon others without working that healing upon oneself is working in ignorance and can be no real healing. There are echoes here of the Apostle Luke, the doctor in the New Testament, who has Jesus recalling the words of the proverb: 'physician, heal thyself'.[21] Bach was later to take this as the title for his book: *Heal Thyself.* Whatever we may think of Hahnemann and homœopathy there can be little doubt but that this inspired Bach with the idea that the first person to be treated with a new form of medicine was the person who discovered it. In other words, physician, heal thyself.

A footnote to Hahnemann's paragraphs on knowledge of medicines may be the most significant of all that Bach read in the *Organon*. Paragraph 117 discusses 'idiosyncratic persons'. As an illustration Hahnemann referred to Emperor Alexius who recovered from fainting when sprinkled with rosewater. This may be an early reference to the use of flower essence therapy. Drops of rosewater were used to help the unconscious Alexius just as Bach was later to use Clematis and Wild Rose. That there might be hidden qualities in plants which would have a curative effect, was mentioned by Hahnemann in the next paragraph (118). Albrecht von Haller (1708-77), professor of medicine at the University of Gottingen, is quoted:

> . . . *a great diversity of strength lies hidden in these plants themselves, whose external features we have long known but whose souls, as it were, and whatever divine element they have, we have not yet perceived.*[22]

This supposed power emanating from plants has a close resemblance to the discoveries which Bach was to make.

One more paragraph of the *Organon* may have been of particular significance for Bach. Hahnemann discussed the preparation of medicines and declared that it is right for the practitioner not only to administer the homœopathic medicine but also to prepare it himself.[23] This assertion by Hahnemann was to cost him dear. Self-preparation brought him into conflict with the *Guild of Apothecaries*; they took him to court and succeeded in having his medical licence revoked.[24] What can we say? Here were the drug companies of the mid-nineteenth century striking out at a practitioner who threatened their monopoly. Bach, too, was to fall foul of such vested interests and had extended correspondence with *The General Medical Council.* His offence? Advertising new remedies, new uses.

The traditionalists of Hahnemann's day remained impervious to the ideas of the *Organon*. When Bach addressed the British Homœopathic Society in 1928, he ended by quoting his own words from 1920—'the attitude of the profession today is one of regard towards homœopathy'[25]—but the sense was more ironic than hopeful. Although his work with vaccine therapy continued until 1929, Bach failed to gain support and acceptance from the allopaths for the essentially homœopathic work he was doing. This must have been a disappointment. A paper published in the January edition of *Medical World*[26] was Bach's last attempt to interest his allopathic colleagues in nosode therapy. His tone is assured, the information detailed and precise, the methodology simplified (he had developed polyvalent vaccines which were more universal in their application) and the whole statement designed to appeal to the practitioner who could diagnose and prescribe in a straightforward way. But the essay was marked as the work of a homœopath pointing a lesson to members of the allopathic school. It was a lesson that they chose to ignore.

This was the time of expansion and discovery for Dr Edward Bach, the time when his ideas and intuitions were confirmed. The pathway that led him to the discovery of the flower remedies was three-fold. First, he was increasingly dissatisfied with orthodox medicine. Secondly, he was convinced intellectually by homœopathy. Thirdly, he was following the insights of his personal spiritual development.

Orthodox medicine, then as now, saw only the material world: its science was materialistic. It regarded the human being as a mechanism and its mechanics could be discovered through the science of disease (pathology). The study of the diseased body was supposed to teach about health just as the study of the dead body (necropsy) was supposed to lead to discoveries about life. When looking for the cause of disease it saw only material agents: germs, bacteria and viruses, physical infections. While a knowledge of bacteria might appear to be useful, Bach thought that it merely aroused fear in people since they believed themselves susceptible to invasive forces. He spoke of this at length in *Heal Thyself*, noticing that 'materialism forgets that there is a factor above the physical plane'.[27]

The turn of the year, from 1927 to 1928, was the crossroads for Bach. He was resolving ideas and about to take his final steps out of the mainstream of medicine. At the time, when Alexander Fleming was at work at the London medical school of St Mary's Hospital, about to discover penicillin, Bach was sketching out the first draft of his new remedies. It is a significant coincidence. Fleming's work, as we know only too well, was to launch the new stream of anti-microbial therapy. It led directly to the antibiotics which are used so universally today. Did Bach offer an alternative to antibiotics? It is a question that need not be answered. He was looking at a larger and more complex picture of human life.

On the second count, homœopathy was immediately attractive. Bach developed new techniques for preparing his nosodes using homeopathic principles. It is likely that the idea for the type remedies came from homœopathy. According to Weeks, it was at a dinner party that Bach saw how people might be grouped according to their personality and behaviour rather than their illness.[28] This moment of inspiration is somewhat legendary in Bach circles. It neatly illustrates the way that a skilled observer can understand a person through the gesture of the body: your body speaks its mind. But it is essentially an idea borrowed from Hahnemann who observed the patient as well as the disease.

As to the third aspect of this three-fold pathway—Bach's own life quest and spiritual development—little can be said for certain. He was careful to avoid specific references to any one philosophy or religion. He embraced a universal spiritual teaching which includes the Lord Buddha, Mother India, Christ, the Great Masters, the great band of the White Brotherhood. His references to 'Higher Self', 'Divine Guide', 'Immortal Life', 'Soul' and 'Grand Design' may give clues to the exact school or tradition that he belonged to. Some ask the question, did he meet Rudolf Steiner? Others see a connection to the Theosophists. We are told that he had a strong connection with Freemasonry. But even a thorough trawl of his writings fails to give a definite address for his schooling. Yet the statements are there in almost every paragraph indicating that the primary focus for his thinking was the spiritual context of human life.

Dr Bach was about to leave London and abandon his medical career, setting out on a new path in life. As any explorer would, he had looked at the maps, studied the past reports and learned what he could of the land which lay before him. But the journey begins, as they say, not with books but with the first step upon the road. There is a strong feeling that Bach was beginning the real journey of his life: the journey of his soul's purpose, the journey of destiny.

Looking at the development of Bach's ideas, from medical school, through the years of hospital work and on to his later research, one thing is clear. He travelled a road of increasing sensitivity: from surgery, through bacteriology, immunology, to homœopathy and flower remedies. To Aesculpius, the Greek god of healing, son of Apollo, is ascribed the aphorism: *first the word, then the plant, lastly the knife*. Bach had begun at the last of these, with surgery. But he went on to assert the primacy of spirit over matter. For him the pathway was to lead to just this place where the medicine of materialism was abandoned in favour of the plant-healers from nature. Yet both are given up in favour of the word, the logos of the Spirit.

2 · Down by the Riverside

L ATE IN SEPTEMBER 1928, Dr Edward Bach was walking along the bank of the River Usk between Abergavenny and Crickhowell in South Wales. It might have been his birthday, the twenty-fourth of September. He had left London upon 'a sudden urge'[1] and without the pressures of his work at the Park Crescent Laboratories, he spent some time in the country. He was continuing his research into plants. He took with him the only laboratory he now needed—himself. We know that he had formulated the outline of the emotional types for his new scheme. That was started after the Masonic dinner which Nora Weeks

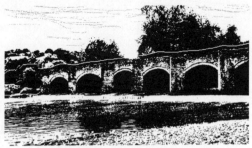

River Usk at Crickhowell

reported,[2] the dinner where he recognized the different gestures and behaviour of the people who surrounded him. As he watched the other guests, he realized some of them shared mannerisms, as if they were from the same family. There were types of people, related emotionally by their common fears, irritability, indecision or aloofness. Combine this with his idea that illness began with emotional rather than physical problems and Bach recognized the components of his new remedies. Now he had to try to find plants which would be equivalent to these human types.

Most of us, if we are doing research, begin by looking up the relevant material published previously. For Bach there was none. Herbals and pharmacopoeias alike spoke only of the physical effects of plant medicines—how we can take a particular substance for a particular disease. Bach was looking for an effect upon the emotional or mental behaviour of the person. This fact alone would explain why he made his search not in libraries but in the fields, not in the pharmacy but within himself. But it is not just the lack of previous information which led Bach to walk the fields in search of new ideas: he switched attention from the outer cause and effect to the inner cause and effect. This means that he looked at the person, not at the disease. And not just any person, but at himself. For the point cannot have been lost upon Bach that if every person behaves in one of the characteristic ways which he supposed, either fearful or dreamy, impatient or uncertain then he himself must behave in one such way. If everybody belonged to one such category so too must Edward Bach. So he made the decision to start by finding a remedy for himself.

What kind of man was Dr Bach? What we know of him comes from Nora Weeks,[3] and while it is clear she loved Bach she tells us little about him personally. But there are gleanings. Bach preferred to work alone, he was clear about his life aims and had a dislike of 'set hours for work, of rules and regulations'.[4] He had great energy and liked to do things for himself (like making his own furniture); he was not an easy, social person, rather a loner, certain of himself and impulsive, determined and with strong convictions. He was quick to make up his mind. Bach reckoned to be able to tell the nosode type of any patient crossing the consulting room to sit down. The body type and the way of walking, the gesture of the person, gave immediate clues to their type. Look at a photograph of Bach. What can we detect about his type?

Two doctors, C. E. and F. J. Wheeler, and Bach's colleague Victor Bullen gave more personal impressions.[5] They wrote that he had a quick and original mind, was courageous, fearless, altruistic and generous. All fine stuff. But more significantly, perhaps, he was irritated by wearing a hat, making 'small unconscious shakes and jerks'[6] as if trying to shake it off. F. J. Wheeler called him direct and said he refused to argue or convince others of his reasoning. He was quick to decide, quick to act and quick to anger, sometimes impatient at the slowness of others. Bullen also spoke of his quick anger which was quickly over but stressed his compassion, gentleness and inspiring confidence.

From this information it would be easy enough now to say that Bach was an Impatiens type. The positive aspects: gentle, balanced and relaxed. And the down side of the personality? —tense, irritable and impatient. So if Bach was looking for his own remedy, this at least is a beginning of a profile for the human side. What will be the profile for the flower?

Edward Bach did actually begin by detailed observation of plants. Nora Weeks reported of him that he 'spent the day long examining a great variety of plants, noting where they grew, what soil they chose to grow upon, the colour, shape and number of their petals, whether they spread by tuber, root or seed . . .'.[7] He spent hours sitting to study 'the habits and characteristics of each flower, plant and tree' and had told her that she must learn to recognize each of the remedy plants at every stage of its growth. Just how Bach made use of his observations is not clear from any records he published.

There is no doubt Bach was intuitive.[8] He may have been a psychic clairvoyant. However, psychism simply removes to another level the question of how anyone, Bach or his spirit guide, could find the plant whose qualities were being sought: a counterbalance to the emotional type or group to which he belonged. If some other being gave Bach the answers it makes no difference to us; neither can be asked today. So we can only face the plant and ask the question. What he might recognize at the subtle, invisible level must also manifest the same truth in the physical form and vice versa. In that respect we are, I believe, in the same shoes as Bach when he walked along the riverbank in 1928. This is the man, this is the plant: how do they correspond?

Impatiens glandulifera, or *Impatiens roylei* (*roylei* after Royle, professor of botany)[9] as it was originally named, is an annual. It grows from seed each year, germinating in the spring. By July it can be more than two metres tall, given favourable conditions. It likes the loose, damp soil by water and thrives on any kind of fertilizer. The seeds are heavy and remain lodged in the banks of silt after winter floods. Once germinated, they cover the bare soil with a vigorous growth. So a colony of plants develops, choking back any competitor with superior growth and numbers.

Impatiens

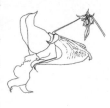

Impatiens is the Himalayan Balsam, introduced into Britain in 1839. Its colonization of British waterways is an astonishing success story; it is one of the most prolific aliens in the British flora. Although there are a few other *Impatiens* that have naturalized in Europe none is as successful as *I. glandulifera*. In the Himalayas, at heights from 1,800 to 4,000 metres (quite some altitude) it is equally dominant. F. S. Smythe in *The Valley of Flowers* (1938) wrote that once these plants 'get hold of the ground, pastureland is permanently ruined'.[10] This tall balsam covers acres and acres in a sheet of bloom—a wilderness of flowering balsam.

It is not a popular plant in Britain since it dominates the local species, lining the riverbanks and canals. An advertisement in *The Hereford Times* a few years ago called for volunteers to walk the banks of the River Wye to slash down and destroy the Impatiens. In Worcestershire a local wildlife trust also goes out balsam bashing on marshland reserves.[11] In the garden of a private house in

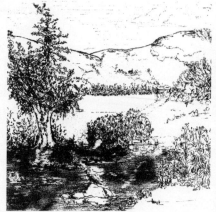

Impatiens growing on the river bank

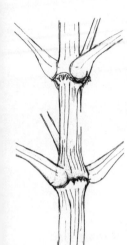

Essex, a neighbour crept in at night to destroy Impatiens growing there. This is a plant which people react to!

Compared to most annuals its growth is rapid, maybe twenty-five millimetres a day, so that speed is a quality to note. The structure of the plant is simple. The stem, like a bamboo, is constructed in segments with structural rings to strengthen it. It is fleshy and hollow, the whole plant being heavy with water. If the stem is cut or damaged the plant quickly droops and collapses. The stems are tinged with red, a copper-bronze, denoting the presence of metals. The leaves are dark green, strong in chlorophyll. The side stems rise at an angle of sixty degrees to the main stalk, which is round, like the shaft of a spear. The leaves are elegant, large and lanceolate (spear shaped) with a broad midrib. The pattern of growth is erect, cardinal, directed, strongly structured. On the main stem we can see the energy lines drawn on the surface like the straight, stretched muscles which hold the stem erect.

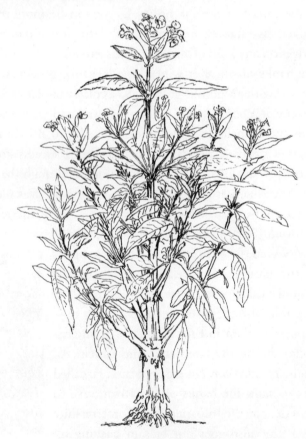

Impatiens glandulifera

Already we have information about the plant which is describing it in a language that corresponds to the human state. To pick out a few of the key words : rapid, speed, strength, spear-shaft, structure, tension. An image is beginning to appear. What is being suggested here is that the language used in description gives information about the gesture of the plant. More than that, the picture of the plant is equivalent to the picture of the human emotional state. We have the gesture of the person: the gesture of the plant.

At the top of the stems we see the flowers hanging on individual stalks (peduncles). They are a strange exotic shape, giving rise to the common names of 'policeman's helmet' and 'poor man's orchid'. The flowers are five-petalled but you wouldn't know it, as these five are fused together to form the open mouth of the helmet (or bonnet?). Into this mouth the bees crawl seeking nectar. Each flower hangs freely, anchored at the top, on the point of balance. When a bee arrives it carries pollen which has been transferred on to its furry back. As it alights the flower tilts, drawing the pistil down on to the bee's back. So as it enters, the pollen is transferred. It is a neat device which ensures cross-pollination. In part it is this device guaranteeing almost one hundred per cent pollination which accounts for the success of the Impatiens species. The whole pollination process takes place in the shelter and protection of the inside of the individual flower.

That description emphasizes the uniqueness and individuality of the Impatiens type; so different to the general run of flowers—and people. The balance of the flower, as it hangs from the stem, points to the ease and grace which are part of the Impatiens character, like Bach's gentleness, compassion and inspiring confidence. It is in contrast to the rather tense, angular gesture of the plant generally. And specifically it is in contrast with the tension that we see in the swelling seedpods which appear from within the flower as the petals fall away. Smooth and glistening, the pod stretches away at right angles to the stalk. Lines of tension are visible along its sides.

Now, a strange thing happens with the Impatiens plant. When the pods are ripe the seeds are shot away from the plant with an explosive force, like bullets from a gun. You can experience this if you touch the pods or if any movement nearby triggers them. The sides of the pod break open, drawing back like a coiled spring, and all with such force (action and reaction being equal and opposite) that the seeds can be fired several yards. You hear them splattering like lead shot on to the leaves nearby. This explosive tension is very illustrative of the Impatiens type. Remember Bullen's comment on Bach—'quick to anger, but quickly over'? This is the sparky irritability of the Impatiens which shows itself in unexpected outbursts of energy. Clairvoyants who see auras, the colourful energy fields that surround the physical body, speak of the constant sparky explosions of irritation and tension in such people: small bursts of fire which accompany the irritation of 'Oh for goodness sake! If you can't do it properly give it to me.'

Bach may not have seen all this in detail as he walked along the river bank that fateful day in September 1928. But he certainly met Impatiens. What led him to the plant? Go back for a moment to his intuition.[12] Intuition is the process of apprehending something without reasoning it out, finding an answer from incomplete or even misleading data.[13] This is glorified guesswork at worst; at best it is inspiration, the use of some unknown mental function from the non-rational part of the brain. But there is a more direct process which explains the matter without recourse to either mysticism or left brain—right brain theories. All living things possess resonance; they can vibrate with a particular pattern of energy. Any two bodies which carry the same vibratory pattern resonate together (like the acoustic resonance of a violin which will pick up the vibration of another instrument played at the same pitch). Bach carried in himself the vibratory pattern of the Impatiens mental state. There was a natural resonance between Bach, the man, and Impatiens, the plant. He recognized it.

We have an account of this process in action when Nora Weeks described the moment when Bach found another remedy plant, Water Violet. That was in June 1931 when he was completing the set of the first twelve remedies which he called *The Twelve Healers*. Her account opens with the statement that Bach 'was shown' the remedy.[14] But how was he shown it? During that morning he had behaved in a Water Violet way (quiet, aloof, withdrawn) and then announced that they were going to find the flower which would help such a person. He said he had the person in mind very strongly. He was resonating the emotional state of this particular woman. Weeks goes on to describe her temperament. Then they went out together, found the Water Violet growing in a stream and Bach 'gently placed his hand' over the plant. Contact with the plant eased his state of mind, bringing a sense of peace, calmness and humility. Later he found Water Violet flowering elsewhere and prepared the remedy.

This *sympathetic resonance* was again described when Bach wrote to a friend telling how he found some of the new remedies. He was lying on the riverbank by the Thames at Marlow 'when this message came through'. He wrote down the message and 'instantly noticed by my side a gorse bush in full bloom'. This flower was to become number thirteen in the sequence of Bach's remedies. His letter continued: 'I got up and went straight to a woman I knew about . . .'.[15] He described the woman and her mental state. He then asked her what was the most beautiful sight she could imagine. Her reply? Mountains covered with the flowering Heather. Heather became the fifteenth remedy in the series. There follows a telling remark from Bach: to many people, this would have meant nothing but to this 'brother' to whom he was writing it showed the way we can be led by everyday affairs.

It shows the way that sympathetic resonance works in everyday life. In the Water Violet case Bach was thinking strongly about the person he wanted to help. He actually began to feel the way that she felt. This is an internal process but one which he was aware of. Then he turned his attention to the outside world and looked for a plant which resonated with that feeling. He was attracted to the plant, which had a similar vibratory quality. He tested this by placing his hand over the plant, but could equally just have visualized it as the Heather lady did. This process of attraction is crucial because attraction is being drawn by pleasurable emotions. When Bach found the plant whose vibratory pattern resonated with the emotional state he was experiencing then the response occurred: he felt the pleasure of peace and calmness. Attraction draws like to like.

Bach's experience of this resonance developed as he made progress with finding the remedies. At the beginning, in 1928, he was, presumably, not so aware of what was happening as he was in 1931 (Water Violet) or in 1934 (Gorse, Heather). The clarity of the process grew upon him. In September 1928 he went twice to look at Impatiens and to make a remedy from the flowers, and again in September 1929.[16] This looks like return visits to check a finding. At this stage he was preparing a standard homœopathic trituration* 'with *sacch. lac.* by hand for twenty-one

---

* A homœopathic trituration involved the grinding of the plant material in a pestle and mortar with *sacch. lac.* or sugar-milk.

minutes in a glass mortar with a glass pestle'.[17] In strict terms this was a homœopathic remedy and not what we would now call a Bach flower remedy. A Bach flower remedy is not homœopathic, but is prepared by the sun method, discovered in May 1930.

Having prepared his homœopathic remedy of Impatiens, Bach returned to London and began to use it with his patients. If he took Hahnemann at all seriously we must believe that he first took the remedy himself. This is the basic process of self-proving and Bach could not fail to have been familiar with it.

His first account of the remedy published in February 1930, therefore, showed how he experienced it at that time. The description was some distance from the fully-fledged account of the Impatiens type he was to give in 1936. In every one of the first nineteen remedies, Bach's description of the emotional state evolved; it changed as his ideas changed. The 1930 account stressed that Impatiens was a remedy for acute pain: 'acute pain of the nerve type', 'intense headaches, sciaticas, acute neuralgias, *tic douloureux,* and acute pain in malignant disease'.[18] This might appear to be in contradistinction to the idea of a type of person or emotional state as he conceived it at the Masonic dinner, and in contradistinction to the idea that Bach set out to find a remedy for himself. But it isn't!

Bach was still beginning his exploration of what a type remedy might mean. What type of person was he anyway? He thought of himself as a person in pain. In conversation with Nora Weeks he said: 'all my life my body has suffered in some way from pain and discomfort and distress'.[19] She commented that she had seen him walk for miles in great pain from leg ulcers, headaches and *tic douloureux.* This last, now more generally called trigeminal neuralgia, is severe facial pain. Bach mentions it specifically in the Impatiens description quoted above because he suffered from it. In 1935 he wrote notes for an essay on pain.[20] Weeks reported him as saying 'I must know what pain is like . . . to have an understanding of what others suffer'.[21] There is the passage where he explained how a leader must be an expert in his branch of knowledge: perhaps a part of Bach's special knowledge was pain, both physical and emotional.[22]

So Dr Bach was looking for a remedy for himself, a remedy which he could test upon himself to see if it worked. He was looking for something to ease the pain. And Impatiens does it. His earliest description for Impatiens said: 'the indication for use is excruciating and very acute pain, no matter what the cause…'.[23] We might ask why the remedy that in 1934 he described as 'for the irritable, cross, peevish, impatient'[24] should act to relieve pain. It is because physical pain is associated with emotional pain and tension. Relieve the tension and emotional pain and that may relieve the physical pain. Here the theory of *Heal Thyself* begins.

The stages through which Dr Bach developed the flower remedies make a fascinating story. It is easy to follow it in *Collected Writings* through the different published versions.[25] To extract the sequence for just one remedy illustrates the point. In 1930, in *Some New Remedies and New Uses* we have:

IMPATIENS ROYLEI

A native of Kashmir, rarely found growing wild in the British Isles. Mauve flowers only used.

Three different series have been prepared: two on separate dates in September, 1928, and one in September, 1929. Although all have been effective, the most active is the last obtained, which is the one now stocked by Messrs Nelson and Co.

It is indicated in acute pain of nerve type, and it not only often gives rapid relief, but in many cases apparently effects a cure of the nerve condition. It has also a beneficent action, and patients frequently report, in addition to relief of symptoms, a much improved mental state with loss of depression and fears, a generally brighter outlook being obtained.

Amongst cases successfully treated may be mentioned intense head-aches, sciaticas, acute neuralgias, tic douloureux, and acute pain in malignant disease.

The indication for its use is excruciating and very acute pain, no matter what the cause; in some cases it has given relief after morphia has failed.

In *Some Fundamental Considerations of Disease and Cure*, 1930:

IMPATIENS
THE ENTHUSIAST

This remedy is for acute pain, no matter what the cause: it is the severity of the pain which is its indication. In some cases it has given relief after morphia had failed.

It is also for acute mental suffering: again the intensity being the guide.

It is useful in those people who (no matter their apparent status) are making a great effort to overcome some adverse quality: hence the intensity of the suffering when they fear failure.

In addition the remedy brings peace, and a definite mental uplift, of which the patients are usually very conscious.

In *Free Thyself*, 1932:

IMPATIENS

IMPATIENCE	FORGIVENESS

Are you one of those who know that deep down in your nature there is still a trace of cruelty; when buffeted and harassed you find it difficult not to have a little malice? Have you still left within you the desire to use force to bring another to your way of thinking: are you impatient and does that impatience sometimes make you cruel: have you left in your nature any trace of the inquisitor?

If so, you are striving for exquisite gentleness and forgiveness, and that beautiful mauve flower, Impatiens, which grows along the sides of some of the Welsh streams, will, with its blessing, help you along the road.

In *Twelve Great Remedies*, 1933:

10. When there is impatience, severe pain, fretting to be quickly well, anxious to be up and about again, impatient with those around give IMPATIENS.

In *Twelve Healers*, 1933:

IMPATIENS is pain of severe type caused by the blocking of a channel which should be admitting spiritual light and truth. It is often some cruelty in the nature which causes this.

In *The Twelve Healers & Four Helpers*, 1934:

IMPATIENS   IMPATIENCE

At all times when there is impatience. Impatient with themselves, wanting to hurry things, wanting to do things quickly, wanting to get well at once, to be out and about again. Impatient with others, irritable over little things, difficult to keep their temper. Cannot wait. This state is common and often a good sign during convalescence, and the restfulness this remedy brings hastens recovery. There is often impatience in severe pain and so Impatiens is of great value at those times to relieve the pain and calm the patient.

In *The Twelve Healers & Seven Helpers*, 1934:

IMPATIENS
For the irritable, cross, peevish, impatient.

In *The Twelve Healers & Other Remedies*, 1936:

IMPATIENS
Those who are quick in thought and action and who wish all things to be done without hesitation or delay. When ill they are anxious for a hasty recovery.
They find it very difficult to be patient with people who are slow, as they consider it wrong and a waste of time, and they will endeavour to make such people quicker in all ways.
They often prefer to work and think alone, so that they can do everything at their own speed.

Since 1936 the ideas of what makes an Impatiens type have been developed and extended by others. Naturally, those using the Bach remedies have confirmed his findings based upon case studies where the mentality of the person has been noted. In some instances this has led to over-elaborate psychological profiles where long lists of behaviour replace a sympathetic understanding of the individual. But observation of the person is only half of the equation. Observation of the plant provides the other half. All too often in the study of Bach flower remedies people have looked at Dr Bach, looked at the remedies and their action and forgotten to look at the flowers. In order to understand the Bach remedies more fully, we must go back to the flowers.

Going to the flowers was the first essential step taken by Bach. *Impatiens glandulifera* still grows along the banks of the River Usk where he found it in 1928. No longer 'rarely found growing wild in the British Isles'[26] it has become one of the most common wild flowers. Possibly there is a connection between the increasing population of this species and the increase in the tensions of contemporary life, what is generally called 'stress'. The efficiency of the plant in pollination, and the explosive force with which the seeds are propelled to ensure successful propagation, have already been noted. But more can be learned of the Impatiens remedy by directly comparing the gesture of the plant and the gesture of the person.

Impatiens people lead with the head, they are up and out of the chair as soon as they have the idea to move. It is their nature to be unrelaxed, tense, always on the edge of their seat, always jumpy. Like a coiled snake, they are ready to strike. This sense of anticipation, of kinetic energy, is in the plant. There are few plants which can trigger physical responses in this way; most are passive. It is emblematic of the reactive nature of Impatiens people, who use their energy to act upon the outside world. They are not receptive and sensitive by nature. And yet the delicate and balanced quality which will ease the tension is there in the flowers as well.

It is a quality illustrated by contrasts: compare the easy relaxation of a cat stretched out asleep in the sun perhaps and the tense vigil of a dog ready to leap up barking if a car goes by. It can be seen in people, if somebody is asked to relax—anyone really relaxed would flop to the floor as when fainting. We see it in people who can't sit still, who itch or fidget, who are restlessly tense. Such people look settled, but they might jump up at any moment: touch the Impatiens seedpods and you cannot be sure which will burst.

The contrast is also there in the flowers: some hot claret-crimson, others pale mauve, almost white. Bach was specific, right from the start: only the pale mauve flowers should be selected for their therapeutic quality, not the red, although the red outnumber the mauve by ten to one. Consider this from the point of view of colour alone and it seems most probable that the red flowers are heating, the mauve cooling. Carmine red is in your face, the colour of fire, blood, pepper and alarms. The mauve of these flowers has the tranquillity of amethyst, the distance of mist and atmosphere, the quiet of age; it is calming and gentle. Individual responses to colour may be subjective, but imagine a room painted in pale mauve and then one painted in red and ask yourself how the colour would affect your feelings.

So far, comment has only been made about what may be seen and felt of Impatiens. But the impact of the remedy plant upon consciousness is more; it extends to all five senses and beyond. Touching the plant leads to the discovery of the exploding seeds but the flowers, leaves and stems can also be felt and more information obtained. The smoothness of the 'skin' is most striking—being filled with water, the stems are cool to touch. Yet for all the boldness of the growth, the plants are rather delicate and crush easily. Impatiens gains protection by growing *en masse* and lacks the fibre and woody strength of other plants. Could this point to the need of the Impatiens type to live and work alone where they avoid the bruising challenge from other people?

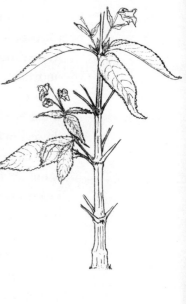

The smell of Impatiens grows stronger when it is touched. This scent is unusual: strong and pungent rather than sweet, like a spicy tar, not unpleasant but warding rather than attracting. Again, there is a sense of isolation rather than joining as this scent dominates the area. The smell seems to be in all of the plant and not produced in any one gland. The Latin name *glandulifera* is supposed to refer to the glands which secrete the scent. But since the Latin word *glans* means 'nut' or 'bullet', *glandulifera* might be interpreted as 'bullet carrying', considering the seeds!

Impatiens does not attract contact. Animals do not eat the leaves; a taste is enough to learn why. The jagged edge to the leaves is antagonistic. Saw-toothed edges look as though they would cut—a visual cue to keep away. Look for the sound of the plant (fanciful, perhaps) and the leaves suggest it: rough, clicking or strumming, the scraping noise of the strigil, (the skin scraper used by the ancients in bathing). Or better still the rasping stridulation of a violin bow as it presses too hard on tense strings.[27] Crush the stems and they sound like crunching of cane, a hollow pain as the fibres are torn.

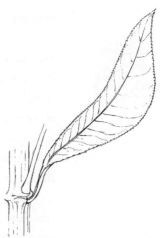

Such details confirm the picture of the plant and its relation to the picture of the Impatiens person. Seen in contrast with the behaviour of other remedy plants the distinction becomes more pronounced. The very upright stance of Impatiens is in contrast with the casual slouch of Clematis and the myopic Scleranthus clinging to the earth. In the detail of the gesture, character can be read. But beyond the five physical senses where we see, touch, hear, smell and taste there is still the sixth sense, the capacity to perceive the invisible quality of the plant. This can speak to us directly of the pattern of life force that informs the physical. Going back to Bach and his use of sympathetic resonance—resonating the emotional state of the person then trying to match that to the vibratory pattern of the plant—we can learn from the plant by resonating with it. Things are learned from the plant which cannot be explained in terms of ordinary understanding. The woman who thought the mountain covered with heather the most beautiful sight, making her believe it possible that there was a God, has been there; she knew the blessing of calm and relief the flowers make manifest in the world.

What of Impatiens? To be with the plant is to sense the gentle easing of the mind, the peace of forgiveness, restfulness, the release of mental tensions and desperation, the admitting of spiritual light and truth—all phrases which describe what Bach felt about the remedy in its positive state. The positive aspect, often forgotten in the mass of negative indications, is what the plant shows of itself. This is the plant's consciousness, perceived with our sixth sense.

Clematis

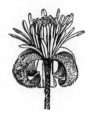

Without a clear record from Dr Bach we cannot be sure which remedy he came to next. It may have been Mimulus or Clematis. Both grow along the riverside between Abergavenny and Crickhowell. Nora Weeks says he prepared Clematis *from the seeds* later in 1928 but that doesn't mean he did not find the flowers in September. Bach wrote that he made 'three separate preparations' of Clematis, as he did with Impatiens.[28] It is simply not possible to be sure what happened when, and it would be wrong to attach too much significance to the matter either way. Clearly Bach made several visits to Abergavenny in these early years and it was there that he later found the Heather and Rockwater remedies.

Today, if the road is taken which runs alongside the river between Abergavenny and Crickhowell, wild Clematis can be seen growing among the trees, straggling over the hedge and fences, just as it did in 1928. Curiously, it grows there in only a limited area where the soil is more alkaline due to a local outcrop of limestone. Bach noted that it grows on chalk and in this he was right since it naturally prefers calcareous soil.* For this reason he later remade the Clematis remedy when he was staying in Norfolk in the late summer of 1930. But the all-important first sight

---

* 'The plants themselves act as most useful indicators as to whether soils are calcareous or not . . . of the more conspicuous plants my own evidence would suggest Traveller's Joy, *Clematis vitalba . . .*'. *Wild Flowers of Chalk and Limestone,* Lousely, J.E., Collins New Naturalist, 1950; p. 15.

of the plant, when he first recognized its gesture, was in the autumn of 1928 a few miles from Abergavenny.

Clematis is the clear antithesis of Impatiens. If Bach was looking for his own type remedy in Impatiens, it is perhaps an indication of his genius that he could imagine something so different at one and same time. Bach may have been a dreamer in that he imagined a better future, an easier life, but he was not apparently touched by the negative attributes of the Clematis type, whom he described as 'having little desire for life'[29]— requiring many hours of sleep at night with a sluggish constitution, a pale and muddy complexion. Bach lived by the bedroom maxim 'time to turn over, time to turn out'[30] and was, as an Impatiens, eager for the day and what it might bring. Just the opposite of the Clematis types as he described them 'wishing there was not another day to face . . . how good it would be just to go to sleep'.[31] Yet presumably he had formed a clear picture of the type of person who might need such a remedy. And his earliest description of Clematis bears this out, since it is almost fully formed and all the main attributes of the type remedy are there from the first. He wrote of the Clematis people as:

- having little desire for life
- day-dreaming types
- content to be left alone
- imperturbable
- having little ambition to survive
- 'the severest type of sleepy sickness'[32]

This last observation is particularly acute since Bach must have been aware of the strange and inexplicable outbreak of a type of sleep sickness in the 1920s—it was an illness without aetiology and certainly without cure.

Encephalitis lethargica had first been observed in the Britain in 1918 and was possibly linked to the influenza epidemic which occurred at that time. It affected five million people around the world and was widely known about. It was, so we are told, 'an interesting example of a serious disease that has appeared from nowhere and mysteriously departed like some of the plagues of antiquity'.[33] By 1928 there were no new cases reported, yet Bach's direct mention of it confirms that he had such patients on his list. The new Clematis remedy (still in homœopathic form, remember) 'proved effective' in treating them. This sleepy sickness was extraordinary in that the sufferer simply appeared to lose interest in life and withdraw, as it were to another place inside themselves.

It was Bach's observation that some people behaved like this in their general approach to life: not necessarily ill, but indifferent, without an interest in present circumstances. It is tempting to suggest that Bach himself had some experience of this state of mind. One reaction to pain is to drift away from the body. In any event, it is evident that he was able to resonate the mentality of the Clematis type and in that way to attract a plant which would 'bring them down to earth',[34] as he put it, bringing them back into life.

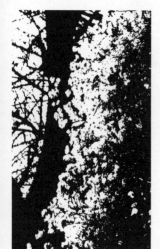

Bach began his work with Clematis by making a trituration from the seeds and perhaps the seed is a good place to start when looking at the plant. Many of us know Clematis best as the 'old man's beard' that hangs, fluffy grey, on the hedge right through the winter. Often arriving late in summer, the creamy-white flowers of *Clematis vitalba* almost escape notice. But when the leaves have fallen and the trees are bare then 'the traveller's joy' (as John Gerard the herbalist named it in 1597) shows like a low cloud or smoke hanging in the lanes. The amorphous, grey mist is, in reality, the feathery plumes of Clematis. On each seed head there are about twenty individual black seeds, each with an awn, the silvery tail some forty millimetres long. This tail is designed to help carry the seed upon the wind, drifting it away from the parent plant.

In the seed some details of the Clematis state can be seen. Where Impatiens shoots out the seeds with explosive force as soon as they are ripe, with Clematis the plant holds on to the seeds through winter, letting the wind tear them free and tumble them into the future. The Clematis seed, which has a striking resemblance to an individual sperm, carries the future, yet it is held by the past, 'but always trying to be blown away and start again'.[35] Hairs on the diamond-shaped seed help to drive it into the soil once it has landed. Held above the earth for so long, the pointed seed is designed to dive downwards to take root.

Yet the gesture of the plant speaks of the attempt by Clematis to get away from the earth. With multiple long stems, often ten or twelve growing from one root, it explores all directions to climb up and away from the ground. Where a tree has a strong trunk or Impatiens has one main stem, Clematis lacks the upright strength and 'backbone' to make its own movement in a vertical direction. It is somewhat like a tree without a trunk. As a climber or vine, it climbs up over and through others to gain height and get to the light. That is why it flowers later than most of the trees which support it, because Clematis must first clamber its way into the open air. It is a perennial, of course, and takes many years to grow out across the hedgerow, up the trunks of trees and out around their branches.

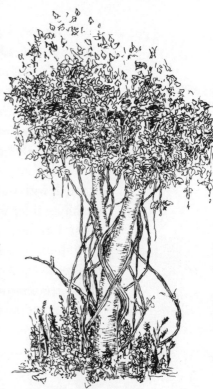

If Impatiens people are described as on the edge of their seat then a Clematis person is laid back—literally. The lack of tree-trunk structure makes these people loose-limbed, like the scarecrow in *The Wizard of Oz*. Like the hanging stalks of the Clematis they may sway in the wind, drooping at the shoulders. But as Bach said, 'the mentals are the important character'[36] and, like children unaware of the wider world around them, they live within the compass of their own minds. With

Clematis stems entwine a tree

their heads in the clouds they carry the air of juvenile detachment. Trying to bring them into the dimension of the living we might well say 'Hello! Is anybody there?'

It is the lack of involvement or indifference which characterizes the Clematis type and represents the life lesson or the soul lesson, as Bach would have it. He described how such people are drawn towards death, perhaps by a person who has died and tries to 'call his partner over'.[37] As Clematis hangs like ropes in the trees the idea of drawing and being drawn is easy to see. Or else these people find so little interest and enjoyment in life that they desire death as a means of escape. In winter the seed heads do give a misty, otherworldly appearance to Clematis and the stalks appear dry and almost dead. There is actually so little life in the stalks that if sections are broken off they can be smoked like cigarettes—hence the familiar name of 'gypsies' bacca' or 'boys' bacca'—the sap drains out from the plant in winter leaving it dry and full of air. The fibrous bark crumbles and peels off in strands, as if the wood were rotten, like old rope.

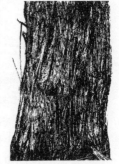

The rough bark of Clematis

The ropy stalks of the Clematis, hanging like lianas from the branches, make a picture for another aspect of the Clematis remedy. Bach said that this was the remedy for unconsciousness,[38] a condition when we are losing close connection with our physical body, as in sleep (some authorities say that Clematis contains a narcotic).[39] In such circumstances it is said that we are tethered to the body by a silver cord so that even if we do actually leave the body (as in astral travelling) we remain connected. This cord, like the umbilical lifeline of a baby or an astronaut, keeps us supplied and in touch with the mother ship. If the cord is severed we cannot re-enter the physical form. Clematis as a remedy helps to bring us back safely into physical reality.

In the plant we can picture this return to physical reality as we follow these individual stems back towards their root. The root in a plant speaks of the relationship to earth, how it is anchored in the world and how the species draws nourishment. Clematis roots are really hard to find. Take one stem and follow it back through the undergrowth and it may lead away to another place altogether, where the root lies hidden. Often, feeling a way along the stem, it is difficult to know if you are moving towards or away from the root. There is no obvious focus to the structure for this plant: that is indicative of the diffused mentality of the Clematis type. When the root is found, it is thick, knarled and stumpy. With the many stems of up to thirty metres in length, and considering the extensive branching structure, it is no surprise that the root eventually digs deeply into a soft rock like chalk.

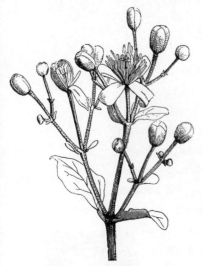

Clématite des haies. (*Clematis Vitalba.*)

It appears that the plant embodies the negative gesture of the emotional type. If so, are the positive aspects fully expressed in the flower? Yes and no. It would be wrong to see the plant as positive/negative (actually it would be wrong to see any of the remedies that way). Rather, the form of the plant is a representation of the whole thought form. It is true that in the flower we can see the focus and concentration missing elsewhere. The flower is constructed of a small, rayed calyx like a tight-banded stippling brush. The sepals fold back, revealing rings of stamens which surround the pistil, and the creamy-white flower stays open as the seeds develop within. When the flower head grows to seed head over some weeks, new blooms appear

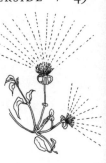

irregularly elsewhere on the stalks. They are like little stars of converging light; it is hard to say whether the energy is raying out or raying in. The small Clematis flowers commune with space.

Bach chose the wild clematis, *Clematis vitalba,* not the colourful garden hybrids. It is a flower without colour and without petals. It is the petals and their colour which, on other flowers, seem to mediate the emotional world, acting as a receiving dish for energies of a certain kind. A petal's colour shows the part of the spectrum which is not absorbed. With white, *all* the light is reflected back, while blue flowers absorb all wavelengths except the blue portion of the spectrum. So white Clematis flowers reflect all the light back, absorbing nothing, as if otherworldly, pure and untainted by the coloured metals of the earth. There is also a quality particular to each of the Bach flowers which do not have petals, such as Clematis, Scleranthus and Wild Oat. In each case the lack of petals suggests that something is missing from the emotional being. It correlates to a remedy state where there is a detached mentality, an indifferent or confused process of thinking about oneself, also a certain emotional dryness and lack of warmth.

When looking at Clematis flowers one is likely to be looking up. Some plants stretch across a bank, lying lazily in the sunshine. But for the most part Clematis flowers above one's head. In July and August the small, white flowers cover the trees like a mantle, a white cloth of lace thrown carelessly across the landscape. Look from a distance and the white flowers of Whitsun appear to be blooming for a second time, so Clematis can be deceptive, not quite what it appears. It makes strange connections, surfacing in unexpected places across the white-chalk downland landscape. The mantle is also like the mantle of sleep that is thrown across the land by the last good fairy in the story of Briar Rose. Clematis does this: it draws into the imagination, to the land where tales are told.

If Clematis draws out, leading the consciousness from the physical to the metaphysical, how important this remedy must have been for Bach. Here was the practical man of medical science, the Impatiens person, who begins to investigate aspects of the subtle, invisible world. The idea of sympathetic resonance is easy enough in theory, but experiencing it can lead to a Clematis state where the ties holding us to the physical world of mundane reality are loosened. So Clematis would have acted as a counterweight for Bach in his discovery of these new ideas, helping him to stay grounded. Clematis helped him to find the other remedies by making his dreams real. It helps the visionary to bring a new idea into the world 'and so enables them to fulfil their work in the world'.[40]

Bach spoke of making the first potencies on site,[41] whether Impatiens, Clematis or Mimulus and we can imagine him sitting by the flowers, pestle and mortar in hand, grinding the mixture of plant and milk sugar the required twenty-one minutes. It was an exact methodology, one borrowed directly from homœopathy,[42] and Bach was familiar with it. Yet we cannot escape the idea that he was making a remedy which was different. He was making not just a mixture of physical material, but a combination of physical and metaphysical forces; more than can be measured by chemical and physical analysis. That may be true of any homœopathic preparation, although homœopathy in the 1920s had become rather orientated to the physical, material world. But Bach wanted to capture some of the indefinable quality, the consciousness and gesture, of the plant, not merely the carbon, hydrogen and oxygen atoms of the leaves or flowers. This is implicit in his comments when he discussed these first remedies of 1928:

> There is much to learn of the gathering and preparation of herbs; many points require consideration if the maximum, instead of the medium result is to be obtained: the natural habitat, age, condition and particular part of the plant; the planetary influences; the time of day, and, by no means the least important, the mental attitude of the physician, which should be one of wholehearted devotion to the work in hand in the cause of humanity.[43]

So he was thinking about particular qualities in the plant, the person and the preparation itself. Bach has told us what the mental attitude of the physician should be but, picturing him there beside the river, in the field, among the trees, there is something else. The physician needs to sense the harmony of nature and see the whole picture of what the plant is. Such a physician needs 'whole-hearted devotion to the work', yes, but that leads to whole-hearted love of life. Any mere mechanical grinding of the potency would make a mechanical remedy. For Bach, his imagination drawn upwards to the light by the Clematis, this devotion contained an overview, a perception of the whole: the cause of humanity.

His choice of the Clematis seed at the first making was deliberate because the seed illustrated the focus of attention and return to earth for the visionary Clematis people. The feeling remains that he was trying to find a way to distil the whole of the plant's energy and that is the seed.

Why else make the first potency on site and return twice to remake the same remedy?

> *At present our knowledge on some of these points is sadly small, but we must do the best in our power, and as we proceed, greater experience will make the task simpler.*[44]

And earlier in the same passage he wrote:

> *We have much to discover, but we must not be afraid of the task.*

And thereby he nods at the third of his flower remedies, Mimulus.

There is a picture map, probably drawn by Nora Weeks, showing the exact spot where Bach made Mimulus.[45] We have no date for the picture and it was probably not 1928, the year when Bach had first found it. More likely it was the summer of 1930 when Nora had been travelling with Bach around Wales, staying for a while in Abersoch, where he wrote *Heal Thyself.* In the 1930s Mimulus and Impatiens grew 'to perfection near Crickhowell'[46] and 'on the edge of streams and marshes where the water is clear'.[47] The place can still be found. It is by the bridge over the River Usk and the footpath along the river bank. But the playing fields of Crickhowell High School, built in 1983, have since occupied part of the meadow, and the marsh area has been drained and ploughed. Mimulus grows there no longer!

Mimulus

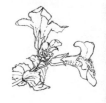

Although Mimulus will grow on damp, marshy ground it is more commonly seen where the water flows swift and clear. When sitting by the plant, preparing a remedy, the most striking perception is often the noise: the sound of water as it streams over rocks or through a millrace. The water must be crystal clear for Mimulus to grow happily. The scum of detergent or invisible nitrate-run-off from farmland will kill the sensitive plants. They must have well-oxygenated water to survive. This is another reason why Mimulus has largely disappeared from Crickhowell. The water there is now too polluted.

These two things, sound and the purity of water, combine to show first aspects of the Mimulus remedy. In his earliest description, Bach spoke of Mimulus types as having 'a marked desire for quietness, aversion to talking and to being questioned'.[48] Later he mentioned 'fear of . . . crowds, of noise, of talking . . . of being alone'.[49] This has been extended to indicate a generally nervous disposition and a desire for tranquillity. Mimulus people are hypersensitive to their environment, and avoid conflict. Their delicacy and sensitivity lead them to shy away from the rough and tumble of life. It conjures a picture of a child covering its ears and running away from fireworks, seeking protection. They are like delicate flowers. Yet here is a plant which lives in mountain streams, often overhanging the water, on the edge of rocks, or tumbling down a rock face. Perhaps it is driven to the edge.

As much as anything it is this fact, that Mimulus lives dangerously, which speaks of the inner nature of the plant. Other plants, with less of a firm hold on life, might be swept away by the flooding stream in winter. Other plants choose to live securely in the hedge or shelter safely at the edge of a wood—not Mimulus. It can be found clinging precariously to a ledge in the water-shoot of a mill wheel, where the driving force of the millstream pours constantly across its roots, splashing the stems and flowers; the roaring of the cascade ever present. Or it grows next to a limestone swallow-hole, where the water plunges into the ground.

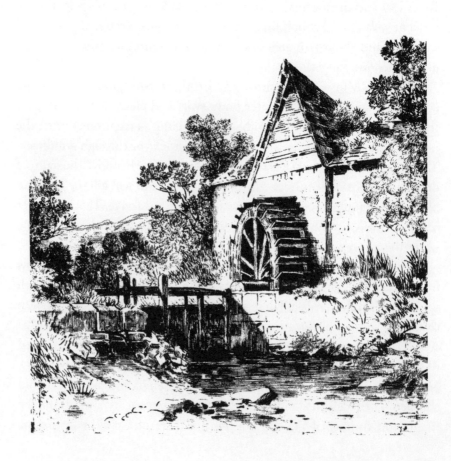

Buffeted by such a flood, then by wind and rain, the stems can be broken and bruised. Sometimes they fall horizontally on to the surface of the stream for support, turning upwards at the end to lift the flowers

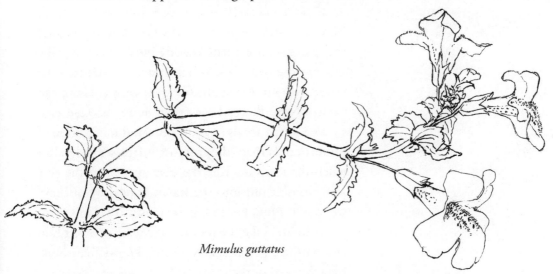

Mimulus guttatus

out of the water. So resilient is this plant that one writer who found Mimulus growing 'in a quick stream hurrying down a valley in Wiltshire', tells us that 'I took some home, and learned something else about monkey-flower, that though its flowers are tender, it picks up wonderfully well in a bowl of water, and will last for weeks, opening single blossom after blossom, and spreading a good feeling through the house'.[50] That good feeling is the positive force of the Mimulus energy: strong, positive, laughing and clear.

Mimulus guttatus, the monkey flower, came from the Pacific states of North America, introduced into Britain in 1812. The word *Mimulus* is from the Latin, a mimic or little actor, and the flowers are supposed to resemble a mask or monkey's face (*guttatus* means spotted, since the flowers are spotted with red). There could be something here about laughing at our fears but not every flower has such literal naming as Impatiens. Like Impatiens, Mimulus has a clever system to encourage cross-pollination as the bees, entering the flower, first have any pollen scraped from their backs by the pistil and then find the anthers have dusted new pollen on them as they crawl forward. Darwin conducted some interesting experiments upon *Mimulus luteus* (the Latin name was later changed from *luteus* to *guttatus*) and proved that plants which cross-pollinate develop stronger offspring than those which are self-fertile.[51] No haphazard strategy then

for the Mimulus plant: it has a developed intention to grow stronger in
the future generations.

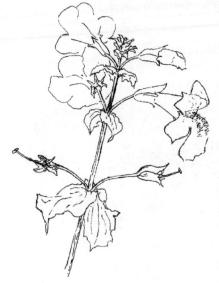

And yet, when it comes to seeds, Mimulus has the
most careless or carefree attitude to propagation. With
Impatiens and Clematis we saw how seeds illustrated
the gesture of the plant/remedy type. This is equally
true for the Mimulus, which casts its seeds into the
water without a thought for their future. Once the
petals of the flower have fallen away the seed case
swells and the sepals grow to surround it, a gesture of
protection. Perhaps they act to keep the seeds dry. But
when the seeds are ripe the case opens and the tiny
seeds tumble out into the water. Foolhardy or brave
we might think, but rather, remember that this plant
trusts to life. Like the mother of Moses who left him
among the bulrushes, this mother knows that somehow the seed of the future will be saved.

The seeds are small, less than half a millimetre across, and they float
on the water for a few days before becoming waterlogged. They then
germinate underwater.[52] Later, as seedlings, they surface again and float
to a place where they can take root and grow. It is a journey fraught
with risks. 'Cast your bread upon the water' it says in the Old Testament
Book of Ecclesiastes—the wise king Solomon is commending a belief
in Divine Providence. Bach clearly had the same thought, since in *Heal
Thyself* he wrote of fear:

> *Fear in reality holds no place in the natural human kingdom, since the
> Divinity within us, which is ourself, is unconquerable and immortal,
> and if we could but realise it we, as Children of God, have nothing of
> which to be afraid.*[53]

It is faith, therefore, which casts out fear.

Yet the Mimulus plant has more to tell of the matter. It is true that
the seeds of cross-pollination bring stronger offspring, but it is a risky
venture. So Mimulus also manages a clever system of vegetative propagation. By autumn the plants begin to look ragged and the stems are often
shredded and weak. They seem beaten and exposed.
But a closer look reveals that small roots are now growing from each node on the stem, like bedraggled hairs.
As the winter floods tear at the plants, so exposed and

vulnerable, small sections of stem break off as they are rubbed against the rocks. Some of these torn stems will be carried by seasonal floods and left in a suitable place, away from the main stream. There the ready roots will find a finger-hold between stones or grip firmly into mud and grow. The plant uses the flood to find a place on higher ground away from the river. That is how Bach found it growing in marshy land at Crickhowell, a hundred yards from the bank.

Those plants which lived beside the riverbank, or lodged in the stones midstream, would be totally submerged during the winter floods. So, like a diver holding his breath, Mimulus can survive for some time under water—another reason why the water must be pure and well-oxygenated. The Mimulus type can be associated with breathing, or rather the lack of it. They stop breathing when frightened (now take deep breaths, we say) and generally breathe in a shallow way, filling only the top part of the lungs. Like the Mimulus plant, these people learn to survive in the flood of feelings, overcome and swept away. It is remarkable; they are both delicate and determined.

So what we observe of the plant we can observe of the person. We see the gesture of the plant: we see the gesture of the person. The Mimulus types, then, are not so much shy and nervous, as we are told, but rather courageous and even inventive. Of course the negative aspect of the remedy state is easily seen and caricatured as the timid mouse. But Bach saw it well enough. Mimulus people are afraid, yes, but they 'go bravely on',[54] have the 'ability to stand up and face the difficulties of daily life'.[55] What then is the great lesson, the soul lesson as he was to call it, for the Mimulus? Bach suggested that these people are learning sympathy and pity, since their own circumstances give them tenderness and the compassion to understand. It is somewhat akin to the proud Water Violets, who also live in the water, as will be seen.

A part of the Mimulus quality can be seen in the colour of the blooms: a bright, golden yellow. Yellow is the colour of intellect.[56] This tells us how to overcome fear. We look at the facts and view them objectively. In practical terms it works like this. If a dog, which frightens me, jumps into the road as I am walking by, fear will root me to the spot—almost hypnotised, as Bach observed.[57] At such a moment I cannot think what to do, I am so frightened. The golden strength of Mimulus will not make the dog disappear. The dog stills snarls and gets ready to leap and bite. But if I can shift my attention from feeling to thought I can prepare my best defence. From the clear space in my mind I can decide what to do; fight the dog, shout at it, call for help (finding again my voice), run away and climb a tree—whatever will best serve to keep me safe! Courage is not the absence of fear. Courage is clear action in the face of fear. So Mimulus helps to utilize our intelligence. It develops a pathway to the mind where we can assess our fears objectively.

Provings

So Bach prepared these three remedies by homœopathic trituration and took them back to London, where he used them in his practice during 1929. He treated a considerable number of cases[58] and in the *Homœopathic World*, February 1930, he appealed to physicians using the remedies to 'help with the work of completing the provings'. Proving is the 'controlled experiment in which medicine is administered to a healthy individual to ascertain what changes (signs, symptoms, behaviour) the medicine produces on the body and the mind'.[59] Bach was probably using the word rather loosely to indicate any testing of the therapeutic effects on patients. At this stage the efficacy of the remedies must have been limited. A Bach flower remedy made by homœopathic methods of preparation cannot be truly effective as a remedy. Bach said that the third making was 'more active' than the first. But he had yet to discover the sun method of potentizing. So there was some lack of definition about the whole business as he struggled to resolve the equation of person, plant and preparation.

In a paper read to the *British Homœopathic Society* in November 1928, Bach said nothing directly about the new remedies he had recently found.[60] He was giving a talk on the seven bowel nosodes which he had discovered earlier, the Bach nosodes. Winding up the lecture he remarked:

> I wish it were possible that we could present to you seven herbs instead of seven groups of bacteria, because there always seems to be some reticence in the minds of many to use anything associated with disease in the treatment of pathological conditions . . . . We are making every endeavour to replace the bacterial nosode by means of plants and have, in fact, matched some of them almost exactly; for example, ornithogalum in its vibrations is almost identical with the Morgan group, and we have discovered a seaweed which has almost all the properties of the dysentery type, but there is yet one thing lacking, and that one point keeps us checkmated in the effort to avoid using bacterial nosodes. This vital point is polarity. The remedies of the meadow and of Nature, when potentized, are of positive

polarity, whereas those which have been associated with disease are of the reverse type, and at the present time it seems that it is this reversed polarity which is so essential in the results which are being obtained by bacterial nosodes.[61]

So we see the focus of his work: he was intending to replace bacterial nosodes with plant nosodes. The polarity problem he spoke of could relate to the experimental provings in homœopathy: in provings he might have expected to see the plant material induce the symptoms in a healthy person which they would heal in the sick. Would Mimulus, acting on this homœopathic basis, exacerbate fear? This remained an unresolved question for Bach. However, he abandoned the whole matter completely in 1930 when he left London to look for new flower remedies and the new method of potentizing: the sun method.

It was the sun method, the original way of preparing the Bach essences, which was to make these new remedies distinctly non-homœopathic. Homœopathy relies upon methods of preparation which incorporate a portion of the physical plant or material. This material is treated in a particular way which leads through a series of dilutions to a point where none of the original physical material is present, although the energetic pattern remains. After each dilution the liquid is succussed or repeatedly tapped or drummed. During this process the polarity of the material could be said to be reversed. This means that a substance which, in its normal physical

Methods of preparation

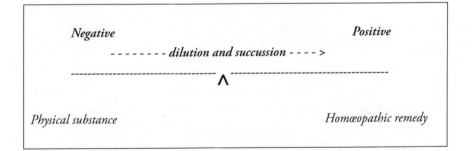

form may be a poison, can become not just non-poisonous but actually therapeutic in quality. Thus arsenic, a poison, can be homœopathically prepared to a dilution of, say, one part in 100,000 when it becomes *arsenicum 5x* the homœopathic remedy. Arsenic produces a set of symptoms if it is taken internally. But *arsenicum* can be used to help a sick person in whom such symptoms appear.

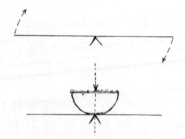

At a certain point the nature of the material changes from negative to positive, from poison to medicine. This point, which is a fulcrum, a point of balance, can only be located in a theoretical way. But if we consider physics we can observe that at the fulcrum there is no turning moment. The forces are only acting vertically. By working with the vertical forces at the fulcrum Bach successfully avoided the polarity problem.

By the winter of 1928, we could say he had found the right question to ask—how to deal with polarity of homœopathic provings. The answer would come in response to his statements at the end of the lecture:

> Perhaps at some future date a new form of potentizing may be discovered, which will be capable of reversing the polarity of the simple elements and plants, but until that time comes we have no alternative.[62]

In the event there was no need to reverse the polarity because that new form of potentizing was the sun method.

3 · The Sun Method

WRITING IN 1930, Bach gave his first account of how to make remedies by the sun method:

A glass vessel, as thin as possible, was nearly filled with clean water, preferably from a spring. Into this were placed sufficient of the blooms of the plant to cover the surface completely. A cloudless day was chosen, and the blooms picked after they had had about two hours' sunshine upon them. The vessel was then placed in the sun and its position changed from time to time so that the sunlight passed directly down the orifice as well as bathing the whole.[1]

By 1932 it was slightly elaborated:

Take a thin glass bowl, fill with clear water from a stream or spring for preference, and float enough of the blooms of the plant to cover the surface. Allow this to stand in bright sunshine until the flowers begin to wilt. Very gently pick out the blooms, pour the water into bottles and add an equal quantity of brandy as a preservative.[2]

And in May 1933:

Method of preparation. The remedies should be prepared near the place where the plant grows, as the flowers should be put straight into the water after gathering, whilst they are quite fresh and full of life.
A thin glass bowl is taken, filled with clear water, preferably from a pure spring or stream. Sufficient blooms of the plant are floated on the water to cover the surface, as much as can be done without overlapping the blossoms. Then allow to stand in bright sunshine until the blooms show signs of fading. The time varies from about two to seven hours, according to the plant, and the strength of the sun. The blossoms are then gently lifted out, and the water poured into bottles, with an equal quantity of brandy, added as a preservative.[3]

His description of this process did not change substantially thereafter. It told us little enough, although he did say that readers should not be deterred by the simplicity of the method.[4]

It is at once a very simple process—Nickie Murray used to say, 'there's nothing to it'*—yet it is a matter that invites the deepest consideration. Flower remedies raise two great questions: how do they work and what factors influence the quality of the remedy? Both these questions could be directed towards the moment of preparation of the mother essence.

First, let us deal with the matter of terminology. As in homœopathy we speak of the 'mother' as the first level of dilution, the original making. So the water from the bowl, potentized by the sun, is the mother essence, or mother tincture. The same names are given to the material after brandy is added since the brandy becomes an essential part of the process of preparation. Subsequent dilution of this mother tincture to the second level is called 'stock' and to the third level dilution is called 'dosage' strength. We should note that none of this dilution is related to homœopathic dilution since no shaking or succussion takes place.

Nora Weeks reported that Bach found inspiration for the sun method by chance when walking through fields one morning in May (1930). She said he saw dew on the flowers and thought that the dew must hold a condensation of the properties of the plant: 'the perfect and uncontaminated power of the plants'.[5] At first he tried to shake the dew into small vials but found it impractical. It was some time later that he hit upon the idea of using glass bowls.

It has been suggested that Paracelsus had known about the special properties of dew in the early sixteenth century. The possibilities of tracing a connection to Bach through alchemy, the Rosicrucians, Freemasonry and other occult and esoteric traditions are tempting. Certainly Paracelsus studied alchemy and had remarkable insights into many new avenues of knowledge; he is even thought to have anticipated homœopathy. There is evidence that he gathered dew, not from plants but as a part of some alchemical process. There is an illustration showing cloths wet with dew being wrung out into bowls.[6] And it is possible that Bach would have read of it. But Paracelsus did not make flower essences as we know them: there was no secret process handed down through the centuries waiting to be discovered by Bach.

Perhaps there is a clue to how the sun method developed, if we go back to Bach's own words: 'take a thin glass vessel'. Maybe this refers to

---

* Nickie Murray succeeded Nora Weeks at the Bach Centre, beginning in 1962 and worked there for twenty-five years preparing the essences. She retired in 1987 and lived first in Crete and then in California before her death in January 1998.

some piece of laboratory equipment such as an evaporating dish. But we know that he sold all his laboratory equipment when he left London at the beginning of 1930.[7] It is more likely that he was referring to glass finger bowls brought to the dinner table for rinsing your hands after eating lobster or asparagus. Such bowls, five inches across and two-and-a-half inches high, were definitely used by Nora Weeks to make essences in later years. Curiously, glass bowls are mentioned as being suitable for table decoration by the doyenne of Edwardian household management, Mrs Beeton.[8] She illustrated 'floating flower bowls' in a chapter on table decoration. 'These are wide, shallow bowls of crystal . . . only a little water is placed in the bowls and the flowers, having their stalks cut off quite short, are floated on the water'.[9] Mrs Beeton illustrated fancy glass bowls but the idea of floating flowers on water is clearly there. Using plain glass finger bowls is a logical step to simplifying the matter. Fine, hand-blown glass is a thing of the past, of course. But such bowls can still be found in antique shops and they are decidedly the best for making remedies. They are very delicate and beautiful. Filled with water, they become reflective, magnifying and concentrating the light in a magical way, lens and prism combined. To see them, with light dancing in the water, is to understand instinctively how they could be used. Is it possible that Bach was familiar with these finger bowls from his time in London when he attended Masonic dinners, like the one in 1928 that Nora tells us about?[10] In any event there is no great mystery here as to how Bach moved from gathering dew to setting the bowls out in the sunshine with spring water. But there was inspiration.

Describing the sun method, Bach commented:

> *Let it be noticed in this that the four elements are involved: the earth to nurture the plant: the air from which it feeds: the sun or fire to enable it to impart its power: and water to collect and to be enriched with its beneficent magnetic healing.*[11]

Again, the idea that the water is there to collect and to be enriched is visually apparent in the 'thin glass bowl'. Water is receptive to the light; the light is taken up by the water. In some respects the sun method is a way of holding the light in a liquid form. Homœopathy induces something akin to a magnetic charge in the physical material that is being succussed or beaten into it, a charge that has polarity. In the sun method, by contrast, the charge, if we can call it that, is just the presence of light in the water.

The water used came from a nearby stream or a 'spring for preference'.[12] Although it would appear that any clean water would suffice, the idea of using spring water must be significant. Spring water of a particular kind is used in the later remedy Rock Water (pages 162–170) and it plays a vital part in the making of Bach remedies. Water that comes from the darkness within the earth is reborn into the light. Like any newborn it takes up most strongly the imprint of whatever it contacts first. Just as the infant coming from the womb bonds with the first contact from the mother, so the nascent water from a spring is most ready to absorb the quality of what it first encounters. In our case, the flowers and the sun.

To obtain the best results a cloudless sky is needed, with uninterrupted sunshine for the morning hours while the mother essence is being prepared. In England there are not so many sunny days that qualify. In 1999 and 2001, in the area of the Welsh borders there were less than twenty such days between April and September. There were about twelve in the year 2000, with only one in May and none in June. There may have been one or two more in the south-eastern counties but there are few enough suitable days available in any year. And a week of perfect weather in July is no help if the plants needed to make remedies are at their peak in May. Such fine weather is almost invariably associated with high pressure over the UK. The constant strength of the sun is important and when clouds cross the sun, even for a short time, the remedy must be poured away and remade on another occasion. The actual making of an essence begins the day before, therefore, when we anticipate the weather may be clear the following morning. Satellite pictures from the Internet are useful.

Selecting a good location to make a remedy also requires forethought. We have to find and identify the correct species of plant. Then we must find plants growing in a place that is conducive to their strength and well-being: away from the towns, industry and industrial farming. We need a place where the land might be said to be less trammelled by human interference; a place away from every kind of pollution: atmospheric, chemical, electro-magnetic, noise or historical. The earth element that Bach says nurtures the plant must be suitable for just that, nurturing. There is the old argument of 'nature versus nurture' in the sense of what is the strongest influence upon character. With remedy plants the matter is clear, both are needed in equal measure. The nature of the species is essential in the growth of those characteristics which are unique to the plant; yet the plant needs to be nurtured in conditions which instruct and inform the patterning of the qualities required. An essence made from the right species will not be effective if it lacks the living character of the remedy. Genetic mutation is a physical expression of only one of the problems which can distort the metaphysical qualities of plants.

For the best results, the group of plants from which the remedy is made should be at the height of flowering. We can make an essence from the last few flowers but it is always better to find a day when perfect weather coincides with perfect flowering: the day when the tree is ablaze with light, the fields are full of flower, the blooms in their freshest and brightest hue. Of the individual flowers we choose those newly open, for the moment of opening is when the flower is ready to be pollinated. It is

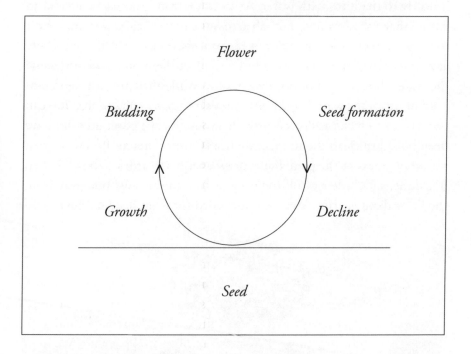

the apogee of the growth, when the plant reaches furthest from the earth and its seed origin. Once the flower is pollinated it begins to close off its receptors, change its chemistry (often changing its colour) and, as the process of seed formation begins, it starts into the cycle of decline.

So, assuming the flowers are right and assuming the weather is right, it is time to begin. On a making day, dawn is always bright and clear. The sky is azure and the day fresh. Bach wore clean, white clothes when going out to make remedies, probably his laboratory overall.[13] Clean, white clothes are a reminder that we should not colour the essence ourselves but stay reflective and clear of the process. First call will be to the spring to gather fresh water which must be carried, along with the glass bowl and bottles, to the 'cooking field', as Bach called it.[14]

It is necessary to find a good place to set the bowl. It must be on level ground close to the plants, but not in such a position that shadows will fall across it as the sun travels around. Begin the essence before nine o'clock, after the sun has been shining for some time upon the flowers which will then be opening fresh for the day. This is not a mechanical process and so it is not possible to be prescriptive about choosing a place. The best place must be where it seems best, all things considered.

Taking out the bowl, which can be wrapped in a clean white cloth, fill it nearly to the brim with water. At all times from now on be careful to ensure that a shadow does not fall across the bowl. Again, it is important to keep our own patterning out of the process. Picking the flowers, a few at a time, bring them back on a leaf and place them on to the surface of the water. Impatiens flowers always sink, while the sprigs of agrimony hold off from the water—pick just enough to cover the surface. You can use scissors to pick the flowers provided they, like the other utensils, have been boiled to clean them. Pick the heads from different flowers so that the whole mass of the plants may draw energy towards the bowl. When it is done, sit a little way off to be a guardian to the bowl but away from the immediate vicinity. You are not needed for what happens next.

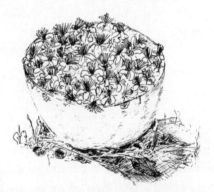

Clematis prepared by the sun method

It takes three hours to make most of the remedies although some give up their energy more quickly. Bach wrote: 'less time if the blooms begin to show signs of fading'.[15] This happens most often with Chicory, which can collapse quite swiftly in certain circumstances (page 104). No two makings are alike, however, and particular results cannot be anticipated. But if the flowers are there and the sun shines the remedy will make. We might wonder, at first, how we will know when it is ready. Observation makes it clear. At the outset a look at the bowl shows the brightness is in the flowers; the water is relatively dull and reflective. As the making proceeds, the light begins to enter the water, bubbles form on the inside of the glass bowl and the flowers begin gradually to fade. The light transfers downwards into the water. At the end the essence shines brightly, with colours sparkling from the bowl. Most of all, it appears to wink light at you. However fanciful this may sound, it has been observed many times and is unmistakeable.

When the essence is made, when it is ready, take a twig from the plant being worked with and, still being careful to keep every shadow off the bowl and fingers out of the tincture, lift away the flowers. Then, using a measuring jug, pour the liquid into a bottle, adding an equal volume of brandy as a preservative. The flowers from the bowl need to be thoughtfully cleared away and every other trace of the operation removed. The essence remains the only record of the proceeding.

Making of the essence, from start to finish, is a complete and continuous process, a sequence, which like the seamless cloth of the day, is a unique and whole event. The circumstances which are closest to the bowl are also closest to the remedy. But all events, near and far in space and time, subtend the central focused place where the flowers lie in the sunshine upon the water in the bowl. This is not a theory but an observation from experience. The landscape is an integral part of the process. And there is a scale to this which can be more readily imagined when we see a single flower opening to the cloudless sky; each flower and leaf connects to the sun through the light that falls upon it. Each plant, bush and tree is a part of the whole landscape and the whole landscape informs the essence just as it informs the plants. For this reason it is possible, at a later date, to read out the quality and circumstances of a remedy making from the essence or stock, tracing back from the record, as it were, the lines of energy to the moment of recording.

This recording is held in the water. The water takes up the impression of the event just as electronic recording devices record sounds and images. The way the water does this is a mystery, although the experiments of Dr

Jacques Benveniste have apparently demonstrated the 'memory of water'.[*] Water is 'the vehicle for information';[16] it is the sunlight, the fire element, which writes the pattern into the essence. Right at the beginning Bach found that dew which had formed in the shade did not carry the same potency as dew which had formed on flowers growing in the sunlight;[17] it was the sun which made the potency. The exact details which the sun writes into the essence are determined by the flowers on the surface of the water, the filter through which the light shines.

Light

Chlorophyll

$$6CO_2 + 6H_2O \rightleftharpoons C_6H_{12}O_6 + 6O_2$$

PHOTOSYNTHESIS

It would be convenient if there were some scientific illustration for all this, some chemistry that, like the formula for photosynthesis, would explain how the energy transfer is made. But in many respects this is a clear enough picture of what is taking place. Replace the catalyst chlorophyll with the flowers on the bowl: a similar formula could be written.

Light

Bowl

Spring water $\rightleftharpoons$ *Potentized Essence*

SUN METHOD

The elements on both sides of the equations are the same but the energetic patterns are rearranged. It might be noticed that photosynthesis is a reversible reaction and that when $C_6H_{12}O_6$ is metabolized in the presence of oxygen then energy is given off. The equivalent of this in the sun method

---

* In 1984 the controversial experimental work by this French doctor appeared to validate the central proposition of homœopathy that there can be a 'memory' in water although it no longer holds any physical substance. Beneveniste (see his website publications at www.digibio.com and www.homœopathyhome.com) speaks of a molecular signal which can communicate like a radio signal or similar even though the physical

is when a person takes the remedy; the patterning of energy is released into their energetic body. To give a name to this process, the transfer of the patterned energy that is in the essence, as well as the transfer that occurs in the sun method itself, we might borrow a term from photosynthesis and call it resonance transfer.

The resonance which is transferred in the sun method can only be a form of light. It is light which falls upon the bowl, light which enters the spring water and light which enlivens the essence. In plant life we see the more general transfer of light into physical form through photosynthesis. In photosynthesis there is the means to compound light energy into starch and sugar to form physical nourishment for other life forms. But here, in making the remedy, the light does not pass into physical form: that is why there is no chemistry involved, no measurable changes. In the resonance transfer of the sun method we can make use of light more directly, not as a source of physical nourishment, but as succour and nourishment for the light body we possess.

In the sun method we have a process which utilizes some of the light that otherwise falls generally on to earth. Light is concentrated and focused into the patterning of flowers of the specific type choosen: Impatiens, Clematis, Mimulus. Light energy is passed through the filter of the flowers and into the water. The water, since it is newly born from the darkness of the earth, is receptive and impressionable—it takes up the resonance of the light with the specific quality of the flower employed. This resonance transfer induces visible changes in the spring water: bubbles form, there are slight tinges of colour and taste. Bubbles which form in the water must indicate the release of gases, such as would be seen if water were heated in a kettle. The transforming element of fire, in the form of light, has entered the water.

---

material is absent. He proposes 'that water is capable of carrying molecular information (biological messages) and that it is possible to transmit and amplify this information, as can be done with sounds and music'. During experiments he observed that although a substance was diluted in water 'to a degree where the final solution contains only water molecules . . . this highly diluted solution initiated a reaction, as if the initial molecules were still present in the water.' His written account of the signals which are exchanged between molecules reads, to a layman, as at least parallel to the explanations of resonance theory in textbooks of science. One comment is particularly apt: 'What about water in all this? It is the vehicle for information'. A balancing account of Benveniste's experiments and claimed results is given in Philip Ball's $H_2O - A$ Biography of Water, Weidenfeld & Nicholson, 1999; page 287ff. We might conclude from this that the results of experiments can be influenced by the thoughts of the experimenter.

It might be argued that if the light has entered the spring water we could expect to see the light in the essence subsequently. Well we do. True, this is not the light which shines physically like light from a candle, but it is the light that can be seen metaphysically, or felt by the sensitive. This light or energy is the potency of the remedy and is unique to each making and each individual essence. It is difficult to describe it if you do not see it, although there is nothing special about it since it is universal: the light of life. All our culture is based upon the idea that there is a difference between light and darkness; thereby we acknowledge qualities which belong to the living. This is the presence of the light body which interpenetrates the physical. It exists around all living forms in varying degrees: rocks, plants, animals, people. When an essence is prepared this light body is released into spring water, the resonance transfer, which gives a particular quality to the essence.

Once made, the essence holds the resonance. And the resonance is transferred from mother tincture, to stock, to dosage as the liquids are diluted. It has already been suggested that Bach used sympathetic resonance to match his emotional state to the plant (pages 36–7). It is equally possible to use sympathetic resonance to match the remedy to the person. Many people use this in dowsing, muscle testing and so on. Then, when it comes actually to taking the remedy, a further transfer can be experienced: from the essence to the person. As the resonance enters the being it lifts the tonal quality, elevating the emotional state, brightening the mood of the life.

Describing that experience, Bach wrote in 1930 of people taking the first sun method preparations. He spoke of the specific qualities of the remedies but observed the general elevation of mood that they bring:

> . . . the remedy brings peace, and a definite mental uplift, of which the patients are usually very conscious.[18]
> . . . the remedy brings sunshine into their lives and helps them to cheer others.[19]

And a little later, in February 1931, he wrote:

> The action of these remedies is to raise our vibrations and open up our channels for the reception of our Spiritual Self . . .[20]

In general terms it is the life-affirming qualities of light in the essence which enhance the mental state of the person—bringing about a change in the light body. The specific therapeutic effect of any one essence is more detailed and that detail is determined by the patterning of the plant species.

Having completed the preparation of an individual essence by the sun method it is necessary to label and store the mother tincture. It is kept in the dark. The integrity of the essence is not inviolable and it is helpful to consider what circumstances will least interfere with it. The circumstances which applied to making also apply to maintaining, so that heat and light may change the quality. Electrical and magnetic forces may interfere with the patterning. A strong emotional charge may also have an effect upon the remedy. More general environmental influences may also need to be taken into account. While it is not helpful to be overprotective, care is needed. This is a subject which requires some study and careful thought.

Once back from the expedition, the utensils need to be boiled in a large pan of water for fifteen to twenty minutes. This has the effect of breaking the patterning from the essence preparation and leaves the bowls clear and ready for re-use. Apparently Bach destroyed the bowls after each making,[21] preferring to use new materials on each occasion. But he had previously described the necessity to sterilize utensils when making homœopathic remedies[22] and we may assume that he or Nora reverted to that procedure at some stage. That Bach broke the bowls illustrates his sense that this process was based upon resonance transfer: the bowl takes up a part of the patterning, if only to a limited extent, and it could transfer that resonance to a subsequent making. Nora also tells us[23] that Bach washed his hands 'to remove any trace of the first remedy before touching the next'. Was this merely a precaution against physically contaminating one essence with another or was he using the hand washing to electrically discharge himself? The more we look into the details of the procedures, the more it becomes apparent that we are dealing with subtle energy and not physical material.

HEAL THYSELF

An Explanation of the Real Cause and Cure of Disease

By

EDWARD BACH

M.B., B.S., D.P.H.

LONDON: THE C. W. DANIEL COMPANY
Forty-six Bernard Street, W.C.1

4 · Heal Thyself—Free Thyself

SOON AFTER HIS DISCOVERY of the sun method, Dr Bach went to stay in Abersoch (in North Wales) and wrote *Heal Thyself, An Explanation of the Real Cause and Cure of Disease.* It is not a long book, less than 12,000 words in all, but given the few weeks involved in writing it must surely have been gestating for some time. It was written during June and July, according to Nora, who was there with him at the time. Her account of *Heal Thyself* in chapter ten of her own book *Medical Discoveries* stands alongside Bach's text.

What is to be made of it? *Heal Thyself* is a challenge, even in its title. One cannot avoid the somewhat messianic style. It is a polemic in favour of the Soul, the Higher Self, Love, Unity and the Divine Creator. Truth to tell, the material is not well organized, the arguments repetitive and poorly-constructed, so that it is difficult to tell if we are in the beginning, the middle or the end. But the message is unmistakable. Bach shouted out his Truth: belief in a greater reality than the growing materialism of his day. If his published work to date had been careful and slightly academic, he now threw caution to the winds and declared himself. He was coming out—as a man with faith in the spiritual reality of the created world.

Looking at *Heal Thyself* today, we might think that it tells us more about Bach than anything else. It is a statement of his beliefs, a picture of how he understood himself, his life and the world in which he lived. In order to avoid any misunderstanding, let it be said that many people share his world view. But the book can still be read as a personal commentary on his life work. It makes clear statements of how and why people get sick and how they may get well. He said, without ambiguity, that illness is meaningful and that each and every one of us can profitably examine our lives with a view to understanding that meaning. He was most taken up with the need to ' be ourselves' and not allow the domination of others—a theme he returned to in *Free Thyself*—to find our true calling and follow that at all costs. If we follow our hearts in that way (our Higher Self, or Soul, as Bach would say) we cannot go wrong. Perhaps he was reinforcing his own conviction that he *needed* to leave London and search for the new remedies and that it was the right thing to do.

It seems certain that Bach felt he was guided to that conviction. He referred, repeatedly, to the responsibility which lies with the 'older brother' or the wise physician, the responsibility to help others to understand themselves. So it might be assumed that he was helped by such a one, as well as informed by his own wisdom. Those who have been helped, in turn help others. But it is in the nature of such things that we do not always know who those 'brothers' might have been. It is clear that, in his view, the priests had abnegated their responsibility for guidance in spiritual matters. That left a vacuum of teaching into which he felt the physician should be called. He imagined that, in the future, we would come to understand life through our understanding of illness and disease. Indeed the central statement of *Heal Thyself* is that disease is generated by our inability to listen to the voice of our soul, a voice which would lead us to understand the individual meaning of our life.

As with Bach's discovery of Impatiens as his own type remedy, it is clear that for him the meaning of his life was to understand 'the real cause and cure of disease'. It does not matter that his understanding was incomplete. His message was not so much in the ultimate cure as in the current understanding: *Heal Thyself* is about Bach's understanding, at that time, of the nature of human life on earth. Some readers might have preferred to supply their own philosophy—'give the facts and we can work out what it means'. That was precisely how Bach had started out when publishing information about the new remedies. He just told it how it was: make the remedy like this, take it like that. But it was so easy for misuse and misunderstanding to creep in, as they had when allopathic doctors wrongly prescribed homœopathic medicines.[1] Perhaps, for that reason, Bach was reluctant to offer his newly discovered flower remedies to the world without the commentary of the metaphysical reality from which he derived them. And this remains a dynamic for us today as we consider the relationship between the spiritual aspects of healing and the materialism of contemporary science and medicine.

If Bach had not written these things, what might have happened to his new remedies? Without his commentary on the reality of the soul and higher self, and the part they play in health and disease, would things have been different? Or, putting it another way, does the efficacy of Dr Bach's remedies depend upon the philosophy behind them? In *Free Thyself* he made it clear that the remedies 'have a definite healing power quite apart from faith'[2] which is independent of the person who administers them. So he appeared to give them independence from himself and his personal magnetism. But it is reasonable to wonder how true that actually was. Does motivation have a part in the process? Weeks cites a number of occasions when Bach's healing gifts came into play, and the healer cannot easily be separated from the healed. These are speculative questions, of course, but there is a tension between the philosophy and the product on the shelf, as it were. Equally it might be asked if there is any value in helping someone towards health if they fail to appreciate the lessons involved. Bach said that healing the body alone, without resolving the cause of the illness, was a serious problem and at best a lesson deferred.[3] There is no suggestion that he withheld remedies from those who did not share his vision for life. But if he had withheld that vision would there be any point in taking the remedy?

In 1930 an article by Bach was published in the magazine *Homœopathic World*, entitled *Some Fundamental Considerations of Disease and Cure.*[4] Written at the end of the summer (he had by then made the last of the sun method remedies for that year, which he listed in the article), it is a shorter and more succinct account of the ideas in *Heal Thyself.* Nora Weeks and other writers have largely ignored it. But it is interesting and positive, even if outspoken. It probably led to trouble. J. Ellis Barker, the editor of the magazine, wrote that 'Dr Bach's assertions are staggering' and he could well understand that the medical profession received them with 'ridicule and derision'. Dr C. E. Wheeler, his fellow researcher from the 1920s, was to comment ' I have not been able to follow his thought easily in these later years and he thought me, I fear, slow and reactionary'.[5] Was he referring to this material? It seems likely.

In the article Bach proposed that if we are to understand disease we must first understand the nature of human life:

> To understand disease, its object, its nature, and its cure, we must in part comprehend the reason of our being and the laws of our Creator in relation to us. It is essential to realise that man has two aspects, a spiritual and a physical; and that of these two, the physical is infinitely the less important. Under the guidance of our Spiritual Self, our Immortal Life, Man is born to gain knowledge and experience; and to perfect himself as a physical being.[6]

Next, he asserted that we must say 'yes' to the lessons of life since learning our lessons is an integral part of life's purpose:

> . . . we learn slowly, one lesson at a time, but we must if we are to be well and happy, learn the particular lesson given to us by our spiritual self. We are not all learning the same lesson at the same time. One is conquering pride, another fear, another hate, and so on, but the essential factor for health is that we do learn the lesson set for us.[7]

Then comes disease:

> Disease is the result of a conflict, when the personality refuses to obey the dictates of the soul, when there is disharmony, disease, between the Higher or Spiritual Self, and the lower personality as we know ourselves.[8]

The physician, said Bach, must recognize the signs and symptoms of this disharmony. According to the individual life lesson that we are having trouble with:

> . . . so on the physical plane does a definite mentality develop, with its consequent results both on the patient and those associated with him. It is this mentality which teaches the physician the real fundamental cause of the patient's trouble, and gives to him the keynote of successful treatment.[9]

'The reason for disease', said Bach, 'is to cause us to cease wrong actions':

> And so disease is sent to us to hasten our evolution. Cruel as it may seem in our narrow outlook, it is in reality beneficent in its nature. It is the method adopted by our own Fatherly Loving Soul, to bring us to the path of understanding.[10]

This must have caused a bit of a stir—disease is good because it offers a chance to understand life? Suffering is a privilege? Disease is the result of mental error? The blurb on *Heal Thyself* said that Bach 'comes directly into the practical politics of medicine' but this was hardly practical politics, it flew in the face of everything that the science of medicine stood for.

Bach was truly swimming against the tide. Although he appealed to his colleagues to give a fair hearing to his ideas, we may be sure that he was at odds with most of the research work that was then being done.

Vivisection he regarded as misguided; 'gland-grafting' was black magic,*
'ten thousand times worse than any plague, for it is a sin against God,
man and animal'.[11] Spare part surgery was not known in his day but
what would he have said about organ transplants? Or worse, what of
the present day issues of genetic manipulation and cloning? He avoided
direct criticism of his contemporaries but pointed to the art of healing
in ancient India where medicine was so advanced that they were able
to abolish surgery.[12] 'The scientific efforts being evolved to obtain reju-
venation, prolongation of natural life and increase of sensual pleasures
by means of devilish practices'[13] were only just beginning at his time. It
seems that Bach was not personally interested in preserving his own life
at any cost. When he was dying, in the autumn of 1936, he 'called in the
profession'[14] only to avoid 'complications, inquests and so on'. There were
worse things than dying, apparently.

Bach is not a hero just because he met his own disease and death head
on; but it is important to point up the fact that he lived what he said.
He had first-hand experience of serious illness from his cancer operation
in 1917. During the nineteen years from 1917-1936, he was struggling to
make sense of his own experiences; trying to discover the cause of disease.
It is unconvincing when someone who has never been ill tells us what
they believe to be the cause of illness. For Bach his own illness was the
forge for his creed: a creed he recited in *Heal Thyself* and other writings.
We do not have to believe him. But, what if we 'come a little further along
the road', as he invited the homœopaths in 1931?[15] What do we find? First
and foremost that Bach had an urgent need to share his conviction that
our real life is not limited to the body we inhabit on earth. That body is
just a vehicle. While we need to take care of it, the physical body is not
important compared to the soul, the 'superphysical' being that we are.

Bach used the issues of illness and health to illustrate the relationship
between body and soul. If we properly understand the purpose of our

---

* In 1928, Bach contributed to an essay on *The Gland-Grafting Operations of Dr.
Voronoff* in *Medical World*. Dr Voronoff had made a name for himself by attempting
to graft apes' testicles on to humans—his cry was 'I call for children of genius. Give
me such children and I will create a new super-race of men of genius'. Bach's concerns
centred on the assurance given by medical authorities of the day that simian characteristics could not cross the species barrier. (CJD has answered that question if we were in
any doubt.) This subject requires an independent study, but it is interesting to record
that Bach was active in the debate on medical ethics and the scientific advisability of
such reckless experimentation.

life, by listening to our soul, there would be no need for illness. In short, illness is there to tell us the way we misdirect our lives. The purpose of our life is to evolve, as it is the purpose of all life. This means that we explore our potential, move into every possibility as air expands to fill every space. This is not the simple evolution of the physical body, not the evolution of the neo-Darwinian school, which considers the adaptation of physical forms as an explanation for life on earth, but the evolution our Higher Self, of spiritual consciousness. And this spiritual consciousness evolves only through the struggle of learning and the overcoming of life difficulties. If there were no difficulty there would be no change. So long as a life encounters no resistance it continues in the same way, repeating itself, expanding the *quantity* of experience without changing the *quality*. But when there is resistance, an obstacle to overcome, there is a need to consider how we continue with life and how we may need to change—how to evolve a new form of activity, to behave differently. It is like a plant which grows in an easy soil and then comes to a rock or dry place and must change the pattern of growth in response—like Mimulus, learning to live under water.

If we encounter the changing circumstances of life and successfully explore our potential, all is well. We learn our lessons and continue with life. If we avoid the lessons of life or react against them in some way, then we are avoiding what life offers. At first 'our Fatherly Loving Soul' will whisper a word of advice, pointing out our best advantage for continuing our schooling here on earth. If we choose to ignore the message then comes a stronger warning. At last, the voice of our soul must break through into the physical world to be heard. Thereby we encounter the process of disease: 'the terminal stage of a much deeper disorder'.[16]

Disease, in Bach's experience, has the useful purpose of pointing out to us, not just the need to change, but even the way we need to change. Although he did not mention cancer he listed some illnesses and the reason for them.[17] He went on to assert that even the affected part of the body was an indication of the 'error' that needed to be understood and learned about.* It is credible therefore that, sick with cancer at the age of thirty, Bach was being given a specific opportunity to change his own

---

* Louise L. Hay has developed this idea and speaks of her own cancer in *Heal Your Body, the mental causes of physical illness and the metaphysical way to overcome them*, Heaven on Earth Books, 1984. Cancer, she puts down to 'deep hurt, long-standing resentment, deep secret or grief eating away at the self, hatred.'

way of living. The exact details are unknown, but his survival showed that he took the opportunity. Then, as he worked with a passion to develop and fulfil his destiny, answering the call of his soul, he held the illness at bay, in remission if you prefer, until such time as he had completed his life work.

It is not always as straightforward as this. Bach's own case illustrated how disease can be neutralized by responding to the life lesson that needs to be learned. But for others (and maybe for Bach) the issues can become more complex. We have to take account of other people and entities which may be involved (Bach's wife, friends and family, his past life), processes working through lifetimes, the part played by chance, or the way an individual responds to circumstances beyond control. But, however the drama of life is experienced, it is sure that, willingly or unwillingly, everything in life is a part of us. With Bach we may draw some few conclusions from this. We must not be afraid. Especially we must not be afraid of death. It will sour life if we are. We must act upon our heart's desire and live freely, provided that we do not curtail the freedom of others in doing so ('to gain freedom, give freedom'[18]). We must support others as we may: the old commandment to love your neighbour as yourself.

Fear, materialism, the modern disease of boredom, self love, worldly amusements, sensuality, resignation, pretence, enslavement, pride, cruelty, hate, ignorance, instability and greed—all these and more were mentioned by Bach as 'the real primary diseases of man'.[19] The symptoms of conflict which he saw as 'adverse to Unity';[20] the unity from which we come and to which we are making our return. The general picture of such emotional states was given a sharper focus when Bach described how each person comes into this life with a particular lesson to learn: a soul lesson which gives the opportunity to transcend the limitations of that particular emotional state and develop the positive virtue which is associated with it.

Doubtless, the nature of the lesson is determined by what an individual needs to learn. If the past life was careless we learn concern; if we were previously cruel then we learn through the experience of pain; if we were downtrodden, we learn to stand up for ourselves. However the wheel of fate deals with us, we enter life with one such predisposing theme which needs to be worked upon. As Bach observed, this is like an astrological type[21]—the essential quality of the life. It does not determine all; it is rather a point of departure, the place from which we begin to learn about ourselves.

In his early work he saw how the body's immune system retained a record of previous microbial invasions—that was the basis for vaccine therapy. Now Bach was suggesting that as an individual developed the virtue which was needed for a life lesson—as courage is developed to overcome fear—then 'once and for all' there would be 'immunity against the adverse quality'.[22] The model for the process of learning and growth in the emotional world is paralleled by the physical world. As an individual learns about the quality of a life lesson that knowledge is retained. Also, certain emotional states are pathogenic, just as certain bacteria are pathogenic. And in both cases we can overcome the pattern of disease by introducing some therapeutic substance. For smallpox we used the smallpox vaccine and that triggers an immune response which the body remembers. For the treatment of an emotional pathogen:

> . . . the work of the physician is two-fold, to assist his patient to correct his spiritual failing, and to give him such remedies as will help him to effect this on the physical plane; so that the healthier mind will effect a cure of the body.[23]

In this process Bach states as axiomatic the principle that 'the mind must be healed first and the body will follow'.[24]

The superior part played by the mind is not easy to prove. The analogy can be drawn of how architects draw a blueprint before a builder constructs the physical form. But that does not constitute evidence. Here it must be admitted that Bach's personal belief carried him across the desert of scepticism. He has little or nothing to say about evidence. Using the Platonic model, which points to the world of ideas and not the Aristotelian model which builds through perceived evidence, he simply stated his view:

> Truth has no need to be analysed, argued about,—or wrapped up in many words. It is realised in a flash, it is part of you. It is only about the unessential complicated things of life that we need so much convincing, and that have led to the development of the intellect.[25]

In this Bach was placing himself in the mystical tradition and taking leave of both logic and science. Not everyone will continue with him on the journey.

Bach wrote *Some Fundamental Considerations* and *Heal Thyself* at about the same time in the late spring and early summer of 1930. He had begun work with the sun method and found the first in the new series of remedies. He was in the midst of a ferment of ideas and discovery. This was reflected in his rather restless crossing and re-crossing of the country from London to north Wales, to south Wales, to London, and from London to Cromer, in Norfolk, through the summer months. He was working on several levels simultaneously. He was finding the new remedies, then testing them and writing an account of the provings. He was attempting to construct a philosophical basis for the fundamental principles of his 'life lessons'. He was, as any one of us might, trying to integrate his new ideas with his personal life, learning and loves; then to integrate his professional experiences as a doctor and medical researcher with the new ideas and the thinking of his colleagues. He was endeavouring to integrate the revelation ('realized in a flash') with the more mundane.

Ye Suffer from Yourselves, a lecture read to the British Homœopathic Society in February 1931, was his attempt to speak directly to his colleagues and share his vision for a new future in medicine and in homœopathy. The opening paragraphs gave fair warning of what he intended:

> *In coming to address you this evening, I find the task not an easy one. You are a medical society, and I come to you as a medical man: yet the medicine of which one would speak is so far removed from the orthodox views of today, that there will be little in this paper which savours of the consulting room, nursing home, or hospital ward as we know them at present.*[26]

As he got into his stride he made it clear he did have a very different view of medicine. Speaking once again of the purpose of disease as a corrective measure adopted by the soul, he dismissed 2,000 years of science as 'entirely wrong' because it 'has regarded disease as a material factor which can be eliminated by material means'.[27] Even Hahnemann had an incomplete conception of the truth. Perhaps it was the strength of his experiences which led him to be so forceful in his expression. A few people must have had a word with him afterwards and suggested that he tone it down a bit; he was likely to alienate his professional colleagues with his assertive style.

Yet Bach was leaving his colleagues, friends and London professional life behind him for good. He wanted nothing more to do with the trappings of doctoring: the white coats, the 'stethoscopes and tappings to impress upon the patient's mind the nature of his illness. No constant feeling of the pulse . . .'.[28] In his hospital of the future he said that there would be no place for disease, only those things that are 'uplifting and beautiful'. *Ye Suffer from Yourselves* is a valediction.

Before he finished his lecture, however, he tackled the question of how to achieve this future. With regard to the training of physicians this meant that we must know ourselves and be familiar with the voice of our soul before attempting to help patients; even more so before attempting to assist them to correct their spiritual failings. No other qualifications would do. Bach said the main task for study was the understanding of human nature and the divine state of man. Then we would need to dedicate ourselves to service and be willing to become an instrument of the Divine Plan. He must have been aware that he was speaking of a distant dream, a prospect for the golden future which *might* be realized. His vision was for the true physician;[29] no longer just a doctor, not quite a priest and yet more involved than a philosopher. His advice for training was there:

> *The way to set about to do this work is to practise exquisite gentleness....*
> *The most that we can do is, when we have a little more knowledge and experience than a younger brother, very gently to guide them. If they will listen, well and good: if not, we must patiently wait until they have had further experience to teach them their fault, and then they may come to us again.*
> *We should strive to be so gentle, so quiet, so patiently helpful that we move among our fellow men more as a breath of air or a ray of sunshine: ever ready to help them when they ask: but never forcing them to our own views.*[30]

This was what we should do while waiting for the world to change.

But will the world change? Was Bach expecting too much? Was he alienating his audience with his *Ye Suffer*... message? Would *We Suffer*... have been an easier pill to swallow? From the perspective of a new century it begins to be clear that Bach was intent upon two separate purposes. On the one hand he had discovered a new set of remedies and he wanted people to use them. They came to be the well-known Bach flower remedies. On the other, he was the herald for a new world, a voice crying in the medical wilderness of materialism and ignorance. The second purpose is easy to forget and hard to accept. The two became separated at an early stage, maybe well before Bach died. The message from spiritual reality became subsumed into the opportunity for people to avail themselves of floral healing. *Heal Thyself* remained in print but it stood apart from the remedies. There have been people who read that book with enthusiasm and never took a flower remedy and many more who have taken a remedy but had no idea that *Heal Thyself* was the message behind it.

The spiritual truth revealed to Bach continued as the hidden power which guided 'the work' through the decades, always implicit but not seen for what it was. Nora Weeks told us that Bach destroyed all the early versions of his work sometime in 1936, making a bonfire in the garden at *Mount Vernon*.[31] It was a strange action, but one which effectively prevented enquiry about the process by which he found out what he did. At the time, he was living with Mary Tabor at *The Wellsprings*, in Sotwell, and it was from this address that Bach wrote many of the letters which have survived from his last years[32] (*The Wellsprings,* Sotwell was given as his address on his death certificate). These letters illustrate the continuing conviction with which Bach lived his last years, inspired with a sense of revealed divinity and self-realization. In one piece he wrote: 'All TRUE KNOWLEDGE comes ONLY from WITHIN OURSELVES, in silent communication with our own Soul [his caps].'[33] In another he speaks of the crusade, the mission to bring hope to the people.

However, looking at what he wrote in 1936, it is clear that he became careful to tailor his thoughts to fit the occasion. In his last two lectures there are two contrasting positions. In the *Wallingford Lecture*, given before a public audience, he focused on the tradition of herbal healing and then in simple practical terms talked about a few of the remedies. No mention of soul and no mysticism. In the *Masonic Lecture* he was speaking to a group of Masonic brothers and sets the perspective from a higher horizon line: the 'Divine Spark' in mankind.* He delivered an account full of the spiritual language characteristic of his earlier writings and lectures. It is apparent that by 1936 he had developed two different versions of the story. One was for the initiated, or at least for those who might respond to his visionary approach, the other, a simpler account, spoke to the caring, good nature of the ordinary person. These ordinary,

---

* The idea of the Divine Spark may well derive from Plotinus (c.205-270) and the neo-Platonists. Plotinus saw the created worlds as illumined by divine light which comes from the Unity or the One and penetrates to the distant darkness of the outer edges of material existence. This divine spark is present in us all and offers the potential for individual union with the higher levels of existence, of the soul with unity. If we read on in *Free Thyself,* where Bach speaks of truth being realized in a flash, he comes to the thought that there are 'moments where there is a spiritual union'.

unqualified people might want to help the sick but lacked any medical training; they were to become the recipients of Bach's legacy.

Having offered the big story to his medical colleagues and been rejected, Bach gave the remedies to the general public as a simple self-help, self-heal methodology. He did not change one part of his system of belief but hid it away from the hard stares of others. Nora Weeks knew what he believed in but, in part, softened it and in part decided to gloss it over. Mary Tabor wrote a book, *To Thine Own Self Be True*, a novel which leans heavily towards Bach's ideas. But she disappeared from the story and went on with her own life. At the end we were left with Bach's short texts of *The Twelve Healers* and the opportunity to find out for ourselves.

Bach's decision to give the remedies to the people began in 1932. In *Free Thyself*, a clearer and better-organized version of *Heal Thyself*, he made some key remarks about how we may help ourselves (without medical supervision) and how we may all take part in the glorious process of healing and helping one another:

> Should any difficulty be found in selecting your own remedy, it will help to ask yourself which of the virtues you most admire in other people....
> We are all healers, and with love and sympathy in our natures we are also able to help anyone who really desires health.[34]

This self-treatment and healing from those who are not medically trained was introduced in keeping with the belief that there is no need to know the name or the nature of the disease: 'our physical illness is of no consequence whatsoever'.[35] By 1933, in an article entitled *Twelve Great Remedies* Bach wrote: 'I am endeavouring to make the prescribing so simple that [the remedies] can be used by lay people'.[36] And he continued with that intention until the end of his life.

Custody of the remedies was given to the public, across the world. No patents, no trade secrets, no trademarks. Bach remedies were there for all of us, whoever cared to pick up *The Twelve Healers* and learn about them:

> Moreover, it has pleased Him to give these Remedies to the people themselves; for such is their simplicity that the people may find and prepare their own medicines and heal themselves and each other of their adversities.[37]

The inner teaching was given into the hands of the small group of his friends who had worked with him. Letters from Bach make this purpose apparent; one written in October, a month before he died, set out his plan explicitly:

> *Dear Folk,*
> *It would be wonderful to form a little Brotherhood without rank or office, none greater and none less than the other, who devoted themselves to the following principles:*
> *1.   That there has been disclosed unto to us a System of Healing such as has not been known within the memory of men; when, with the simplicity of the Herbal Remedies, we can set forth with the CERTAINTY, the absolute CERTAINTY, of their power to conquer disease.*
> *2.   That we never criticise nor condemn the thoughts, the opinions, the ideas of others; ever remembering that all humanity are God's children, each striving in his own way to find the Glory of his Father. That we set out on the one hand, as knights of old, to destroy the dragon of fear, knowing that we may never have one discouraging word, but that we can bring HOPE, aye, and most of all, CERTAINTY to those who suffer.*
> *3.   That we never get carried away by praise or success that we meet in our Mission, knowing that we are but the messengers of the Great Power.*
> *4.   That as more and more we gain the confidence of those around, we proclaim to them we believe that we are divine agents sent to succour them in their need.*
> *5.   That as people become well, that the Herbs of the field which are healing them, are the gift of Nature which is the Gift of God; thus bring them back to a belief in the LOVE, the MERCY, and the tender COMPASSION and the ALMIGHTY POWER OF THE MOST HIGH.*[38]

5 · Not the Right Remedy

WITH THE BONFIRE at *Mount Vernon*, in which Bach is said to have destroyed his papers, much of the evidence illustrating the stages by which the remedies were discovered was lost to us. His idea was that when the house is built you take away the scaffolding. But anyone who has bought a house knows the value of a set of blueprints and information about the alterations made by previous owners. One way to come to a deeper understanding of Bach's work is by re-examining the way he made his discoveries. This is an interesting exercise as we know for certain that Bach made a series of changes to the list of remedies, particularly in the early days.

At the outset there lay before him the whole created world: he could look for therapeutic substances in any material—animal, vegetable or mineral. Remedies, he said, can be looked at in the context of the 'evolutionary status of the material'.[1] Metals were not appropriate for treating humans. The dismissal is easy to appreciate. Metals had enjoyed medical favour in the days when chemistry was a novelty but have since been shown to carry no direct curative value for us—metals are best mediated through the plant world. Bach said that animals should not be used, since that would entail cruelty. No animals in healing means much of contemporary medicine must go: vaccines and drugs are often developed in guinea pigs. Bach's objection was on ethical and practical grounds: 'it is essential that the remedies chosen should be life-giving and uplifting; of such vibrations that elevate'.[2] Any process that limits the freedom of the animal would be counter.

And so 'we are left with the vegetable kingdom'. Chosen by default, he gave scant attention to the real qualities of plant life:

> *Just as God in His mercy has given us food to eat, so has He placed amongst the herbs of the fields beautiful plants to heal us when we are sick. These are there to extend a helping hand to man in those dark hours of forgetfulness when he loses sight of his Divinity . . .*[3]

He divided plants into three categories:

a.   Primitive varieties—below man.

b.   Food—on the same relative scale as man.

c.   Healing plants—those on as high or higher than average mankind.

In the first category, the primitives, he includes seaweeds, cacti and the parasitic dodder; then plants 'which have been used for wrong purposes' (what purposes he did not say), some of which are poisonous; he mentions plants like henbane, belladonna and orchids. There are some problems with this analysis. Essentially, Bach seemed to be grouping certain species in a category where they lack the healing quality he seeks, rather than because of some collective negative quality. Some cacti have remarkable energy patterns which act to clear and order. But, perhaps, they do not act with appropriate resonance for what Bach was seeking. He described this first group as 'lowering the vibrations of the body'[4] and worse, making the body unfit 'for the habitation of the human soul'. Well, that is one way to describe the action of poison.

The second group, plants used as food, is not that much clearer, unfortunately. Several of Bach's remedy plants have been and can be used as food: Oak (acorns), Wild Rose (rosehips), Olive and Vine. It may be that Bach was making a specific rejection here, however. It is characteristic of most food plants that they lend themselves too readily to hybridization—the *Brassica* family has been adapted to produce cabbages, sprouts, broccoli and cauliflower.* As such they do not possess a dependable and exact species pattern. They cannot be relied upon; they might be useful or might be damaging, it would depend upon conditions for that individual. This is an important consideration since there is concern about the dependability of so many plants at this time. Those that hybridize most readily are the weakest metaphysically: the patterning of the subtle body is uncertain and that informs the physical

---

* Lawrence D. Hills of The Henry Doubleday Research Association, in *Save Your Own Seed*, wrote: 'One of the many differences between cabbages and men is that we have the genes that carry our inherited qualities in forty-six chromosomes, and they have eighteen. Broccoli, cauliflowers, most kales, cabbages and kohlrabi are all descended from the wild *Brassica oleracea* from the cliffs of Britain and they all have eighteen chromosomes. So has the Charlock, a bright yellow weed of the wheatfields, and all of them can meet, join and change partners in the dance of life as easily as all races do at a Fourth of July party at an American Air-base in Hawaii. For men and cabbage are alike in sharing their qualities, good and bad, because they have no chromosome difference.'

body with distortions, like distorted signals or like corrupted electronic messages. It is a lack of integrity. As we shall see, this becomes important when we choose plants for remedy making: cultivated vines, for instance, are likely to carry less of the clear patterning than original, wild plants (page 173).

Bach's third group still apparently offered him about two thousand species which might be suitable, in Britain alone. Except that it is not known what qualified a flower or tree as being suitable, in Bach's mind. His idea of a 'power to elevate our vibrations, and thus to draw down spiritual power, which cleanses mind and body and heals'[5] sounds wonderful but lacks definition. Weeks noted that Bach spent many months walking in the countryside examining prospective remedy plants but fails to explain how he discriminated between one and another. The bonfire might leave us thinking that the choice was absolute, voiced like Mosaic Law. But the facts tell a clear and different story.

Of the fifteen plants which Bach chose and published as remedies between 1928 and 1932, only twelve made it through reselection; they became *The Twelve Healers*. Impatiens, Clematis and Mimulus remained first team players even after Bach changed the method of preparation to the sun method. But two other plants chosen in 1929 were to be dropped. Cupressus made only one appearance, in *Some New Remedies,* while Cotyledon was selected a second time for the listing in *Some Fundamental Considerations.*

Cupressus has a remedy description which is entirely physiological and is immediately seen as useful—but in the old way. It was dealing only with bodily symptoms. Bach does not tell us exactly the tree he chose from the *Cupressus* family, which has twelve or more members. One of them, *Thuja occidentalis,* is listed as a herbal cough remedy by both Mrs Grieve and Potters Cyclopaedia.[6] Parkinson mentioned it as being tried experimentally for 'purulentous cough', although not until recent years has Thuja been seen as a treatment for bronchial catarrh.[7] Perhaps Bach was on to something, experimenting with a new constitutional remedy for the catarrhal type. But where did the idea come from? Was he making an association between the use of the herbal remedy and the type of person who might benefit from the medicine? The irony here will not be lost upon those who have been accused of inventing new flower essences merely on the basis of a traditional herbal association: Bach did it as well, apparently. Or at least he considered the possibilities!

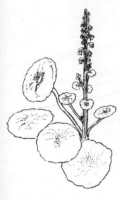

Cotyledon umbilicus (the plant is now named *Cotyledon rupestris*), was, at first, nominated by Bach as a remedy for epilepsy, hysteria and the after-effects of treatment with bromide. He noted that it had a positive benefit 'restoring the natural brightness of the patient'[8]—the brightness that had been dulled by bromide presumably. Cotyledon (its common name is Wall Pennywort, or Navelwort) had no known medical action and is not referenced in any herbal text or pharmacopoeia. Therefore, Bach's selection was original so far as we can tell. It grows commonly upon dry-stone walls in Wales and the south west of England and can

Cotyledon umbilicus be found readily enough in the Abergavenny–Crickhowell area, which is probably where Bach found it, along with Impatiens, Clematis and Mimulus. Bach prepared Cotyledon by homœopathic trituration and we might suppose that he learned the plant's qualities by homœopathic proving: observing the effect when eating some of the raw plant. Recently, when I conducted such an experiment it produced a definite disorientation, a drugged sensation, but no hysteria.

At the beginning Cotyledon appeared to fit within the scheme of things for Bach, as one of the archetypes or soul qualities he had planned. He called this one 'The Hysteric'. Such a person lacked emotional stability, 'they are excitable, nervous: useless in emergency: they become flustered over trifles'.[9] Bach appeared to be working upon a typical emotional picture, one that may be consistent with the instability of the epileptic: 'many cases of hysteria: hystero-epilepsy: and paralysis come into this group'.[10] But he must have decided that 'this group' was not one of the clear type remedies that he was looking for; it was not the kind of soul lesson that one is born with. It seems that he was still unsure whether to base the new remedies upon ordinary medical observation or upon the great soul lessons. He was to decide upon the latter; that is why Cupressus and Cotyledon both had to go.

Different doubts surrounded the discovery of Centaury. This was one of the twelve great types and it was one of the first made by the sun method. But Bach's description in *Some Fundamental Considerations* is perplexing: it is exactly opposite in tone to the description he later settled upon. Centaury people, he said, are noisy, impatient, demanding, over-bearing.[11] He gave them the archetype of 'The Autocrat'. Those who have learned their Bach remedies will recognize that this description is out by

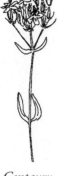

Centaury 180 degrees. How could this happen? What does it tell us of the process

that Bach was undergoing? Is it another illustration of the problems of polarity?

Thinking back to resonance theory this dichotomy is easier to understand. We now recognize the way Centaury types allow themselves to be dominated and often live in a symbiotic relationship with another person who enjoys being dominant, the autocrat. In other words, a Centaury type must be a servant to something, not just a servant in the abstract. In resonating the idea of Centaury, perhaps Bach thought of the dominant character in whose shadow the Centaury person cowers. But, whichever side of the coin we look at, we can see that the soul lesson concerns power. Power tops the list of seven principal errors* which Bach wrote about, the 'seven main divisions into which we have to place our patients'.[12] Centaury people are learning about power. Bach has already told us that these lessons arise through the learning process which the soul experiences over lifetimes. Like the combination of Fear and Courage or Impatience and Forgiveness he saw the whole picture of the Centaury type as Weakness and Strength. In chapter seven of *Heal Thyself* and chapter four of *Free Thyself* Bach wrote about the process of listening to the voice of the soul. Sitting quietly in meditation, he allowed the first clear perception to guide him to the meaning of his experience or answer to his question. Resonating the quality of Centaury in this way he must have misheard, or misread the situation which he was picturing in his mind, the picture of the autocrat and the soul lesson of service.

Another remedy plant which he discovered and then abandoned was *Sonchus arvensis*, one of the Sow Thistles. Sonchus is a bright yellow flower of the daisy family (a *compositae* like dandelion). Bach found Sonchus in August 1930 when he was in Norfolk. He called the remedy Arvensis (the Latin word means 'of the fields') and gave it the archetype of 'The Destroyer'. 'These people,' he said, 'are in the depths of gloom; no light; no joy; no happiness'.[13] It is a description that is like

---

* These seven are:
  1. Power
  2. Intellectual knowledge
  3. Love
  4. Balance
  5. Service
  6. Wisdom
  7. Spiritual Perfection

both Gorse and Mustard—remedies he was to discover later on. Curiously, Mustard uses the same species name *arvensis*: it is *Sinapis arvensis*. Both these later remedy flowers are also yellow and we cannot avoid the thought that yellow flowers have a quality, like the sun, which brightens the person and brings light into life.

At this stage Bach was intent upon finding plants which would fit within the framework of twelve types. Yet here again the kind of brooding depression which he associated with *Sonchus arvensis* is an emotional state which may develop in life without being essential to it. It does not carry the quality of a soul lesson which a person might be born with. As such Arvensis was short-lived as a remedy in the Twelve Healers series, despite the statement from Bach that these 'are certain types'.[14] When he had finalized the twelve basic type remedies in *The Twelve Healers*, the place of this pessimistic personality, who looks always on the dark side, was taken by Gentian (pages 128–131).

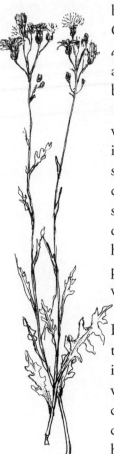

Sonchus arvensis

By choosing remedies which were later either changed or discarded, Bach revealed much about the process he was working with at this time. There are moments when it appears he was acting according to instructions, as if the voice of some other authority was telling him what to look for and the message was wrongly interpreted. If Bach was clairaudient then a message concerning a yellow flower might easily be confused. His account of how, when 'a message came through' (page 37) he turned to the Gorse bush next to him, is indication enough that he made spontaneous assumptions in these matters. Yet these assumptions were subsequently checked empirically. It may be that he destroyed his notes out of vanity, not wishing it to be seen that there had been either doubt or contradiction in the process of discovery. But seventy years later it is easy to accept errors as a positive part of the journey of discovery. Equally, we can see that Dr Bach was changing and modifying his selection of remedy plants in the light of experience. This entailed a rebalancing of the whole set as each new plant was found. Those selected formed a harmonic group which were tuned, as it were, to each other. Or, like the geometry of natural forms he saw in plants, the structure of the set of remedies fell into a natural configuration.

Bach was thinking of great soul qualities and felt that they needed to be named: Love, Sympathy, Understanding and so on. It is as though he had taken a piece of paper and written down the titles or headings for the type remedies he was looking for: there needs to be a remedy for Fear, a remedy for Balance, a remedy for Power. When he asked himself, how many types, did the answer come—why, seven, like the days of the week, the seven planets or the seven wonders of the world; or twelve, like the twelve months, the twelve apostles or the twelve tribes? The appeal may be more to symbolism than to practical value. Combine this theoretical structure with the real practical work of walking in the fields and sensing the resonant properties of individual flowers and we may come close to a sense of how Edward Bach set about finding his remedies.

6 · Cromer

IT WAS MORE THAN THE CHALK SOIL which drew Bach towards Cromer and the east coast of England in the summer of 1930. Chalk soil gives rise to a different range of plants from those he had looked at in Wales and it was an important factor in the discovery of the new remedies he was to find. But chalk is found in many parts of England. Most likely there was a personal involvement for Bach (was there a woman in it some-

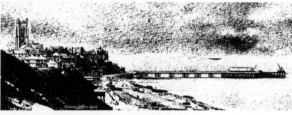

Cromer Pier

where?) for Weeks says that he went there straight from London. As usual, there is that quiet rectitude of Nora's biography that leaves one guessing as to who or what attracted him. There is a photograph of Bach on the beach at Cromer;[1] a group of people sitting somewhat separately, two men and five women. Who was taking the photograph? Of them all Bach looks the most relaxed; no doubt he liked Cromer.

It was during this year that Dr Bach had taken to walking. He walked extensively in Wales and 'he would often take his stick and tramp the fields and lanes around Cromer from morning until night. . . .'[2] This was a change in behaviour for the medical man, used to hospital wards and town life. Walking, however, is a particular way to learn. Mostly, we walk with an end in view and that purpose occupies the mind. But to walk without a purpose is to allow ourselves a freedom to slip between the outer meaning of things. It is a form of meditation. Bach used walking as a way of learning, not so much learning in the sense of accumulating information but learning about the natural rhythms and patterning of life forms. This is not something to be understood in an afternoon: it requires repeated practice over a period of time.

In many different and detailed forms this practice is described by Carlos Castenada in the *Don Juan* books[3]—Castenada repeatedly encounters the problem that he cannot empty his mind of questions, despite the walking. Robert Louis Stevenson wrote about walking alone: ' . . . and then you must be open to all impressions and let your thoughts take colour from what you see. You should be as a pipe for any wind to play upon . . . so long as a man is reasoning he cannot surrender himself to that fine intoxication that comes of much motion in the open air, that begins in a sort of dazzle and sluggishness in the brain and ends in a peace that passeth all comprehension'.[4]

The point here is that after walking repeatedly, day after day, Bach would have come back to town and the people of Cromer with an eye both fresh and clear. The effect of such an exercise was to sharpen his perception so that he might recognize the emotional state of an individual, person or plant. Walking had the effect of emptying him out, clearing away the personal patterning, leaving him open to the impression of external patterning. This is in contradistinction to his earlier method of amplifying his personal remedy state, as he did with Impatiens. Thus, if in the evening he went to have a glass of beer at the pub, he would have met people there whose emotional state resonated clearly upon the still sounding board of his being. If in the morning he walked in the fields and saw Agrimony growing among the grasses, the plant too resonated upon the still sounding board of his being. Such recognition would have been unlikely if he had actively sought a plant to use as a remedy for a certain person. The trick is in the way of seeing without looking, finding without seeking.

Agrimony

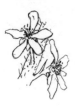

By these means Bach came upon six new remedy plants during August and September 1930.[5] The first of these were Agrimony, Chicory and Vervain. Agrimony as a remedy state definitely belongs to town: these people are sociable, they seek the contact and stimulus of company. It follows that the plant is one which reaches out to touch you, growing in places where it will find company, on the roadside, the field edge, by the paths and tracks where people pass. Yet Agrimony is strangely solitary; even when it grows across a field each plant is distinctly separate, in its own space, interspersed with many other grassland flowers. This is not a plant which builds a massed population of its own kind—it does not grow in a group like Impatiens. Agrimony is dotted among the grasses. Because of its isolated habit it is not even listed as a weed of arable land. Its hold among the population of grassland plants is not strong.

Bach described the Agrimony types as tormented, suffering from restlessness in the soul. The virtue that they seek is peace. Looking back to the words of R. L. Stevenson, it seems to be the same peace which he found in solitary walking: the peace which passes all understanding.[6]

Bach referred to this peace of the soul on many occasions and regarded peace as the first great quality which 'the treatment of tomorrow' will bring to the patient.[7] Quite specifically peace will come from an acceptance and understanding of our individual soul's purpose within life on earth: it is this which the Agrimony type finds hard to accept. To the Agrimony person realities do not stack up. They see and experience the pain of the world (that is their torment) but they feel themselves inadequate for the task of reconciling that pain with faith in life. Rather than face the problem they turn the matter aside with a play of humour. Or they seek to forget themselves with drink or drugs; there is a desire to escape from life.

The mental torment, however, waits within. One can fill the time with banter, with social entertainment, games, with any distraction, but there comes a time of solitude. It was that very alone-ness which Bach sought in his walking. When out walking in that way we leave behind the trappings of appearance, the social meaning of life and may see ourselves as we really are. It might even be framed as a question for diagnosis: 'how do you feel about the prospect of a day, alone, walking in the countryside?' The Agrimony person would at once recognize their vulnerability and plan a defence. An Impatiens type would think about where to go and the quickest route. A Mimulus person would shyly confess the thought of it makes him nervous—supposing there are cows in the fields? A Clematis would be happy to have the time to be alone with dreams. In *The Story of the Travellers*[8] Bach saw the Agrimony person as worrying whether the right road is being taken—later he strides along confidently, free of care, jesting with the others. (Appendix 1, page 287.)

The Agrimony person, however, is a complex character; as a soul type much more than the jester of popular perception. It is as a jester that Bach may have first recognized the type (perhaps among his companions in the *Belle Vue* Bar in Cromer). Bach's various descriptions of Agrimony people showed them as highly sensitive, and the plant illustrates this with a delicacy in leaf and stem, which are both covered with fine hairs. Indeed, the leaves are extraordinarily fine and soft, especially when young. These hairs are a sign of the sensing, receptive nature of the Agrimony. They stand in contrast to the smooth, glabrous leaves of Impatiens, Clematis and Mimulus, each of which are insensitive to the people around them. The leaves are

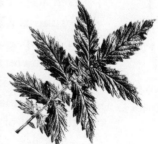

pinnate with leaflets arranged on either side of a common stalk, and they are deeply cut and furrowed. This shows the agitated energy of the Agrimony type, stressed and unbalanced.

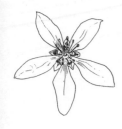

Agrimony flowers, set in a cluster on the stem, look out horizontally, watching the earth, not gazing at the sky. Like radar receivers for terrestrial signals, they scan for messages from the human world around them. In this the Agrimony type is a receptor, absorbing pain and emotional stress from the surroundings. As with Mimulus, the flowers are yellow. This might suggest there is a mental quality to Agrimony, but rather the reverse, the Agrimony state is strongly emotional: it is a flooding of feeling. These people cannot bear to think. One of the reasons they seek company and entertainment is to drown out thoughts which demand attention when they are alone. Now we can see the idea that yellow flowers point to the intellect is too limited: in Agrimony the yellow speaks of more than a mental clarity, although mental clarity is what they yearn for. It also speaks of a soul clarity which can see the world and not be overcome by the pain of seeing. This yellow has the soft, enduring strength of gold, impervious to corrosion. It speaks of the serenity which comes from inner tranquillity, a knowledge of the eternal.

Bach pointed to the 'church-like spire' of the Agrimony 'and its seeds like bells'.[9] He was following the popular plant name of 'church steeples'. These spine-like stems tend to curve over at the end, particularly in warm weather, as if they lose confidence (see Larch page 211). So while there is a certain exuberance it is tentative, uncertain. Nevertheless, each flowering spike is a finger pointing to the sky and as flowers open along the stem there is a ring of golden fire which burns upwards during the summer weeks of flowering. As each flower fades and the petals fall, others open above on the same stem. Progressively the seed fruits form on the stalk, each separate and covered with small hooks, seeking an individual journey to the future; for this is a plant which uses the passers-by as a vehicle for diffusion and propagation. Each fruit has an individual destiny, although curiously there are two seeds in each bell-shaped container—there's an Agrimony joke in there somewhere about never being alone with your self for company. Many authorities, including Mrs Grieve, have noted this habit of catching on to the fur or garments of those walking past:

Agrimonia eupatoria

> It was, Gerard informs us, at one time called Philanthropos, according
> to some old writers, on account of its beneficent and valuable properties,

others saying that the name arose from the circumstances of the seeds clinging to the garments of passers-by, as if desirous of accompanying them, and Gerard inclines to this latter interpretation of the name.[10]

This clearly describes the desire for company felt by the Agrimony type.

Mrs Grieve lists the herbal properties of Agrimony—and they are considerable. She says that it has a great reputation for curing jaundice and other liver complaints. So it is a liver herb: the yellow flowers connect it to the 'yellow system' of liver, bile, kidneys and urine. A part of the liver's physiological function is to cleanse the blood of toxins, specifically the alcohol and other drugs which Agrimony types are apt to take 'to stimulate themselves and help themselves bear their trials with cheerfulness'.[11] As Bach observed: 'frequently they drink heavily or give way to drugs to help them stand the stress'.[12] But the liver is also thought of as the organ that mediates emotions. Just as it functions physiologically to work upon both the sugar content and the toxins of the blood so it functions as a processing station for the building blocks of emotional experience. This processing of emotions can be dysfunctional in the Agrimony type: emotional feeling and reaction is suppressed. These people, said Bach, give up much for the sake of peace and to avoid quarrels and argument. They cannot handle the emotional drama, just as a dysfunctional liver cannot handle the toxins in the blood.

Working in the conventional way of herbal medicine we can read of Agrimony as a treatment for skin disorders.[13] While it is generally agreed that Bach remedies are not linked directly with medical conditions it has been observed that there can be a relationship between the Agrimony type and skin problems. The skin flags up the suppressed emotion, as if to say 'laugh that off your face'.

Agrimony is a perennial plant and stores sugar in a taproot, just as Chicory and Vervain do. All three have things in common with respect to how the emotional life is managed. These are three plants of similar size, growing in broadly similar conditions. In each case the plant and the person both speak of the past life and the way the soul has dealt with life experience—in a similar way we have seen that Impatiens, Mimulus and Clematis each look to the future. Life experience is like the stored starch in the roots of the plant. This starch is used to carry it through the winter (death) to the following spring (new birth). Starch is the result of metabolism of the plant, sugar manufactured through photosynthesis, and it is emblematic of the way the individual soul deals with life lessons, a spiritual metabolism. Just how each soul type works with life experience is illustrated by the gesture of the plant.

Agrimony, then, the plant which stands alone, is both sensing and receptive and, at the same time, pushing energy upwards and outwards. This movement in the energy of Agrimony is important. By nature the plants are pliable and open—we can observe this in the flexible branching structure and the way the stems bend and move following the sun through the day. Yet this very openness allows in pain and that, in turn, causes Agrimony people to push experience outwards and away. Specifically the Agrimony type has insight and some knowledge of the world but does not wish to work with that. In psychological terms, the Agrimony person suppresses emotion and with a laughing face attempts to shrug off the knowledge—knowing, but pretending not to know.

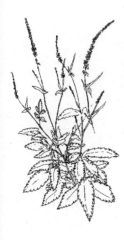

The form of an Agrimony plant is quite variable depending upon local conditions and there is even a difference of opinion in the botanical textbooks as to whether there is a sub-species: *Agrimonia odorata*. This is probably an adapted form of *A. eupatoria*, *A. odorata* being generally larger and more branched. Weeks said that both are suitable to make the remedy.[14] This variety in form illustrates Agrimony the actor, putting on a changeable performance. There is a shifting quality about Agrimony, described as the mask of good humour. But the truth is that Agrimony people feel the need for armour, a protection against the world. They are sad, like performing bears, with neither teeth nor claws. But the real life opportunity offered by Agrimony is this: only through spiritual understanding can we transcend the pain of the world. There is no armour (no thorns and spines on the plant) which can defend us against experience. That is the lesson of the yellow Agrimony flowers with their spire of flame, pointing to the sun:

> *The lesson of this plant is to enable you to hold peace in the presence of all trials and difficulties until no one has the power to cause you irritation.*[15]

With the twelve soul lessons which Bach described the question arises—are there equal numbers of each soul type? Looking at plants, we can be sure that some of the Bach species are more populous than others, just as some plants produce more flowers or set more seeds. Bach wrote of Agrimony in 1933: 'there is such a vast army of these sufferers who so often hide their torment under smiles and joviality'.[16] It is an interesting fact that today Agrimony is not so popular a remedy as Mimulus or Impatiens, although there is widespread pretence of well-being in our society, often based upon the pursuit of drugs and stimulants. Agrimony, the modest and forgotten healer, may be underestimated in its power to help us overcome our anxiety about living.

Chicory was originally named 'The Egoist' by Bach, with the soul lesson of becoming selfless through devotion to others. In his sixth published account of the remedy type he described the Chicory person as over-full of care for others, correcting, and needing family and friends close to them.[17] His first account was more outspoken and called Chicory people possessive, self-centred, hard-natured, spiteful, vindictive and cruel.[18] One is tempted to think Bach knew a particular Chicory type whom he was describing; someone he disliked! Chicory is a remedy state which lacks a certain appeal when we look only at the negative aspect. But Chicory people are not unpleasant. We must focus equally on the positive soul lesson and handle the feelings of these people with care: that is what the remedy is about.

Chicory

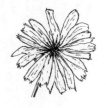

> *The remedy, in addition to relieving any symptoms of this class of patient, stimulates sympathy with others, which is their lesson: hence turns their attention more from themselves, and so, out of sympathy for their victims, they cease their aggression: and may become of service to those they previously devitalised.*[19]

Elsewhere Bach places the emphasis on gaining freedom to serve the world[20] and on another occasion, self pity.[21]

With such a changeable 'indication' for this type we might suppose that this is a variable plant which takes different forms, reflecting the variable qualities that Bach identified. This is true to some extent, since *Chicorium intybus* adapts its pattern of growth to the soil and circumstances in which it is growing. It will flesh out in a rich soil, growing woody and tough in poor, dry conditions. By the same token it can form a loose, open structure or be very upright with bundled stems, straight as a ruler. It used to grow widely in many parts of Britain and Europe but it has become less common in recent years. It has a preference for loose, stony soils with a neutral or alkaline *pH*, particularly chalk. It is the alkaline chemistry which keeps the blue flowers such a beautiful, celestial blue. Where the soil tends to acid, or where the rain is acidic, the blue flowers will be tinged pink.

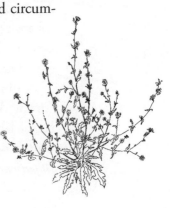

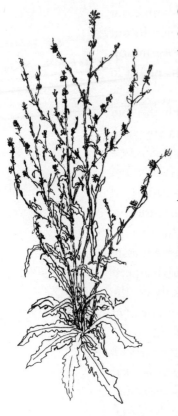

Chicory flowers are an indicator, like a type of litmus, which changes colour according to the acid-alkali chemistry of the water. This obscure detail is delightfully illustrated by a story in Professor Henslowe's book *British Wild Flowers*:

The flowers are occasionally white; and Curtis [William Curtis, of Botanical Magazine] *remarks, that the fine blue colour of the petals is convertible into a brilliant red by the acid secretion emitted by the ant. He says, 'Mr Miller, an engraver, assured me that in Germany the boys amuse themselves in producing this change of colour by placing the blossoms on an ant-hill.' This secretion, which is ejected by the wood ant when irritated, and called formic acid, is very powerful.*[22]

Botanical writers seem fond of such boyhood anecdotes about Chicory (or succory as it is sometimes called). The Rev. C. A. Johns, in his *Flowers of the Field*, tells us:

—Sir James Edward Smith, the founder of the Linnean Society, thus alludes to his early attraction to this beautiful flower: 'From the earliest period of my recollection, when I can just remember tugging ineffectually with all my infant strength at the tough stalks of the wild succory, on the chalky hills about Norwich, I have found the study of nature an increasing source of unalloyed pleasure, and a consolation and a refuge under every pain.[23]

It is certainly true that Chicory has a strong attraction for some people; there are few plants which have such a striking colour. But is there something more in this that draws particular children to remember it? It is an interesting connection that Sir James makes between plants (Chicory in particular) and the pain and need for consolation. One fascination is the brief life which the flowers have, opening at about eight a.m. and collapsing by about noon. Linnaeus, the great Swedish botanist who gave us the Linnaean system of species classification, used Chicory as one of the flowers in his floral clock at Uppsala because of the regularity of its time keeping.[24] Like 'Jack-go-to-bed-at-noon' (*Tragopon pratensis)* Chicory belongs to the extensive *Compositae* or daisy family. This is by far the largest of the natural orders and accounts for nearly a tenth of the world's flowering plants[25] and might be compared to the singularity of *Impatiens,* for instance.

Already much has been learned of the gesture of Chicory. Just as the flowers change colour so Chicory types can change the way they behave, according to the company they are in: charming and pleasant to a visitor, they may be simultaneously heaping emotional garbage upon the family or friend who is out of favour. This adaptable presentation of emotion is also seen in Cerato (page 117) another blue flower which changes hue. *Chichorium intybus* has been adapted for domestic use and has been cultivated as a forage crop and as a salad plant, as well as being grown as a coffee substitute, which is made from the root. The *Witloof* hybrid is well known and was grown extensively in northern Europe in years gone by. Wild Chicory is often an adapted form of the domestic plant that is returning to nature.[26] There is a movement here between the true nature of the plant/person and the assumed character and characteristics of the domestic type. To understand the true nature of the Chicory types we may need to see them outside and away from their domestic environment. Bach noted this when observing that they want to love and bless the whole world but feel constrained by those nearest to them.[27]

Like Agrimony, Chicory is a hairy plant, though coarser and less delicate in structure and form. The hairs, again, show sensitivity but the sensitivity of feeling in the Chicory type is more sensing inwardly, not looking outwards. Chicory asks always the question: 'How do I feel? What are my concerns?' Clearly a contrast to Agrimony. We see this in the powerful domineering structure of the plant that thrusts others aside. Agrimony is more delicate, Chicory tough and dominant. At least, the leaves and the stems are tough, while the flowers are as fine and delicate as could be. This is the contradiction of Chicory: it is changeable, fussy and contradictory.

The leaves are a simple but irregular form, each different, but with a clear mid-rib that gives direction and structure. Chicory is cardinal but pretends to be mutable on the outer surface. Chicory people know what is best for everyone, correcting and criticising those around them. The first leaves which appear at ground level, the radical leaves that sprout from the root, spread out horizontally to prevent other plants from growing; they take the light. The early spring form of this perennial is like a star on the earth. These early leaves tell us how the soul begins the life journey. Impatiens, Vervain and Agrimony grow vertically from the

first, while Clematis branches out, spreading leaves at a forty-five-degree angle to the ground. So Chicory betrays its domineering strength from the start. From the centre of the rosette of leaves stems appear, growing upwards with tremendous strength. In the first year this may be a single stem but by second and third year a family group of three or four, then six or seven stems grow together from the same root. As they grow taller, these stems branch outwards forming a substantial plant—up to a metre or more in height.

Chicory has a white sap; milky-white latex as it is called is often a sign of poison in a plant. The leaves and root have a bitter taste. This milky bitterness is a sad reversal of the sweet maternal milk which children might hope to experience, and perhaps it points to the connection sometimes made between Chicory and the wronged and bitter mother.[28] To point again to the contradictory and contrary nature of Chicory, we have an amusing account from Pliny, the Roman writer, quoted by Henslowe :

> *The ancient Egyptians are known to have used Chicory in great quantities, and Pliny remarks on its importance in the diet of that people. Pliny adds: 'The magicians state that persons who rub themselves with the juice of the entire plant mixed with oil, are sure to find more favour with others'.*[29]

So the Chicory plant has powers to attract!

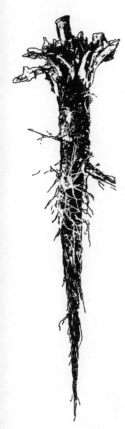

Drawing together these observations on Chicory, we can best look to the plant's root. The root stands for the past, the family and, for want of a better term, karma. As with Agrimony (page 97) the root can be seen as the place where experience from the metabolism of life is stored to supply the force for the future. Sir James Edward Smith was unable, child or man, to pull up Chicory's taproot, because the root was so deeply attached to the earth and to the past. This demonstrates the process of family learning which often accompanies Chicory: where there is a Chicory child you are likely to find a Chicory parent (or grandparent) from whom the child learns this behaviour. Equally this pattern of manipulation carries over from life to life (in plants from year to year) so that these people are bound into a perpetual drama of restrictive relationships.

To see the way this context of root and family works, contrast Chicory with others of the Twelve Healers. Impatiens is an annual, growing from seed: this shows independence, individuality, freedom from family. If a person claims to be Impatiens but still lives close to mum, it's a self-deception. With Clematis it was noted that the roots could not be found: they are lost in space. With Scleranthus (page 120) the root is thin, long and seeking, but it is an annual, so there is no family connection. With Water Violet (pages 124–5), proud, independent Water Violet, the root has no real context for the plant since it floats in water, freed from the earth. So Chicory is a little unusual, or at least particular, with its perennial tap root and store of experience and memories.

The leaves of Chicory clasp the stem, without the usual petiole (stalk) which allows independence from the stem. The flowers have no stalk either, and bud straight out from the axil of the leaves. So the children are bound into the structure of parental behaviour, clinging, smothering, holding and held tightly into the mother plant. It is this grasping and holding which links the Chicory state to Cancer (the star sign) and the tight pincers of the crab.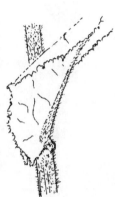

As with Clematis and Impatiens, the seed reveals much about the remedy type. If the root speaks of the past the seed speaks of the future. Clematis drifts away, Impatiens explodes, Agrimony is carried away by catching at a contact (please take me with you), Mimulus is dropped into the water and swept away. And Chicory? Chicory keeps its seeds hidden and in its own time, during the winter, drops them on to the ground, right at the feet of the mother (parent) plant. Chicory keeps the family close by.

Chicory plants produce a large number of seeds: some estimate that a single plant produces as many as 3,000.[30] By contrast, Agrimony plants probably produce about a tenth of that number. Impatiens, with some six seeds per pod and maybe ten flowering heads, each with ten flowers, might manage six hundred. Chicory produces only one seed per flower but since the flowers are composite there are many florets on each flower head. Again we see a picture of individuals brought together, bound into a family relationship.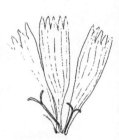

Chicory is a tough plant. As an agricultural weed it earns the following entry in an old book on land management: 'wild Chicory should be attacked by careful and persistent spudding to exhaust the rootstock and prevent seeding or even strong growth above ground . . .'.[31] Spudding is the use of a small, sharp spade to cut the roots of weeds. Bach noted hidden aggression in the Chicory type,[32] and this picture of spudding the Chicory roots indicates a need for people to be free from the dominance of the Chicory person. Sadly, Chicory people need to control others and, if left without the help of the remedy, the victims of their control may strike violently for freedom. In remedy terms, the positive Chicory type gives love without restraint, freedom without binding ties of obligation and the blessing of celestial harmony from the celestial blue flowers.

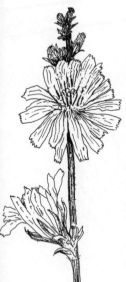

It is the flowers that are so eye-catching, opening like bright blue stars. They are arresting when you see them, bringing you up sharp with surprise and delight. What a gift! For many years, banks of Chicory have grown alongside the M5 motorway in Somerset and passing them in the morning, in July or August, the motorist had a spectacular road of blue. Returning in the afternoon the plants are hardly seen, for the blooms have gone. Everything is put into the brief life of the flower. Chicory gives its energy so fast that it is quickly exhausted. This is particularly apparent when making the essence by the sun method (pages 64–5). If the sun is strong then the essence can be made in forty-five minutes or an hour. Chicory is the fastest to make of all the sun method remedies. Bach spoke of three hours, 'or less time if the blooms begin to show signs of fading'.[33] That is what happens with Chicory blooms: they rapidly give of their vitality to the spring water they float upon, and fade and wilt in the process.

Difficult to describe, Chicory blue is subtle, fugitive, fluid and moving; giving, gentle and receptive. It lifts the spirit, turning our hearts away from the difficulties of human life on earth towards the clear skies of heavenly blue. Insects are frantically attracted to these flowers, drawn by the generous outpouring of nectar and pollen. Chicory has one of the longest flowering periods of all Bach plants, from June until October. So, as in the daily display of new flowers, Chicory people give and give and give. Love will always be there.

Vervain

Vervain is a counterpart to both Chicory and Agrimony. Where Agrimony feels an inner dissatisfaction, Vervain is dissatisfied with the outer world. Both types are distressed by life. But Vervain looks for the cause and for the release by pushing at the external form of things. Bach speaks of this as over-enthusiasm, puritanism, rigidity:

> *The patient may be too stern, too rigid in principle, too narrow-minded in outlook, endeavouring to mould the world too much to his own ideals. Of highest principle, yet intolerant of faults in others; too severe on himself. . .*[34]

Where the Agrimony state is based in the sensing and feeling of a person, the Vervain state is more mental, based upon theories and ideas about how life should be.

Like Agrimony and Chicory, Vervain grows where the ground has been disturbed: by the roadside, on the edge of a cultivated field, by a farm track or in stony soil where grass might find it harder to take hold. There is no doubt that Vervain is a traveller. As an example of how it may arrive in unexpected places, a plant took hold for a while in a timber yard, the seed coming in, no doubt, on saw logs from some woodland and going out again, perhaps, on the wheel of a lorry or in the small debris of a trailer. Where the timber is delivered the seed may be shaken from its lodging and begin a new life.

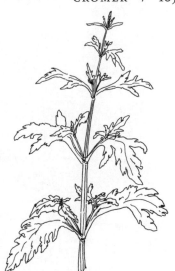

Vervain types like new beginnings and if, like the seed, they find themselves in a new community they will quickly establish themselves as people with opinions and with something to say about daily affairs. In a village, the newly arrived Vervain person will be on the council before two summers have passed. Bach noted this when he wrote of Vervains 'you have within you the power of being a leader and a teacher . . .'.[35] But, in terms of a soul lesson this type needs to learn tolerance, patience and broadmindedness.[36] Vervains need to realize, said Bach, that 'the big things of life are done gently and quietly without strain or stress'.[37]

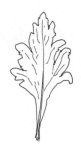

Simplicity, then, must be a keyword for Vervain. Certainly, the plant starts simply enough in its growth and basic structure. The single, unbranched stem has leaves in opposite pairs spaced regularly up the stalk. The leaves are simple with uneven lobes but broadly symmetrical. Then, out of the axil of each leaf another shoot appears with a pair of smaller leaves growing out at right angles. Some of these axillary leaves develop into secondary shoots so that new stems develop on either side of the original stem. Clearly, if each shoot puts out new leaves in turn the single stalk becomes a three-dimensional structure with leaves filling every available space. As if realizing that this upsurge in growth becomes self-defeating if it carries on, the plant has a mechanism of sensing where it may form a new side shoot and grow into clear space: it is self-aware. Then, after growing to a certain height, the Vervain plant modifies the growing tips and, with no further leaves, pushes out a spike of flowers. Just as with Agrimony, these flowers open progressively along the spike throughout the summer months of July, August and September. Since

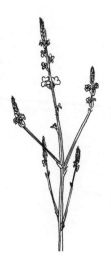

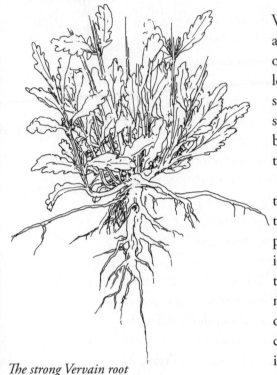

The strong Vervain root

Vervain continues to grow, the flowering spikes are lifted clear of the tangle of leaves at the base of the plant and out into clear space above. The leaves photosynthesize and produce starch to store in the root for the following year. But since the foliage is so dense they also act as a blanket to prevent other plants growing into this clear space where the flowers open.

Because it is a perennial, Vervain repeats this pattern of surging growth each year, with the root growing thicker and stronger and the plant putting out more and more young shoots in the spring. But there comes a point when the whole process becomes self-defeating: the new shoots cannot find a way through the old dried stalks from the previous year. The plant can simply choke itself to death by overgrowing. With this in mind we might find a new sense to Bach's early description of Vervain:

Are you one of those burning with enthusiasm: longing to do big things, and wishing all done in a moment of time? Do you find it difficult patiently to work out your scheme because you want the result as soon as you start? Do you find your very enthusiasm making you strict with others; wishing them to see things as you see them; trying to force them to your own opinions, and being impatient when they do not follow?[38]

There is a small point of distinction here, of differential diagnosis. It is not unusual for people to speak of themselves as impatient and then say 'I'm an Impatiens type', when in many cases they are actually of the Vervain soul type. The problem arises in this way. We see and recognize the irritation, the tension, the self-stressing and so on and think that it is a sign for Impatiens. But it may be a sign for Vervain, at least it is a sign for Vervain when the personality type is mental as opposed to emotional. Impatiens (page 42) works upon the feeling response, Vervain upon the mind set, the idea that we have about ourselves and others. Vervain people work to a scheme, creating an exclusive environment where they are the dominant force. Chicory does a similar thing within the family. Impatiens also wants to be in control but not in control of other people. That is why the Impatiens plants retreat to the river's edge and the bare soil which has been washed down by the winter flood, where there is open space for growth. We can see how it is by looking at the group which Bach allocated to each remedy when he had discovered all thirty-eight and placed them into seven groups (pages 280–1). Impatiens is in the *Loneliness* group. These people prefer to be alone. Vervain is in the *Overcare for the Welfare of Others* group (as Chicory is); they like to be with people. Simple. Vervains like to control others and direct their lives. Impatiens does not want to be bothered by other people at all.

Vervain types are said to be strong-willed, and, just as Dr Rudolf Steiner observed that the human will is in the limbs, so in the plant world we may say that the will is represented by the stalk and the stem. So the will in Vervain people is strong and directed; they know what they want to do. Compare Scleranthus (page 117) to see a contrast. In Vervain the stalk, while pliable and soft at first becomes dry and woody. It is ribbed and more or less square in section, having flat sides. This tough, rigid material is very strong and speaks of whipcord and sinew, the stringy qualities of determination. It is in contrast to the fleshy stems of Impatiens where the water element is dominant and the stems collapse almost immediately when they are damaged.

The flowers express the way Vervain comes to the simplicity and elegance of doing things 'gently without strain and stress'.[39] Pale mauve and five-petalled, like Water Violet (page 126), Vervain flowers are as understated as the foliage is overgrown. Here the plant almost laughs at itself for producing so little after so much effort. As with the Oak (pages 154–5), the smallest flowers come from the greatest strength. The mature plant in flower shows the subtle gesture of Vervain: little stars of light create a picture of electric impulses in the brain, tiny explosions of energy which combine to create concept and purpose.

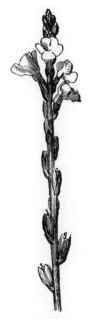

The perennial rootstock, again, shows a link to the past, the family and karma. These Vervain souls have knowledge and experience. In some respects that is their problem; they come into life with a view of how it should be. Bach says 'They are people who have advanced sufficiently to realise . . .'[40] and so gives them the acknowledgement of the beginnings of wisdom. But now they must learn '. . . that big ideals are only attained without stress and hurry'.[41]

Ultimately, we must ask ourselves what are the 'big ideals' of our individual life? In its negative form the Vervain type adopts any purpose that allows the exercise of will:

Vervain.
(*Verbena officinalis.*)

Those with fixed principles and ideas, which they are confident are right,
and which they very rarely change. They have a great wish to convert all
around them to their own views of life. They are strong of will and have
much courage when they are convinced of those things that they wish to
teach.[42]

Vervain plants are tough, deep-rooted and hard to pull out from the
ground. Vervain people are inflexible, strong-willed and do not find it
easy to change their mind (for a contrast see Cerato, page 116). They do
not see that there is more to life than getting their own way. The obstruction of the ego is such that they cannot view themselves objectively. Yet
Vervain, in many respects, is a modest plant, easily overlooked, without
perfume or beauty, the small flowers being lost in the lush verbiage of
summer.

Vervain seeds are small and drop directly beside the parent plant. And,
as these plants grow on waste ground or by the roadside, the seeds often
germinate among the stones and gravel, growing into a strong colony.
A few seeds travel on animals, since they fall with the remains of the
dried calyx intact, and this is easily hooked into wool, cloth or fur. This
sometimes links Vervain to people—the hem of a coat, skirt or trousers
picking up the seeds. As with the Agrimony type, we can read from this
a sociable temperament.

One other aspect of a plant's gesture instructs us about the gesture
of the human emotional state: the way of dying. A perennial taproot
gives continuity below ground and, as we have seen, this may indicate a
continuity through life, death and rebirth. But what happens to the plant
above ground, when winter comes, indicates the attitude of Vervain types
to how they will be seen by others in the future: their reputation and
name in the world. Impatiens dies with the first frost, collapsing quickly
as the water in the stems falls back to earth. They care little for reputation. Like Water Violet people, they are rather individually involved
with the process of self-development, not seen by the world. Mimulus,
too, collapses but uses the broken stems for propagation, leading to a
new life, so there is a connection there to the future, albeit somewhat
random. Vervain and Chicory (and to a lesser extent Agrimony) leave
stems which remain visible through the winter and on into the following spring. Chicory people want to be remembered; they are part of a
family line and will hope to control their heirs, even from beyond the
grave. Family karma, a family pattern if you prefer, is often based upon

a group of Chicory souls who continue through lifetimes together. With Vervain, however, the stalks remain even longer, tough and dry, sticking up when the other plants around have fallen back to earth. Bach saw Vervain people as struggling on 'long after many would have given up their duties'.[43] But we can also connect this to a desire which Vervain souls have for reputation and fame: a desire to leave a lasting mark in the world. This twinning of fixed ideas and ambition is readily seen in politicians, many of whom are Vervain souls. But those who wish to change the world often hope more for posthumous fame and recognition: the stalks may be dead, but they show where the plant grew and will act to support the tender shoots of the next generation. Indeed, it is this intention, to be a guide and teacher to the new generation, which characterizes Vervain types: they try to convert people to their point of view and to use their courage and will to convince others.[44]

Nora Weeks states that after simultaneously preparing Agrimony, Chicory and Vervain, Dr Bach turned his attention to re-making Clematis. He used the sun method and the flowers, not the seeds as he had previously. He also made Sow Thistle, *Sonchus arvensis* (pages 88–90) before coming to Centaury.

Centaury

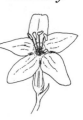

When Dr Bach discovered it in 1930 and described the remedy in *Some Fundamental Considerations of Disease and Cure,* Centaury was presented as being for the tyrant who exerts power over others. Two years later, in *Free Thyself,* he changed this description so that it related to those who became subject to the power of others (pages 88–9). There is no record of the process which brought about this reversal. But, with Centaury in its new role, there is logic and balance in the relationship between these four remedies: Agrimony, Chicory, Vervain and Centaury. The relationship can be seen in terms of the way that energy is used by each of the four.

Vervain and Chicory both act upon the world, wanting to change it. Agrimony and Centaury are passive and accept the world acting upon them. Vervain and Centaury are both concerned with action in the outer world; Chicory and Agrimony are feeling and sensitive to the inner world. Vervain and Chicory are strongly self-orientated; Agrimony and Centaury are more self-less.

Centaury, like the other three, grows by the roadside, by tracks and paths, on a hedge-bank or on waste ground. It was once a common meadowland flower, which is how Bach described it.[45] But these days it is more likely to be seen beside a woodland ride or neglected road, where

```
Vervain                              Centaury



                    Outer
Selfish              ◯               Self-less
                    Inner


Chicory                              Agrimony
```

farming and traffic do not intrude. Equally it will be found on downland and dry, grassy places where there is poor soil and little commercial value to the land. Significantly, Centaury does not grow in rich soils and valuable pastures.

Look up *Centaurium umbellatum* in the books and you will find little useful information: we must learn about Centaury by observation. Here is a plant which lacks the reputation of Vervain (and so lacks the ego), lacks the character of Agrimony (although like Agrimony it can take a variable form and so shows itself to be easily adaptable) and lacks the stature of Chicory (and so does not carry the same intensity in the emotional life). Centaury is a small plant which for most of the year is easily overlooked, if not invisible among the general throng of flowers. Centaury people, therefore, may be seen as good-natured but unassertive. Bach spoke of them as 'doormats', lying there passively while the other children run in, boisterous and noisy. The stem and leaves are entirely without hairs (glabrous) and this suggests a lack of sensing and sensitivity on the part of Centaury types: they do not respond and interact with the world around them in the way that Chicory and Agrimony people do.

Centaury is a biennial plant: the seeds which germinate one year will produce flowers the next. The first movement of growth is so small it is hardly observed. Two oval leaves, no more than a millimetre long, but with a root of twenty-five millimetres or more, are the first sign that the plant has begun a new cycle of life. Everything depends upon the root: if it can find constant moisture then little by little the plant will grow, eventually pushing its way up through grasses to get to the light. The way the seed germinates and begins to grow tells us how the soul type enters life: here it is small, tentative and fragile. As a member of the Gentian family, Centaury shares some characteristics with Gentian (page 129) in this pattern of growth.

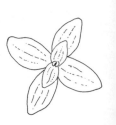

For the first season, Centaury remains as a seedling with a rosette of leaves (thirty to forty millimetres across) hugging the ground. By fanning out the flat, oval leaves horizontally it asserts itself within a small space (compare Chicory page 101) and deliberately prevents other plants from taking the light and water it needs for the future. The territory may be small but Centaury can dominate that part of the earth. Lying flat on the ground, however, the plants are often walked on or driven over. The flat Centaury leaves are slightly cupped so as to incline the rainwater to run to the centre and so to the root. Three veins in the leaf help to structure it to this 'decumbent' shape.

In the spring of the next year a single, smooth stem grows straight up from the centre of the rosette of leaves. In this delayed vertical growth we can see the latent assertion of the Centaury will: they begin to stand up for themselves. It does not reach a great height, maybe twenty centimetres, but with the competition held back by the spread of the basal leaves there is a clear space in which to grow. So exactly does the Centaury plant describe the necessity of the Centaury person:

> *Are you one of those people whom everybody uses, because in the kindness of your heart you do not like to refuse them anything: do you just give in for the sake of peace rather than do what you know is right, because you do not wish to struggle: whose motive is good, but who are being passively used instead of actively choosing your own work.*[46]

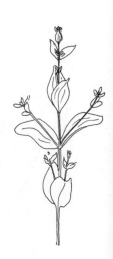

Stem with buds

Centaury people find it difficult to assert their own will and purpose in the face of the dominant presence of others. The plant demonstrates how it is necessary to make a space for oneself to live in. Bach intended that the remedy will help, 'so that you may become an active, positive worker instead of a passive agent'.[47] He saw in this a polarity between weakness and strength. Weakness at the soul level shows itself in a lack of self-assertion, this in turn shows as a weakness of will, this then leads to a weakness physiologically. Bach then went on to say:

> *Those who are weak, pale and have no strength, just feeble and tired, will be much helped by CENTAURY.*[48]

In this description he was tying the remedy to physiological symptoms. But, more generally, he saw here a psychological disposition:

*CENTAURY are the doormats. They seem to lack all power of individu-
ality or the ability to resist being used by everyone. They put up no struggle
whatever to gain their freedom.*[49]

The individuality of Centaury is shown in the flowers, each of which
acts independently on the flower heads, variously opening and closing
according to the strength of the sunlight. On a dull day the small pink
flowers remain folded, closed. As the sun shines some open but not all,
unless the day is really warm and bright. As Henslowe observed:

*The clusters open only in fine weather and before twelve o'clock after which
time they gradually close; and one who was previously unacquainted with
the plant, would suppose that it as yet had but unexpanded buds.*[50]

These unexpanded petals give the appearance that the flower is just about
to become, but hesitating, uncertain. When the flowers do open fully, the
brilliance is wonderful. The soft, pink, five-petalled flowers shine brightly
at your feet. The idea that is spoken by the Centaury flowers is simple:
'It's OK to be me!'

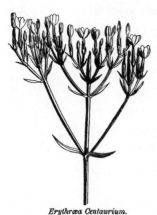

Centaury flowers throughout the summer from June until
early September. The first blooms appear at the head of the
main stalk with lateral shoots growing symmetrically from
the axil of the leaves. Seeds which form from the first flowers
will be ripe before the last flowers have opened. These seeds
are very small, like powder, and they are shaken from the
pods by the wind, so even in this the plant is passive. So
light, the seeds are often washed away by a storm of rain, but
they settle then in some small rut or stony track. Some will
germinate in the late summer, overwinter and flower the next
year. Others will germinate in the spring but not develop a
flowering stalk until another year has passed.

Erythræa Centaurium.

Centaury plays a waiting game and is slow to evolve its unique life
story, believing, perhaps, that 'they also serve who only stand and
wait'.[51] But when, at last, they do find 'their particular mission in life',[52]
Centaury souls have learned this lesson: that the development of their
soul qualities comes not through giving way to others but through the
assertion of their own will. This action of the will is not simply selfishness
but the willing act of service. For these are people, said Bach, speaking to
them directly, who 'are a very long way along the road to being of great
service once you can realize that you must be a little more positive in
your life'.[53]

The uncertainty of Centaury types concerns will. The uncertainty of Cerato types concerns self-identity: these are souls who do not know who they are. Bach gave Cerato the archetype of *The Fool* and in a complex description of the condition he set the positive virtue as wisdom—'wisdom to comprehend the truth: judgement to define right from wrong and encourage strength and ability to keep to the right path when realised'.[54] When someone says to you 'I am not sure of my type remedy, I am quite Water Violet at times but I'm also Impatiens and Mimulus . . .' there is a good chance that this is a Cerato person, if only because of the evident contradiction in the other three. Implied in the statement there is also the question—'what do you think my type remedy is?' Bach said:

Cerato

> *Always asking advice from different people but not following it, never feeling quite satisfied that they have the answer they require. Often wish to do things that seem foolish.*[55]

Cerato was discovered (if that is the right word) by Ernest H. Wilson, Chinese Wilson as he was called, on a plant-collecting expedition in 1907-1908. Wilson sent back seeds of the plant, which were given to Miss Ellen Willmott, 'a noted lady gardener'[56] who had helped to fund the trip. Although neither Willlmott nor Wilson play a direct part in the finding of the Cerato remedy by Bach, twenty-five years later, there is some value in a digression here to consider the circumstances which brought this plant, and a thousand other new species, to cultivation in Britain and North America.

Ernest Wilson made four separate expeditions to China between 1899 and 1911. The first two were sponsored by James Veitch & Sons of Chelsea, a nursery specialising in exotica. It employed Wilson to find new plants for commercial development. One of these was *Davidia*, the handkerchief tree, for instance. Wilson was to become the best known plant hunter of his time but he was one among many who had searched the world for new species throughout the nineteenth century. Wilson's later trips to China were organized by the Arnold Arboretum of Boston and had less commercial intent, being more in the way of botanical research. It was on the third trip that Wilson came upon Cerato, somewhere in the Min valley in Sichuan, central southern China. The expedition was arranged so that those who had contributed financially might expect to receive plants of some particular kind which interested them. Ellen Willmott paid £200 towards the cost, a considerable sum no doubt, but actually less than two per cent of the expenditure. She received for her garden at Warley Place in Essex some seeds of a plant which will carry her name in perpetuity: *Ceratostigma willmottiana*. Although this 'redoubtable Edwardian lady gardener'[57] had other plants named after her (a tulip, wallflower and campanula), all these were bred by nurserymen; only Cerato came from the wild.

It would be amusing if either Wilson or Willmott showed signs of being a Cerato type. We can be reasonably confident that they were not.* But Cerato, having once arrived in England, was to become one of the most famous plants that either of them was connected with. Ellen Willmott succeeded in raising two plants from the seeds sent to her: all the Cerato plants now grown in Britain derive from these.[58] The extensive gardens at Warley Place long ago fell into decay and disrepair. They are now a reserve, part of the Essex Wildlife Trust. The house burned to the ground in 1939. Among the ruins one can see part of the old conservatory, cold frames and greenhouses where Miss Willmott no doubt propagated her collection of plants. If the Cerato seeds were germinated in 1908 then it would have been a couple of years before the plants grew sufficiently to flower. It was 1914 before the botanists at Kew conferred the title *willmottiana* on this Cerato.[59]

Cerato is a perennial, woody shrub, growing to half a metre or more in height. It is only half-hardy; a strong frost will kill it off, or knock it back to the rootstock to regrow. Little is known about how it grew in China, the climate, the average temperature, the winter conditions, and the soil. But, to all intents and purposes, it arrived as a new plant in the UK and we must address our questions here. Bach found Cerato growing in a private garden in Overstrand, near Cromer, Norfolk. *The Pleasaunce* was another grand house with elaborate gardens. designed by Luytens for Lord and Lady Battersea (he an MP, she a Rothschild). The gardens were the work of Gertrude Jekyll, the celebrated lady gardener, who was a friend of Ellen Willmott: that is how Cerato came to be there. Whether

---

* Wilson was rather reserved and even secretive but a strong-willed and purposeful man, who did not suffer fools gladly—probably an Impatiens type. Miss Willmott, if we are to judge from her comments about Wilson's wife in a letter concerning his reluctance to make the trip, was more likely to lead than be led: '. . . it was sad that such a promising man should be hampered by such an ignorant short-sighted wife at such an early stage in his career' [quoted by Roy W. Briggs in *A Life of Ernest H. Wilson*, HMSO; 1993, page 45]. Ellen Willmott died in 1934 while Mr & Mrs Wilson had a fatal car accident near to their Boston home in 1930.

Bach was more than a casual visitor to the house is not known. In 1933 he spoke of it as:

> CERATO is not a native of this country and is only to be found on one or two private estates. It may later be possible to find a British substitute for this.[60]

In 1934, when he wrote *The Seven Helpers*, he noted that it was 'at present' very rare in this country.[61] How long he continued to seek a British replacement for Cerato is not known. Weeks said nothing on the subject, but it tells us something about the uniqueness of this plant that he did not replace it. Curiously, it has become a standard in garden centres in recent years; it is even planted in municipal gardens. The bright blue colouring and long flowering period make it an attractive, low maintenance variety. That it came to be at Overstrand and that Bach saw it there is a part of the mystery which surrounds this oriental immigrant. It had travelled half way around the world for him to find!

We should surely be able to investigate and evaluate Cerato by the same criteria as other plants in *The Twelve Healers*. First: what it is not. Although it is in the *Plumbaginaceae* family, it is not Plumbago. A herbalist once tried to make out that the *Plumbago capensis* growing in the botanical gardens in Sydney, Australia, was Cerato, but it isn't; the flowers are the wrong blue and the whole gesture of the plant different from Cerato. How vital it is to be sure of what we are espousing as the truth: that's Cerato, that is. *Ceratostigma willmotiana* is a deciduous shrub without any direction or structure to its growth; it does not know where it is going, growing outwards in random, bushy fashion. This is a clear variation on the vertical 'will' structure of the previous remedies.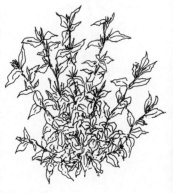

Leaves of the plant are hairy, more bristly than anything, rough and unpleasant to handle. While we might observe that Cerato people are sensitive to their environment, there is a lack of warmth and empathy here. These are souls that do not fit easily into society. The soft hairy leaves of Agrimony, by contrast, speak for people who are popular and friendly; the few tough bristles of Vervain, like the Cerato, make for a more reactive relationship. Cerato leaves are dark green, but begin and end the season tinged with purple—they are changeable. The form of the leaf is simple (Cerato types are unsophisticated) and the flower too is an elegant but simple five-petalled form. As noted with Vervain (pages

108–9), the stalks of last year represent a structure for the future; Cerato also needs to leave its mark and message for the world. Bach said of Cerato people:

> They should be wise teachers and instructors, but they seem to listen too much to other opinions, and be too easily influenced by outside circumstances.[62]

This problem is written in the gesture of the plant, just as it is in the gesture of the soul type. The dry stems which held the flowers and leaves in summer, may or may not be alive come the spring. We can only guess. Flowers will only form on new growth. Gardeners, with this in mind, know that it is better to prune the plant in autumn and so stimulate new growth from the base.

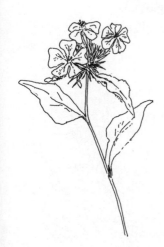

Of all the flowers and trees that Bach chose, Cerato is the only one specifically domesticated here in England. It does not grow wild. For two reasons. First, the plant rarely sets seed—it is propagated by cuttings. Secondly, if it were to grow wild it could not maintain itself against competition with other species. This tells us a lot about Cerato types: as children they need to be protected against others who are stronger. They simply lack the drive to maintain the identity of themselves in life. A flower which fails to produce seed does not know its future. Given that this plant is so far from home, should we be surprised? (Well, Impatiens manages.) The pattern of experience (in the seed) which carries Cerato people into the new life is weak and half-formed. No wonder they appear foolish as they enquire from others how to live in this foreign land. As to the propagation from cuttings, we should note that this plant has now become the possession of nurserymen who even market particular strains of the plant as their patent. Cerato allows its identity to be controlled by others.

Look at the flowers and observe the same depth of blue, the wisdom of deep space, found in Chicory. But in Cerato the flower form is built upon the regular geometry of the pentangle. This formation of perpetual movement, the symbol of time and eternity, shows what deeper understanding can manifest for Cerato people. The name *Ceratostigma* refers to the prominent horn-like stigma which protrudes from the corolla (petals). It reaches out into space, as if searching for meaning, like an antenna.

The flower head of Cerato is composed of spiky bracts from which the flower buds emerge. The structure here is reminiscent of the Clematis flower and speaks of the same need to focus the energy into a centre. This focusing is also apparent on the petals where a herring-bone pathway points to the centre of the flower. With Chicory (page 100) we noted the significance of flowers which acted as an acid-alkali indicator. Cerato flowers, which only last a day, often collapsing by noon in the heat, deepen their colour to purple as they close. Here, again, we see the changeable, perhaps evolving, nature of Cerato. As the petals close and the flower collapses, they twist into a spiral and form a focus of indrawn energy and meaning. This is a plant which wants to learn and understand.

All these considerations can have found scant part in the thinking of Dr Edward Bach when he saw the plant growing in the seaside gardens at Overstrand. Perhaps the plant simply called to him: 'Come and look, here I am'. But even that assumes a self-knowledge on the part of the plant—it is just that self-knowledge Cerato people seek through their experience of life on earth. It is their soul lesson.

Scleranthus

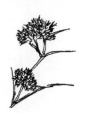

There was one other remedy which Bach found in the Cromer area that year: Scleranthus. The first description reads, in many respects, as an extension to Cerato with the suggestion that Scleranthus people 'are always seeking the advice of others'.[63] But the real nature of the soul type is then apparent as he described first the intellectual quality and then the alternating mental outlook—the weather vane he called it—and we come down to the Scleranthus type balancing indecision and steadfastness.

One of the smallest of the Bach flowers, Scleranthus hugs the ground, a tangle of green stems, leaves and flowers that is of so little importance and stature that is easily overlooked. To those of us who know what we want—what we want for breakfast or what we want to do with our lives—this soul condition of indecision may seem of little significance. But there are those who suffer, silently, according to Bach's observation, 'unable to decide between two things, first one seeming right then the other'.[64] This alternating energy leaves them powerless to act, trapped in an oscillation between left and right, up and down, good and bad, between any polarity of choice. This state of mind paralyses the will and prevents the individual from moving, from acting in life.

Looking back at earlier remedies a contrast can be drawn with Impatiens, or Vervain. With those the gesture, of both the plant and the person, speaks of an active will driven by a soul which knows what it wants to do in life. It is portrayed in the upright stature of the plant, its

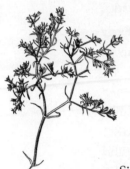

main stem vertical and strong, growing in a clear direction, like a tall tree. This is in contrast to the languid, clambering gesture of the Clematis and the loose, shrubby form of Cerato. These two lack the definition of the 'I' form, the upright stance of the fully incarnated self. The same is true of Scleranthus which grows higgledy-piggledy, tumbling over itself, without main stem, direction or apparent purpose. Mimulus, too, lacks this upright form, draping itself across the rocks, falling out over the water.

Since this quality, this lack of the upright trunk or stem is so much a part of the gesture of Scleranthus, it may be helpful to consider the matter further. It has been noted how the Clematis seeds dive headfirst towards the earth to take root (page 46), just like a child presenting head down in the womb. Once born the child lies on its back. Then, as it grows, it

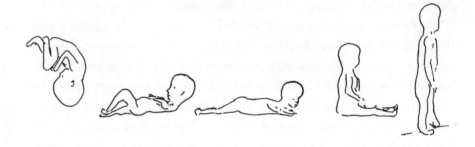

learns first to move its head and limbs, then to turn over, to crawl, to sit up and finally, pulling itself up with the arms, to stand upright, marking the stages in a developing consciousness and involvement with the world. It is useful to learn how different these things are: to experience them by just lying on the floor, then crawling and so on. The changing perspective carries with it a changing mentality. How we live between the horizontal and the vertical is a useful guide to the state of our inner being. The different gestures carry different messages. We are back with Bach's observations on his patients as they walked into the surgery: even so small a gesture as looking up or looking down can express the emotional state of the individual. It is hard to dream when standing up straight. It can be difficult to galvanize the will when lying in bed! To experience and understand the differing emotional states that Bach observed in *The Twelve Healers* we can observe and resonate the gestures of the remedy plants that he chose.

Scleranthus annuus is an annual, except that it is sometimes biennial: it starts with contradiction. The form of the plant varies considerably depending upon the moisture available but it is rarely more than fifty millimetres high. It usually grows in dry, sandy soils and then tends to lie flat over the ground. Old textbooks list Scleranthus as a weed of agriculture[65] and in Bach's day it was commonly found in arable land, growing among wheat or barley. Here it enjoyed the loose soil that came from ploughing. Since the chemical revolution in agriculture however, when farmers began to spray every field with herbicide to eradicate all competition for the crop, Scleranthus has all but disappeared from farmland.

To make this point more strongly, refer back to *Flora*s published 100 years ago for different English regions. Bach also used and recommended these 'local botanical books'[66] which list locations and the frequency with which plants can be found in different districts. Druce, in his *Flora of Berkshire*, 1897, says of Scleranthus 'too widely distributed to need the mention'.[67] By 1968 only a few sites were listed for Berkshire (these included Didcot rubbish tip, hardly the place to make a remedy!)[68] Captain Roe, in *The Flora of Somerset*, 1981, says 'formerly widespread . . . but now very rare'.[69] It would be wrong to give the impression that Scleranthus has disappeared, but it has certainly become scarce.

So Scleranthus is a plant which we have to search for. Here again, we notice something of the gesture of both the plant and the remedy state. Looking for it may necessitate getting down on our hands and knees, crawling over the ground, as it were with a magnifying glass. It is this closeness to the ground which illustrates the soul nature of Scleranthus types. These people become limited in their vision and without a strong vertical connection they do not have a context for decision-making. Bach says 'they rely entirely upon the intellect and not at all on their intuition'.[70] Intuition, he said, is the voice of the soul.[71] At times of choice, Scleranthus people do not or cannot hear that voice of intuition. Without soul guidance it is impossible to make an informed choice about anything—we cannot tell whether something is good for us, nor what is right or wrong, if we have no link through to who we are.

The seed of Scleranthus is a small nut. On germination it sprouts a pair of leaves in a little 'V' and a slender root rapidly extends downwards, deep into the earth. As the plant grows, the recumbent stems move outwards across the ground in all directions. The narrow, pointed leaves grow out in pairs at forty-five degrees, clasping the stem at their base. Where they

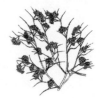

join, axillary shoots appear which send out new growth in all directions. Left undisturbed, a single plant will form a dense, matted tangle of stems. The English common name 'knawel' comes from the German word for 'a tangle of threads'. This undifferentiated growth speaks of a mental confusion and uncertainty in direction, although all the growth focuses back into one point, a single stem as it enters the ground. Like Centaury (page 110) the root is vastly more extensive than the visible plant and even more tangled, forming a web of filaments of great delicacy, searching for water in the dry, sandy soil. Scleranthus people are trying to resolve their inner conflicts by rooting deeply into the material world. As they deal with life's problems with steadfastness and stability they draw experience like water from the earth.

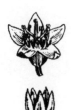

The flowers appear in a random fashion, clustered on short stalks, growing from the leaf nodes or at the end of the stem. Scleranthus, like Clematis, (page 49) lacks petals. This reinforces the image of a mental and not emotional type. The goblet-shape form of the flower is made by five pointed green sepals edged in white. It is the simplest construction and self-pollination inevitably occurs. Every flower leads to seed and every seed is fertile and will germinate: Scleranthus in its strength of soul carries a determination to learn from life and carry that experience, through the seed, into the future.

In the seed there is an indication of the way that Scleranthus resolves its problems. Where other plants allow the petals to fall away, Scleranthus holds everything exactly as it was in the form of the flower: steadfast. It does one thing and it sticks to it. The visible change is only in the colour, turning from green to straw yellow as the stems dry. Within the cup of the sepals the nut forms, but it only grows to fill the existing shape, there is no swelling pod, no metamorphosis of the calyx. As the plant dies these seeds fall to earth and will germinate in the same soil as the parent. In terms of the soul lesson Scleranthus people are not evolving some new principle or discovering some new life aim. They simply need to act with determination and purpose within the world.

The light sandy soil that Scleranthus prefers is also attractive to rabbits. Rabbits and Scleranthus actually have a symbiotic relationship—rabbits dig their burrows and, of course, kick out a lot of loose soil, ideal ground for Scleranthus to grow in. As it grows, the rabbits come and eat the shoots. When these shoots have flowers and seeds the rabbits eat those as well. That is why Scleranthus comes and goes—you can locate it one day and find that it has gone the next. It is the same with the white rabbit in Lewis Carroll's *Alice in Wonderland*; he is always disappearing and then popping up again, unexpectedly. The seed, being a nut, travels unharmed through the rabbit intestines and is dropped, with a convenient pellet of manure, in the local rabbit latrine.* Like most animals, rabbits are careful not to eat from such a place and so the plant may be left, for a while, to grow undisturbed. Rabbits and other grazing animals carry Scleranthus seeds to new sites.

The association with rabbits is also seen in the way a rabbit runs. If ever you chase a rabbit in a car you will see how it runs first to one side then to the other. Just when it seems determined to jump into the hedge it changes direction and leaps back into the road. It cannot make up its mind, dodging from left to right.

The Scleranthus plant and flower is green. Green is the mid point between blue and yellow. Yellow light comes towards us from the sun, blue is the colour of light moving away from us into the darkness of space—the night sky. We see winter as blue, summer as yellow. Where the warm, yellow light falls upon the cool blue surface of darkness there is green of the plant world in spring. Illustrating this, Scleranthus has the green of balance and harmony, the middle way. It represents the fulcrum on the seesaw. The fulcrum is the point where there is no turning moment and all the forces are vertical (page 58). These vertical forces connect Scleranthus to the intuitive voice of the higher worlds. They provide the Scleranthus person with a point of reference to make decisions successfully.

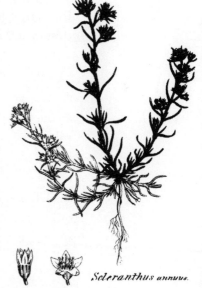

Scleranthus annuus.

In *Scleranthus annuus*, therefore, there is a picture of confused and undirected growth which is anchored at the node between the earth and the deeply penetrating root. It grows across the surface of the ground just as Scleranthus people work over the surface of a life prob-lem. The constant branching of the stems speaks of a mind always at the crossroads of decision; the fork in the road at which they must make a choice. That is why

---

* H. N. Ridley in his book *The Dispersal of Plants,* noted that the seeds of *Scleranthus annuus* had been found in the excreta of cattle in Sweden and red deer in Western America. He provides confirmation of the importance of certain animals in the distri-bution of plants and their seeds.

Scleranthus people are afflicted by the 'yes/no' disease, saying both and meaning neither. They are not perverse but lack the depth or penetration to go one way or the other. Perhaps these are souls that belong strongly to the earth. A contrast with the remoteness and wisdom of Water Violet (pages 124–5) or the experience and certainty of Vervain (page 107).

Bach spoke of the physical symptoms which attend this state of indecision: 'their symptoms, temperatures, etc., all come and go, rise and fall with rapid fluctuations, following the example of the mental state'.[72] While it is true that the mental state will lead to physical symptoms, this is a remedy which has particular importance as guidance for the soul. Looking at today's life circumstances, we might give an additional keyword to the Scleranthus people: discrimination. In the confusion of contemporary Western culture, with its marketing, hype and spin, we need the clarity of discrimination to see what is good for life and what is not. Scleranthus, in its positive form 'brings clearness of mental vision: ability for quick decision: determination and calmness in face of difficulties'.[73] It helps us 'to form correct opinions and be steadfast in following them'.[74] This modest plant, under pressure through loss of habitat, offers a renewed connection to the higher worlds, through intuition and consciousness.

7 · The Last of the First Twelve

IF WE LOOK AT THE REMEDY PLANTS as individuals, observing their gesture in the same way as the gesture and personality of people, the structure of Bach's work and discoveries becomes clear. There are various different plants, growing in a variety of soils and circumstances. These reflect the variety of soul types which he described as his *Twelve Great Remedies*. These soul types, or soul lessons, characterize the opportunities that we have for learning and development in life on earth. According to the way the plant grows we can detect the qualities associated with it, and build a vocabulary based upon simple observations.

Water Violet

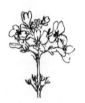

Water Violet grows, not just by the river, like Mimulus and Impatiens, but actually submerged in water. It is thought that life originated in water and later migrated to dry land.[1] But freshwater aquatic plants moved from the land back into water. It follows that such species are more highly evolved. As plant forms they have a longer ancestry of adaptation, reaching back through the geological ages of time. That Water Violet is such an 'old' plant is proved by its unusual and sophisticated system of avoiding self-fertilization. This is called heteromorphic incompatibility.[2] This leads us into the soul nature of Water Violet; a flower which appears simple but has a complex life history.

Water Violet is a member of the primrose family. The Latin name is *Hottonia palustris:* Hottonia after the Dutch botanist Petrus Hotton and *palustris* from the Latin for marsh or pond. All primroses have simple five-petalled flowers and like to live in damp ground, though Water Violet is the only one in Britain living entirely in the water. For much of the year it is submerged. Only in May and June do the stems rise clear of the water, straight and elegant, as they lift flowers into the sunlight. Bach wrote of the Water Violet soul type:

> *These are very beautiful people in mind and often in body. They are gentle, quiet, very refined and cultured and yet are masters of their fate and lead their lives with a quiet determination and certainty.*[3]

This statement is apt as a description of the plant, too. For these are flowers which lead their lives with great precision, clarity and purpose.

Water Violet has always been relatively scarce, growing only in slow-moving but pure water, in ditches and ponds where it will not be disturbed. By nature it is fastidious and cannot abide any form of pollution. Perhaps it does not like competition and that is why it withdraws to water where it can spread out undisturbed. Certainly, Water Violet people will withdraw into their own space and do not like intrusion—like a cat, some say. But the withdrawal from land to a water habitat signals more than a desire for peace and solitude; it is symbol of the transition to a higher plane of being. These souls are older and wiser than the rest of us! This idea is conveyed succinctly in a commentary on medieval cosmology by E. M. W. Tillyard in *The Elizabethan World Picture*:

> *Water is nobler than earth, the ruby than the topaz, gold than brass: the links in the chain [of Being] are there. Next there is existence and life, the vegetative class, where again the oak is nobler than the bramble.*[4]

While such ideas may not sit easily with contemporary scientific thinking, we know that Bach was familiar with them (his reference to combining the Four Elements shows that)[5] and they have a meaning based upon observation. Water Violet is a plant which has only the slightest contact with earth, living in water and pushing a stem to open flowers in the air. After Antony's death in Shakespeare's *Antony and Cleopatra*, Cleopatra recalls how:

> *. . . his delights*
> *Were dolphin-like; they show'd his back above*
> *The element they lived in.*[6]

She is comparing Antony to the dolphin, king of the fishes, leaping out of the water into the air, since he too transcended his element and became thereby more than an ordinary mortal. Water Violet as a soul type has just such greatness and superiority. Bach calls Water Violet people 'great souls':[7]

> *Very quiet people, who move about without noise, speak little, and then gently. Very independent, capable and self-reliant.*[8]

Remembering Chicory (page 102) and the way its root illustrates a connection to the past and to family, this context is precisely absent with Water Violet. Although it is a perennial it has only the frailest of roots—a few fine, white threads which dangle from the green stems. They only serve to absorb minerals for the plant and do not anchor it to the land: Water Violet has freedom. The leaves and stems are 'spongy', containing many air spaces which allow the plant to float, just below the surface. The rosette of leaves, pinnatifid (deeply cut into segments), looks like a green star in the water, delicate and refined, yet somehow inspiring and exciting.

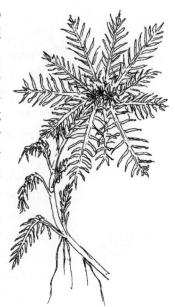

But interesting changes in behaviour occur as the water level drops, if the pool dries in July or August. The roots then play a more important part, anchoring the plant to the mud, keeping it alive by transmitting moisture. In these conditions, the leafy stems grow rapidly and spread outwards to prevent any other plant or seedling from obtaining light and space. Water Violets are capable of asserting themselves and will not tolerate interference from others. Equally, this is indicative of the growth and gain for Water Violet people if ever they fully involve themselves in the physical world. When the water rises again the rooted plant releases the individual stems and leaves through a process called 'stolon budding' and they float upwards to cover the available space.

Bach commented directly on this pattern of growth with unattached roots and freedom to float:

> If so, the beautiful Water Violet, which floats so freely on the surface of our clearest streams, will help you . . . to stand absolutely alone in the world, gaining the intense joy of complete freedom.[9]

And later:

> They do not often form strong attachments even to those nearest them.[10]

This may be the clearest indication yet that Bach was looking at the plants as a literal emblem of the soul condition.

What then is the soul condition for Water Violet types? What is the lesson they are here to learn? The soul difficulty is pride and aloofness; the lesson that of 'perfect service to mankind'.[11] Bach described it as a contrast between joy and grief. His point was this: these are souls who 'know their work in life and do it with a quiet, certain will'.[12] They have experience and know what this work brings—'have you had real losses, sad times and yet go quietly on?'[13] But it can also be inferred that these people come somewhat reluctantly into life. They know too well the vicissitudes of the world and have striven to leave them behind. But simple human duty obliges them to return to assist their fellows, to absorb the flood of grief and work with love to better life. It is the commitment to turn back and become involved in the world which leads to 'the intense joy of complete freedom':[14]

Moreover that little plant will help you to the understanding that so much you think of in life as being cruel and sad, is truly for the good of those you pity.[15]

The flowers are pale mauve, similar to the Impatiens mauve, and both are remedies for loneliness. With a yellow centre, the Water Violet flower points to self-knowledge and the calm assurance of an unemotional understanding. It has knowledge of life, a certain calm detachment. The stem is glabrous (smooth, without hairs) and there is a general lack of that responsive, emotional sensitivity found in Chicory (page 103) or Agrimony (page 95).

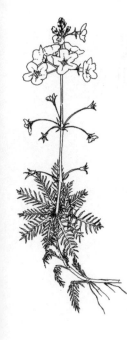

Water Violet is unusual in the structure of its flowering stems. The flowers are arranged in whorls around the stalk, like a coronet of lights that shine with soft intensity. Three, five or sometimes up to seven individual flowers open at the same time, while on the whorl above, the buds are still developing. There are six or seven rings of flowers, depending on the weather in May and June. One can tell at a glance what stage this plant has reached, reading from a clear calendar each stage of life development. This is in distinct contrast to plants like Chicory or Cerato where, looking at a photograph, it would be hard to say whether the flowers were the first or even the last of the season. In its structure, Water Violet demonstrates a clear and straightforward purpose in life.

Because of its dimorphic incompatibility Water Violet flowers do not always set seed. Dimorphic means 'two forms' and each form can only be fertilized by the other. It is a strange system, which ensures cross-pollination and therefore stronger progeny.[16] However, it reduces by fifty per cent the opportunity for an individual flower to form seeds. Being loners, we might think that Water Violet people, like the plants, are less likely to form relationships and have children. But, remember, there is always the standby of vegetative reproduction: as Water Violet grows it branches occasionally and then sections may break off and float away (stolon budding). Without the fixed attachment of a root, this allows for dispersal but not necessarily an increase in the volume of the population—there are more plants but they are smaller. It is anything but aggressive in its reproduction.

The seeds of Water Violet sink to the mud, germinate and then, secreting a bubble of air, the young plant rises back to the surface of the water.[17] So, even at the beginning, these seedlings move freely in the water and do not take root. There is a picture here for Water Violet children. Quiet, self-sufficient, knowledgeable and showing a wisdom beyond their years, they are often independent of their family. It is not hard to imagine that such children, born into a family which fails to recognize and respect their need for privacy and solitude, might become deeply unhappy. There is much to be said for parents who allow their children to develop their own nature rather than imposing adult values and old family patterns of behaviour. Bach wrote of this on many occasions, stressing the need to avoid interfering with the individuality of one's offspring (*Free Thyself*, chapter one; *Heal Thyself*, chapter five). The privilege of a parent, he said, lies in 'enabling a soul to contact this world for the sake of evolution . . . every possible freedom should be given for unhampered development'.[18] Arbitrary control, emotional manipulation and falseness are particularly offensive to the Water Violet person.

Selfish parenting can be seen as a form of emotional pollution. It is paralleled in the outer world by physical pollution. This, as was said earlier, forces Water Violet into retreat so that it is now difficult to find. The

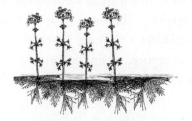

drainage dykes where Bach found it growing in Sussex have been changed by modern farming methods, as have the Somerset Levels. Writing in 1946, Geoffrey Grigson said we need not be surprised or alarmed by the changes taking place:

> *There is less water on the face of Britain. Marshes have been drained, the vast amount of water taken for cities has lowered the permanent water-table. Roads and drains and ditches are better kept, so water hangs about less and runs off quicker into streams and rivers and into the sea.*[19]

Fifty years on we might not be so sanguine: the process of change has accelerated hugely and plants have been among the casualties. But perhaps the loss of flowers like Scleranthus and Water Violet merely reflects the soul qualities which are diminishing in our society.

Gentian

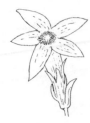

The last two of the _Twelve Healers_ grow on chalk downland in thin, hilltop soil: a contrast to the Water Violet. Bach spent 1931 travelling across the country, from Cromer to Abergavenny on the border of the Welsh mountains, back east to Sussex, then Berkshire and the Thames Valley, where he was walking the Chiltern Hills, then back through Sussex and Kent, walking on the Pilgrim's Way near Westerham. At this point he seems to have been particularly attracted to the higher ground and the plants which grow there when left undisturbed by human activity. It was on the ancient Chiltern footpath, the Icknield Way, that he found both Gentian and Rock Rose and formulated the last of the soul types in the group of twelve remedies.

For some time he had been seeking a replacement for _Sonchus arvensis_ (pages 89–90), the gloomy and brooding type which he called The Destroyer.[20] Perhaps he was uneasy with the idea that a soul lesson could be so negative, although he had observed such people well enough: 'they wallow in all that is morbid and infect and depress others with gloom'.[21] It was a state of mind for which he later found suitable remedies like Gorse, Sweet Chestnut and Willow. But the archetypal soul lesson was different, not so extreme and with an underlying strength in the positive opportunities for learning. This new remedy, Gentian, was given the qualities of Doubt and Understanding. These people doubt their abilities, doubt that they will ever succeed and yet come to the understanding that everything in life is gain, even if we cannot always directly perceive the benefits:

> _The understanding that there is no failure when you are doing your utmost, whatever the apparent result._[22]

The key phrase might be 'doing your utmost', with the implication that these are souls who know what they are to do in life, who find it easy to apply themselves but subsequently become discouraged.

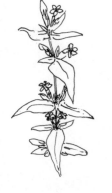

Gentian is _Gentiana amarella_, the autumn felwort. It flowers, as the common name suggests, in August and September. Centaury (pages 110–111) is also in the same Gentain family and they hold in common certain aspects in the pattern of growth. As biennials they have been delayed, as it were, in the journey to flowering. But the Gentian delays for longer and chooses conditions which are more difficult. It is altogether a smaller plant and more vulnerable, less able to assert itself in the face of competition. That is why it keeps to downland where dry, thin calcareous soils (chalk and limestone) make for short grass. On germination, the seedling puts most of its effort into growing a root; during the first year it forms a few pairs of leaves which die back in the autumn. The small, swollen, yellow root cannot be seen but it will produce new leaves in spring. The root contains a mildly bitter principle used in herbal medicine (more usually taken from the related species *Gentiana lutea*). The accumulation of life experience may be stored in the root; this bitterness suggests the disappointment of being let down by life.* We find the same bitterness with Chicory (page 102) which feels let down by others and with Willow (page 221), the remedy for resentment.

Just how a plant grows depends upon the surroundings. The small, square stem of the Gentian begins to thrust upwards in late spring. Despite the bitter taste, it is sometimes eaten away by grazing animals and this causes it to branch, distorting the vertical form of the plant and forcing a dense and stunted growth. If it is a dry spring the upward progress will be limited or delayed. In any event the plant usually stays close to the ground, sheltering in order to retain moisture and stay within the humid layer of dew-laden grass—fifty or seventy-five millimetres from the ground. Such conditions may not be harsh, but they are not easy: that is what characterizes the Gentian soul state. The number of flowers in any one year will depend upon the success of the seed crop two years before and the rainfall in the intervening seasons.

The leaves are lanceolate and dark green, while the stems are tinged with red; both the colour and shape suggest strength of purpose and

---

* Some writers make an assumption as to the 'evolutionary' purpose of such bitterness in a plant. Seeing all poisons and thorns as weapons in a fight for survival they miss a more subtle perspective of meaning. Anthony Huxley wrote: 'Many plants have passive devices such as thorns and poison against predators of various kinds; not man initially, but primarily grazing animals….alpine meadow gentians, whose juicy, bitter roots are prized medicinally, are avoided by cattle above ground and rodents below….' Yet Lousley comments about gentians: 'The bitter taste of the stem and leaves is said to offer protection against grazing, but this is certainly of little value in the face of attacks from the hungry rabbits of the downs. When they nibble the young shoots down to ground level the plants branch out from the base and grow into very floriferous bushy little tufts on which the flowers are sometimes divided into 4's instead of 5's'. This points up the difference between theory and practical observation. Lousley knows what he has seen. His comments are reinforced by other research which has shown that the seeds of *Gentiana amarella* may be found in the dung of cattle and horses (Heinitz, *Food of Animals in Sweden*).
See: Anthony Huxley, *Plant and Planet*, Allen Lane; 1974, p. 282.
J.E.Lousley, *Wild Flowers of Chalk & Limestone*, Collins; 1969, p. 31.
H.N.Ridley, *The Dispersal of Plants Throughout the World*, L.Reeve; nd, pp. 360-361.

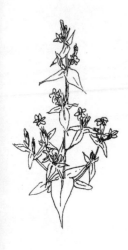

involvement in life. A plant's leaf is the main organ of respiration (it is the lungs) and as such it is the place where the elements are joined to form the energetic force for living. The quality of this respiration is described by the form of the leaf. In this plant it is directed, pointed, smooth and defined: the qualities that are needed by Gentian people. Bach wrote of them:

> *Are you one of those with high ideals, with hopes of doing good . . .*[23]
> *People who wish to do much . . .*[24]

The Gentians may be small but they are capable and resourceful. At their base the leaves clasp the stem and the flowers grow on short stalks

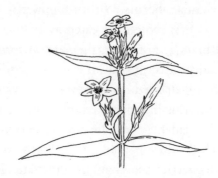

from the axil of these leaves, which have the appearance of providing a platform, presenting them. This gives Gentian a compact and geometrical intensity. Even when it manages only a single flower at the top of a small stalk, the gesture is one of determination, making the best of meagre resources. The flower has a tubular form with five petals opening in the sun and closing when there is rain or a drop in temperature. This response is very pronounced:

> *Autumn Gentian . . . has reddish-purple flowers which open and close with surprising speed, according to changes in the temperature. Since it is warmer when the sun is shining, the opening is generally observed as clouds roll away, and the time taken for the change may sometimes be as little as twenty seconds.*[25]

Was this what was in Bach's mind when he wrote:

> *When success is in your path are you elated, but when difficulties occur easily depressed? If so, the little Gentian of our hilly pastures will help you to keep your firmness of purpose, and a happier and more hopeful outlook even when the sky is over-cast.*[26]

Certainly Gentian flowers only open when conditions are favourable; on a cool, dull day they remain closed. That can mean a long waiting period (and thus a long flowering period) in an English summer.

Gentian is pollinated by insects which push their way through the fringe of pale hairs in the throat of the flower. The pistil is longer than the anthers, and as the insects struggle to climb into the bell of the flower they dust pollen on to the style. On their way out they pick up new pollen to carry on to the next stop. The upright position of the flower presents a landing pad for those flying in: Gentian has a precise system for pollination and it demonstrates a strong link to the world and the future.

The flowers remain attached after flowering, although they wither somewhat and fade. As the seedpod develops, the petals and sepals provide protection. This is important for a plant where the seeds ripen late in the year. This speaks of Gentian's tenacity, holding to a life purpose (see Scleranthus page 120). Gentian people appear to give up easily and become despondent, but the flower says just the reverse. It says hold on, keep making the effort. Visually, the effect can be disconcerting since the old flower pods look like yellowed buds. At first glance it appears that the flowers have yet to open or that they have given up and dried on the stem.

The seeds are many and small; some are distributed by grazing animals but most fall at the foot of the parent plant when it is shaken by the wind. Consequently, Gentian grows as a scattered colony. Since it is a hilltop plant, it spreads down the slope for as long as conditions remain favourable, edging its way into a field below if the farmer does not cultivate the headland. But it is the view from the hilltop which allows Gentian types to take a higher perspective on life's difficulties: 'often they desire things to go too much their own way, instead of seeing the bigger outlook'.[27] This bigger picture can only be seen from high ground. Sitting with this plant on the chalk downs, it is easier to see our place in the world. And while the little Gentian is often burned off in a dry summer or trodden under foot on the pilgrim's path, it has a strength of purpose to keep on going and do really well.

Bach had first seen Gentian growing on the Chilterns, but it was in Kent, on the North Downs, that he actually made the remedy. Weeks tells us that he went back there in the following summer to find Rock Rose.[28] But Rock Rose must have been flowering when he was in the Chilterns the previous year. He saw it but did not recognize its significance until

Rock Rose

later. This is not a criticism but an observation of the complexities Bach experienced in selecting the twelve basic type remedies. It was made more difficult by the fact that, to all appearances, Rock Rose is less of a soul type and more of a 'situation' remedy.

Weeks says that Bach was looking for a plant which carried the same instantaneous healing power which he himself could sometimes bring to people, calming them when they were in deep distress. He had wanted to show people they had the same ability, but he did not know how. So he went looking for a plant, 'a material agent, a herbal remedy which would act in the same manner'.[29] This remedy was to be Rock Rose, for 'those in absolute despair, in terror: who feel that you can bear nothing more; terrified . . .'.[30] Yet Rock Rose is the twelfth remedy and a soul type just like the others. Bach gave it the soul qualities of Terror and Courage.

How can terror be one of the 'twelve primary types of personality'?[31] Indeed, among the majority of people using Bach's remedies today Rock Rose is seen as only a treatment for acute fear, panic or distress (he called it 'the rescue remedy').[32] While it does work in that way, it also has a deeper resonance with a certain type of person: one who lives life mutely under the intense pressure of fear. When this fear is overcome, perhaps such people are able to help calm the distress of others, just as Bach anticipated. It is a particular kind of fear, however, not the nervous fear of Mimulus but rather a deeply hidden fear of life itself. Being hidden it is perhaps hard for others to recognize. Like the secrets of the twelfth house in astrology, the Rock Rose secret is not apparent to the outer world. Only those who resonate with the blind panic of the Rock Rose soul will recognize its quality.

The Little Mermaid by Hans Andersen is a fairy tale which illustrates aspects of the Rock Rose soul condition. A mermaid falls in love with a prince after she saves his life during a storm at sea. She decides to leave her own family and go to live on land in the hope that the prince will love her in return, and thereby she will gain an immortal soul. She visits the sea witch who agrees to make her a potion which will give her human legs to replace her mermaid's fish-tail, but on certain conditions. With her legs she will be the most graceful dancer but each step will pain her as if she is treading upon sharp knives. Then, if the prince marries another, her heart will break and she will dissolve into foam on the water. Lastly, in payment, she must give to the witch the best thing she has: her beautiful voice.

'If you take away my voice,' says the little mermaid, 'what will remain to me?'

'Your beautiful form,' replied the witch, 'your graceful walk and your sparkling eyes: with those you can take captive a human heart . . .'

With great courage the mermaid agrees; the witch cuts out her tongue and gives her a potion. Once on land, in the human world, she drinks the potion. It pains her, burning like fire, cutting like swords, and she falls down in a swoon. She is found on the seashore by the prince who shelters and protects her. She lives in the palace and goes everywhere with him around the kingdom, always in hope and always in pain. In the end the prince falls in love and marries a princess; the mermaid, as was foretold, becomes sea-foam and as pure spirit travels the world.

The story may be interpreted in different ways; the sexual inference is obvious enough. But consider the possible symbolism of the soul incarnating in the physical world. This is the stated intent for the little mermaid; she wants an immortal soul, a human soul; she has lived at the bottom of the sea for her first fifteen years, an innocent dreaming of life on earth. And then, when her opportunity comes, it calls for intense courage, brings constant pain which she cannot avoid if she is to fulfil her life aim (to marry the prince) and leaves her mute, unable to tell her story or, more importantly, to sing the beautiful song of her being. It all points to the soul circumstances of the Rock Rose.

Rock Rose has had a variety of Latin names but is now generally called *Helianthemum nummularium*, the flower of the sun, like gold coins. The golden-yellow flowers are round and flat, lying on the ground like scattered gold pieces that have fallen among the grass. The five-petalled flowers are notably frail with an appearance like creased silk or crumpled tissue paper. They last only a day and the petals quickly fall. It is the extreme delicacy of the petals which shows the tenuous, febrile nature of the Rock Rose type, who have such a loose grip upon life—Bach said that this is the remedy to use when there is an accident, emergency or intense fear in both the patient and the people around. The soul type lives with such a fear throughout life. The strength and hope come from the golden light of the sun, which is reflected in the golden light of the flowers. They brings courage, fortitude and the brave will to win.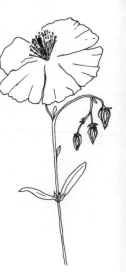

The plant is perennial, growing low to the ground in a massed clump. The sprawling stems are thin and woody with small, dark green leaves in opposite pairs. Rock Rose is evergreen: the leaves stay on the plant throughout the year. The gesture here lacks the vertical, directed growth of the strong will and ego (see Vervain page 107, Impatiens page 43) which expresses a clear and individual purpose in life. Rather the spreading, horizontal growth holds to the earth (see Scleranthus pages 117–8). The Rock Rose souls endeavour to sustain their presence on earth; just existing is work enough. It is an undifferentiated life without the seasonal vertical growth and decline which is usual in plants.

The flowering stems do rise vertically some eighty to one hundred millimetres from the mat of leaves, although the individual flowers, always at the top of the stem, turn 180 degrees to face the sun as they open. As buds they face downwards, but in the sun the stem flexes and turns the opening flower to face the sky. This remarkable reactive strength makes the plants like a weather vane: they hang their heads on a rainy morning but turn, like sunflowers, to face the sun if the skies clear. Rock Rose people have a similar watchful quality; always awake, always observing, always responsive to the environment of life. Like the little mermaid, watching her prince, they say little but see much, waiting for life to respond.

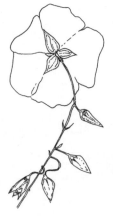

*Back of
Rock Rose flower*

Rock Rose is a common enough plant on chalk and limestone soils and yet it attracts scant attention from botanical writers. G. Clarke Nuttall, one of the few to consider it at any length wrote:

> *Sensitive to a degree, the golden flower of the Rock Rose only attempts to face the world for one short day at most, and even during these few hours its blossoming will not unfold its delicate petals unless the sun be shining. . . . The crumpled look is due to the way in which the petals are folded up in the bud, for there, instead of being neatly pleated or rolled, they are—to quote an old writer's succinct description—'cramb'd up within the Empalement (i.e. calyx) by hundreds of little Wrinkles or Puckers; it is as if Three or Four fine Cambrick Hankerchiefs were thrust into one's pocket'. And they never get properly smoothed out afterwards.*[33]

More generally it has been noticed that when the flower first opens the stamens crowd close to the stigma but that any light touch (from an insect seeking pollen, for instance) makes them fan apart. This 'irritability' as it is called is distinctly unusual in plants and it is not easily explained. While there may be some benefit here in discouraging self-pollination[34] it is, perhaps, another demonstration of how the Rock Rose soul type interacts and responds to the world around. Rock Rose is singularly sensitive.

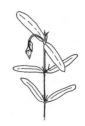

Sensitivity has been linked to the hairy leaves of some plants (page 95). Rock Rose does indeed have a hairy leaf, but the leaf form is simple, ovate and plain. It is a little unusual—hairy and dark green above yet grey and downy beneath. Does this signal a kind of vulnerability? The sepals which surround the bud are also hairy; after the petals have fallen they quickly close up again and protect the seedpod which swells within. The seeds fall from the pod and may be blown or washed downhill to germinate in the spring. Extraordinarily, Rock Rose seeds are often taken by ants[35] into their nest where they are stored, presumably as food. Some that are dropped on the way into the nest germinate in the loose soil which the ants scatter from their excavations. Rock Rose, in consequence, can often be found growing on a tump—the old mound of an ant colony. The germinating seed puts down a quick and deeply-diving root. The root system of a grown plant has been found to be as long as seventy-six centimetres with many side branches and rootlets.[36] This strength in the root shows an inclination to work strongly into the materiality of life in the physical world: common to many plants but more pronounced in Rock Rose.

With the finding of Rock Rose, Dr Bach's *Twelve Great Remedies* were complete. He spent the last months of the year in Cromer and put the remedies to work. At this stage the first cycle of his discoveries was over. He published the full information about these twelve several times: there is no doubt they appeared to him as a complete and finished set of remedies. That Rock Rose, the last of the twelve, was also moving towards a situational remedy and away from a singular type remedy merely served to illustrate the way things were about to develop.

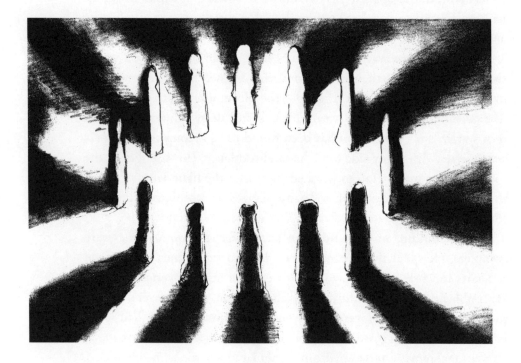

8 · The Architecture of the Twelve Healers

IMAGINE A CIRCLE OF STONES with twelve monoliths marking the twelve points on the perimeter where the numbers stand on a clock face. In the middle of the circle there is an open space. Into this space visualize the outpouring of light from a centre that is beyond this world, in a different dimension. From the bright light of the centre shadows extend, lengthening behind the stones, out into the darkness. One side of each stone is illuminated by the light. It is thrown into relief by the shadow and half-light, the unseen form which has turned, facing away into the dark.

These twelve stand like the twelve soul lessons of *The Twelve Healers*. Each of us, said Bach, is born with the purpose of learning one of these great life lessons.[1] The negative aspect of each remedy state is seen in the shadow, in the darkness and isolation which we encounter when we turn away from the light. Wherever we stand on the circumference of the circle we can look outwards into the darkness and see fear or pain, indifference, grief, or doubt according to the soul lesson that we are here to learn. When we turn around and face the light we meet the positive soul force of that lesson: courage, peace, tolerance, or understanding. Bach lists these qualities in a table:

Failing	Herb	Virtue
Restraint	Chicory	Love
Fear	Mimulus	Sympathy
Restlessness	Agrimony	Peace
Indecision	Scleranthus	Steadfastness
Indifference	Clematis	Gentleness
Weakness	Centaury	Strength
Doubt	Gentian	Understanding
Over-enthusiasm	Vervain	Tolerance
Ignorance	Cerato	Wisdom
Impatience	Impatiens	Forgiveness
Terror	Rock Rose	Courage
Grief	Water Violet	Joy[2]

In reality these positive soul conditions are all one and the same: the experience of love and light, the unity of life. Bach sees these virtues as the attributes of Christ:

> *If we now think of the twelve attributes of Christ which we most wish to attain, and which He came to teach us, we find the twelve great lessons of life.*[3]

In this model we can see that the action of the flower remedies is to turn us around, to turn us from the isolation of a path leading into darkness, to one which leads towards the light. They help to turn us around, for instance, from the path that leads to the pain of impatience and irritation, to the heart-easing path of gentle forgiveness.

With a group of other people it is possible to get a sense for this. Stand in a ring facing inwards and imagine the light entering the world as coming from a sun at the centre. Each face, each person, is lit by that light. Each of us stands with the four elements of the physical world to compose our physical bodies and the four elements of the invisible world to compose our soul. This soul carries knowledge of the life lesson which, individually, we need to learn. For this person it is Gentian, for that one Centaury, then Chicory or the next Vervain and so on. Then, one by one, turn around from the centre and begin to walk out into life. There are still people either side but the further you walk, the more you will walk into isolation. On this path the life lessons, the opportunities to learn and grow, present themselves. We can see them as they stand in our way, illuminated by the light from behind us. At a time of our choosing we turn around and begin to walk back along the path towards the light, to the centre and the ring of people standing together.

With his Masonic background[4] Bach was drawn to the architecture of ideas, to design and number. In his writings he referred to the 'Great Architect of the Universe', the 'Divine Plan' and the 'Grand Design'. He spoke of the temple of the soul, the stones of the temple, the edifice and the new building in prospect. Geometry and the numerical structure of growth and form are evident in nature, particularly in plants and their flowers. Bach saw nature as the ordered creation of life where Divinity is reflected. 'The harmony of the world is made manifest in Form and Number,' wrote D'Arcy Thompson, 'and the heart and soul and all the poetry of Natural Philosophy are embodied in the concept of mathematical beauty'.[5] We can see it in the geometry of crystals, in the numerical pattern of petals, the symmetry of plants and the complex design of life forms: life is developed through natural ordering and not through chaos.

Bach's interest in numbers showed itself throughout his work; in particular he elaborated the qualities of seven and twelve. He chose seven nosodes, seven soul lessons, seven principles; then twelve chapters in *Free Thyself,* twelve failings and twelve virtues, *Twelve Great Remedies, The Twelve Healers* and later *The Seven Helpers.* And having found nineteen remedies by the end of 1933 he began a second sequence of remedies in 1935, of which there were also nineteen. Numerically it all resolved as 12+7=19, 1+9=10, 1+0=1; then 19+19=38, 3+8=11, and eleven, a special number in its own right, resolved 1+1 into 2, indicating the two parts of his work.

It is in this context that Bach chose twelve basic soul types. It linked with the twelve astrological signs (although he said that they related to the twelve moon signs[6] and not twelve sun signs), with twelve disciples, twelve months of the year, twelve tribes of Israel, the twelve Imams; the list goes on. It may well be that there are more of these basic soul types, perhaps hundreds. But Bach started with twelve and held to the idea that each of us might find our essential nature exemplified by one of these. With this limited number of types available he speaks of 'definite groups of mankind, each group performing its own function, that is, manifesting in the material world the particular lesson he has learnt'.[7] In other words, each of these soul groups is responsible for the transmutation of its own life difficulty: it is the task of the Cerato people to bring wisdom into the world, of the Vervain types to bring tolerance.

This idea, where we see the soul type representing an essential virtue which is necessary for the evolution of life on earth, is woven into the fabric of Bach's writings. Listing the twelve great virtues in *Free Thyself* he wrote 'and it is by perfecting these qualities in ourselves that each one of us is raising the whole world a step nearer to its final unthinkable glorious goal'.[8] Each person, he said, 'is of the same importance in the Divine Plan'[9] and can play a part in being the saviour of the world. We are all in the line with the twelve disciples sent out into the world.[10]

Each of us, then, has work to do, in accordance with the nature of our soul group and the unique life purpose set for us by our individual soul:

> *Each individual in these groups has a definite personality of his own, a definite work to do, and a definite individual way of doing that*

> work. These are also causes of disharmony, which unless we hold to our
> definite personality and our work, may react upon the body in the form
> of disease.[11]

It was to help counter this disease reaction that he put the twelve flower
remedies alongside the twelve soul types. The action of the remedies is
to remind us of our true vocation in life: to show us, again, the purposes
of the soul.

Anticipating the problem that people would have in choosing one of
the twelve, Bach says:

> To find the herb that will help us we must find the object of our life, what
> we are striving to do, and also understand the difficulties in our path. The
> difficulties we call faults or failings, but let us not mind these faults and
> failings, because they are the very proof to us that we are attaining bigger
> things. Let us find for ourselves which of the battles we are particularly
> fighting, which adversary we are especially trying to overcome, and then
> take with gratitude and thankfulness that plant which has been sent to
> help us to victory. We should accept these beautiful herbs of the fields as a
> sacrament, as our Creator's Divine gift to aid us in our troubles.[12]

And:

> Should any difficulty be found in selecting your own remedy, it will help
> to ask yourself which of the virtues you most admire in other people; or
> which of the failings is, in others, your pet aversion, for any fault of which
> we may still have left a trace and are especially attempting to eradicate,
> that is the one we most hate to see in other people. It is the way we are
> encouraged to wipe it out in ourselves.[13]

And, if we are unclear as to what we should be doing on this pathway of
life, leading us out into the world:

> Let us find the one thing in life that attracts us most and do it. Let that
> one thing be so part of us that it is as natural as breathing; as natural as
> it is for the bee to collect honey, and the tree to shed its old leaves in the
> autumn and bring forth new ones in the spring. If we study nature we
> find that every creature, bird, tree and flower has its definite part to play,
> its own definite and peculiar work through which it aids and enriches
> the entire Universe. The very worm, going about its daily job, helps to
> drain and purify the earth: the earth provides for the nutriment of all
> green things; and, in turn, vegetation sustains mankind and every living
> creature, returning in due course to enrich the soil. Their life is one of
> beauty and usefulness, their work is so natural to them that it is their life.

And our own work, when we find it, so belongs to us, so fits us, that it is effortless, it is easy, it is a joy: we never tire of it, it is our hobby. It brings out in us our true personality, all the talents and capabilities waiting within each one of us to be manifested: in it we are happy and at home; and it is only when we are happy (which is obeying the commands of our soul) that we can do our best work.[14]

A long quotation, but it neatly conveys Bach's message concerning the way to find and then to follow our life purpose, without interference.

These twelve remedies, *The Twelve Healers*, are at the base of the thirty-eight Bach flower remedies: the foundation of the building. Come back to them as the great soul lessons. Try to see them as different, individual types. Try to see how the form and nature of the flower reflects the nature of the personality. Look closely into the life to observe which is the strong theme for the individual soul, which lesson keeps repeating so that we can see it and change. Learn the twelve types by their gesture, the gesture of the soul, the gesture of the plant and the gesture of the life.

It is quite common for people to look at the twelve and find that they can associate with more than one of the soul lessons. People sometimes do not want to be limited to the confines of one remedy and tell themselves that they are a little like that, but not so extreme. Others find their image of themselves is more complex, more refined, more evolved than one of the twelve basic types. But a person will make better sense of life, whatever stage it is at, having learned these twelve great lessons. If, as Bach suggested, we work upon one lesson at a time in this life, adding that experience to the evolving knowledge of the soul, then already we will have a familiarity with each of these soul virtues at some level in ourselves. We will have met them in previous lives. Or perhaps it is true that we work upon different soul lessons at different times and stages in this one life—a child may start as a Gentian, as a youngster become Clematis, and as an adult Water Violet. Yet this seems less likely. Bach proposed that a single soul is essentially one or the other, even if it takes up the quality of another emotional state for a time. There is always the possibility that we see aspects of ourselves in this or that one of the twelve because we are not looking directly at what is in front of us.* We are not always willing

---

* Dr Bach gave the booklet of *The Twelve Healers* to his sister, asking her to say which remedy she thought she was taking. She considered all of them possible, but was adamant that she was not Mimulus, never nervous and afraid. But that was the remedy he had chosen for her to take.

to look full in the face the lessons of the individual remedy which awaits us on the path through life.

For this reason we can often see the soul lesson if we look back to moments of crisis and trauma in our life story. Bach said, look at the people you dislike or admire; by that he meant the people we have strong feelings about. Equally, we can recall formative events in life and assess our reaction to them—the same strong feelings will be attached there, too. We might consider something specific and personal, or we might look at a more general event from childhood. We look back towards childhood because these twelve types are what we are born with. It is commonly experienced that other emotional states come into play as we travel on the path of our life. We may end in hopelessness and despair. But if that should be the case despair is not a type remedy: we were not born with it. Each of us is born in hope. It is with the hope of the soul's longing for life that we begin.

9 · The Four Helpers

IN NOVEMBER 1932 Dr Bach placed newspaper advertisements in, among others, the *Northern Daily Telegraph*. He offered information on 'British herbs of great value',[1] giving his name, address and medical qualifications. Two days later a letter was sent to him from the Registrar of the General Medical Council, not an enquiry for information but a warning about advertising for patients. Such advertising was then and is now against the ethics of medical practice. Evidently Bach had made a decision. He no longer hoped to persuade his colleagues to convert to his new remedies and was going straight to the general public. Was this out of frustration? It seems likely. It was extremely difficult to introduce new ideas to a closed profession. He had appealed to the allopaths; he had lectured the homoeopaths. Both had responded with mild indifference. They were not interested.

Bach himself had been treating patients with the Twelve Healers although we cannot be sure how successfully. He quoted a few cases in *Twelve Great Remedies*[2] and they suggest that he was able to help people with rheumatism, paralysis, asthma and acute lymphatic leukaemia. He was in an unusual situation: people came to him as a medical doctor and he treated them with new and totally unproven herbal remedies. Today we are careful to say to somebody to whom we give flower remedies that we are not treating them medically; they may also need to consult a doctor. But Bach was a doctor. Was there a professional conflict here? Maybe that was a factor in his decision to advertise his new remedies. With his lecture *Ye Suffer from Yourselves* (pages 79–80) he had renounced his involvement with the homœopaths. Perhaps he was renouncing his commitment to the whole medical profession.

There was another factor, however. It is apparent that Dr Bach had modified his ideas during this time. He started with a clear proposition that it was the soul's condition which lead to illness and disease. Later he moved towards a more general perspective that mood influenced health. It was the difference between theory and practice. His theory still held good that there were twelve essential soul types* and those were the diagnostic framework to be used by the professionals. But in practice he was saying to the general public: look at these descriptions and see which of them fits the mood of the moment. He was working on the two ideas simultaneously. So he wrote: 'If in doubt between one or two, give both; they can be put in the same bottle . . .'.[3] And, 'It will often be found necessary to change the remedy as his case changes and in some cases even as many as half a dozen different herbs may be required'.[4] This last comment was written in *Twelve Great Remedies,* a magazine article published in February 1933. He began it by writing:

> *The twelve remedies which I have been working on for the last five years are proving so wonderful in their curative results and they are bringing health to so many so-called incurables, even where homoeopathic treatment has failed, that I am endeavouring to make the prescribing so simple that they can be used by all lay people.*[5]

The methodology was simplified in order to assist even those without medical training.

It was safe to give the remedies into the hands of lay people because they 'never give strong reaction, since they never do harm, however much is taken . . .'.[6] We can see the logic here. If they are truly safe there can be no harm in taking several remedies either together or in sequence (this was in contradistinction to both allopathic medicine and homœopathy). Accurate prescribing was no longer the imperative. So Bach eased the stricture in his method of diagnosis; getting it wrong would not result in harm. He noted: '. . . if the wrong remedy is given, no bad effect will follow, but when the right one is given benefit will be obtained'.[7]

Nonetheless, as Bach himself employed the remedies therapeutically he deepened his understanding of 'how simple it now is to prescribe with accuracy'.[8] He found it easy to recognize the different soul conditions and their corresponding remedies, and easy to follow the changing mood of a patient. But in some cases, he concluded, people are not obviously one of the twelve. The soul type appears to be obscured by another emotional state, one of long standing, a chronic condition:

> *It will be found that certain cases do not seem to fit exactly any one of the Twelve Healers, and many of these are such as those who have become so*

---

*There has been a suggestion (in the video presentation *A Further Understanding,* The Dr Edward Bach Centre, 1993) that some of the Twelve Healers are 'mood' remedies and not type remedies. This is an invention and not based on Dr Bach's work.

used to disease that it appears to be part of their nature; and it is difficult to see their true selves. . . . [9]

Bach was speaking of a different range of emotions exhibited by people in a 'state of stagnation'.[10]

Such people have lost much of their individuality, of their personality, and need to be helped out of the rut, out of the groove, in which they have become fixed before it is possible to know which of the Twelve Healers they need.[11]

Remember that the Twelve Healers are still about turning us around to face the light; giving the insight to the individual which will enable that person to recognize the life lesson which must be learned. But now Bach was suggesting that we may need one of these new helpers to bring us to the point of recognition. Lift the chronic condition, he was saying, and you will see the essential type beneath:

When they have progressed so far, their individuality will have sufficiently returned so that it will be possible to know which of the Twelve Healers will be required to bring them back to perfect health.[12]

These new remedies, the Four Helpers, are to 'get us over this stage' of being resigned to our illness or problems and 'bring us into the range of the Twelve Healers'.[13]

Bach said of these Four Helpers that each indicates a kind of lost hope, because the people concerned have accepted into themselves the idea that they cannot change. Each of the four remedies, Gorse, Oak, Heather and Rock Water, looks like a type but is not. Often they are erroneously referred to as type remedies, the Heather type or the Rock Water person, but this is just the point Bach was making: the Rock Water state so overlays the essential self, has become so much a part of the personality, that 'the abnormal state of mind or body is regarded both by themselves and others as part of the character'.[14] It is not. The purpose of the Four Helpers (and later the whole group of the Seven Helpers) was to lift the chronic emotional state to reveal the real person and thereby the soul lesson he had described in *The Twelve Healers*.

The Four Helpers started with Gorse, the remedy which shakes and *Gorse* reawakens the mentality of someone who has long been ill and has become resigned to fate. It challenges the assumption that nothing can be done, however hopeless the situation may appear. This chronic condition builds up over time like a slow suffocation or mental decay. Bach must have seen it often enough amongst patients who had stopped making the

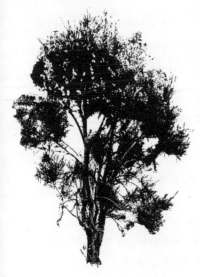

effort to improve in health. 'Of course, in all healing there must be a desire in the patient to get well', he wrote in *The Four Helpers*.[15] This remedy was needed for those whose desire to become well had not only faltered but stopped.

In his description for Gorse, Bach said nothing of the plant and looked only at the state of mind, adding some notes on the physical appearance of Gorse people (sallow complexion, dark rings around their eyes). Nevertheless, the plant succinctly describes the remedy, reflecting exactly the gesture. To raise the energy of the Gorse state, to prick the person back towards life, a powerful plant is needed, with a ferocious will to live; something brilliant, resilient, tough and tenacious, a flower that is sensitive and delicate yet strong and ablaze with light. Bach left no clue as to how he made his choice (except the 'message' received on the bank of the river Thames at Marlow, see page 37). But examination of the Gorse plant and its conditions for living shows a precise correspondence to the message of hopelessness and renewal.

Gorse grows on open hillsides, on wasteland, on heaths and commons. There is the occasional single plant, but it generally grows in massed clumps, often covering acres of neglected pasture. It is the collective strength of the species that is needed to lift the energy of the Gorse state; it lacks the individuality of the earlier type remedies. Look at a bank of Gorse and you will find it hard to see individuals either in the stems and branches or among the flowers. As one writer observed, it is a landscape plant.[16] Its golden-yellow flowers, offset by the vivid green stems, blaze with colour, painting the hillside. As with Heather, another of the Helpers, there is a sense that the Gorse bushes draw down the light and burn like flames upon the land.

Bach's Gorse is *Ulex europaeus,* a woody shrub growing to about two metres in height. It flowers over a long period from November to June. It has a smaller counterpart, *Ulex gallii* (not Bach's Gorse), which flowers in the second part of the year. Together they form an annual cycle for this type of plant which flowers throughout the year. Hence the oft quoted 'when Gorse is out of flower, then kissing's out of fashion'. Mabey, in *Flora Britannica,* links this idea to the fact that Gorse grows on common land and offers those hidden places where couples may go for illicit sex. It points up an interesting link between the Gorse state of desolation and

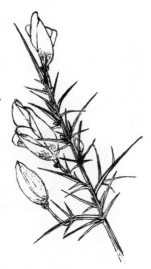

the life-affirming act of making love. The same idea links to Wild Rose (page 267).

Ulex europaeus grows exclusively in north-west Europe between about forty-five to sixty degrees North. It begins to flower shortly before the winter solstice at the tail end of the year when the vitality in most other plants has declined (the first flowers may appear in October). In this part of the world, as we approach the shortest day around the twenty-second of December and the sun is at its lowest in the sky, this is the season for death, dormancy and hibernation. Yet the light is promised to return. In pre-historic times the people of this land waited for the light of the sun to fall upon a marker stone to show that the longest night was over and the new year begun.* The flowering of Gorse marks just such a cycle of renewal and rebirth. It continues to bloom through the frosts of January, the wind and rain of March, bud after bud developing in the axils of the leaves. Building to a crescendo of golden light, it reaches a peak at Easter and the Spring Festival. Easter is a Christian feast day, but it is significantly a celebration of death and resurrection, the qualities of Gorse.

It is not until the warmer days of April that Gorse bursts into full flower. The exciting scent, a cross between coconut and vanilla, calls to bees and other insects searching for early pollen and nectar. Stand in the midst of Gorse in April and every sense is awakened and stimulated, just as the flower remedy stimulates the life force. See the brilliant colour, hear the sound of insects and smell the scent. Also, feel the sharp touch of the spikes and spines, for it is impossible to walk among Gorse without being scratched and jabbed at by these needle-pointed leaves. They quickly draw blood and this is emblematic of the arousal caused by Gorse, pointing to the lifeblood. Gorse people 'are resigned to their infirmity, they do not even complain. . . . [They] have lost the heart to try any more'.[17] The little swords that cover the bushes jab at this resignation, forcing the person to another effort.

---

*In *The Myth of the Goddess*, Anne Baring and Jules Cashford (Viking Arkana, 1991), describe how New Grange in Ireland (dated about 3200 BC), was constructed so that the sun's rays could only penetrate the darkened interior on the few days around the Winter Solstice. 'The ritual enacted must have been one of the sun fertilizing the *body* of the earth and so awakening her after her winter sleep to the renewed cycle of life' (p. 98).

It is given out in some botanical textbooks[18] that Gorse has spiny leaves to deter foraging animals and/or to help it to withstand drought—an extension of the idea that apparently lies behind the cactus. However, plant forms are not determined merely by physiological functions. The idea behind Gorse is very different, the aim and life form of the plant being more in service than in competitive survival. When the leaves first form from the bud they are soft and juicy and attractive to eat, so much so that Gorse was formerly used as a fodder crop for cows and horses.[19] The stems were cut and bruised in a mill; penned stock ate them with relish. In the field, Gorse is often ignored by animals because these young shoots grow in early summer when there is grass a-plenty. The idea of drought has little relevance since Gorse only grows in the moist climate of north-west Europe and not in the drier Mediterranean.

So why does Gorse have these spiny leaves? They express the gesture and the life pattern of the plant. The spiky leaves are symbolic, a picture of the life force, the subtle energy and strength. There is also another explanation. Gorse grows naturally in exposed conditions, where the turbulence of the wind disturbs and rocks the shrub. The spiky leaves interlock, stem-to-stem, branch-to-branch so that a woven mat provides a network of support (see Holly page 237). It is noticeable that people in a Gorse condition must be supported in just this way; they cannot be left alone.

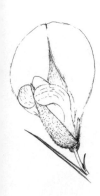

Young stalks of Gorse are ribbed for strength and show clear lines of energy in the plant. Although barely visible to the naked eye, these stalks are covered by fine, straggling hairs as if pointing to a fragility, in contrast to the angular structure of the spiky leaves. The flowers, too, are delicate with the sepals covered with a soft down. Gorse has the flower of the pea family. The sepals and stigma are protected within the cusped form of the five petals in such a way that they are only revealed after pollination. Holding back and waiting for warm weather, the flowers show their colour but are slow to open fully. They give the impression of a shielded lamp.

Gorse has an unusual device to ensure pollination. When the pollen is ripe it falls into the 'keel' of the flower (two joined petals which form a boat shape). When an insect lands it triggers the release of the stigma and stamens which also lie sheltered in the keel. The pollen is then thrown up by the explosive force and dusts the abdomen of the visiting bee. This display of mechanical cunning leads to the flower being called 'explosive' or 'excitable'. Another explosion occurs when the seeds are ripe. As the pod dries on a warm summer day it splits open, shooting the seeds away from the parent plant. It is a reminder of Impatiens (see pages 35–6)—certainly that is a remedy type which has a strong involvement in life. This explosive character reinforces the idea of Gorse needing to get the energy moving again. Just as the spines draw blood, these explosions are like fire crackers to make the person jump, like an electric shock, a jolt to restart the heart.

Of Gorse people Bach said 'they look as though they need more sunshine in their lives to drive away the clouds'.[20] And the strongest impression from Gorse is the radiant strength of the golden flowers: it is a sun flower. But all the brightness and lively energy is on the surface, on the outer edges of the plant. Look beneath and inside the bush; there are brown,

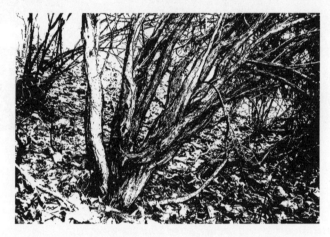

dried stalks, dead shoots and the dry debris of fallen leaves. The bark of the main stems is flaky, rough and without visible sign of life or energy (see Clematis page 47). Gorse takes four years or more to reach maturity and then, as it grows outwards, away from the root, it seems to die within. Like the people in a Gorse state, whose vitality has ebbed away, the plant appears to be dying: the green shoots and golden flowers a last effort for life.

It is not old age which kills Gorse, however. Rather the extremes of drought and cold. The geographical limits on *Ulex europaeus* show this. It cannot withstand a prolonged frost and will die back towards the root if the soft growth on the periphery is damaged. Gorse thus shows another aspect of its character: it can appear to be dead and done for and yet still shoot again. It is a kind of rebirth and resurrection. This was illustrated on one occasion by the harsh treatment meted out to some potted Gorse

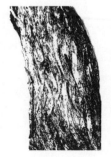

plants left unwatered through a dry summer. They could only be dead it seemed. Yet, put into the ground and watered, several of them came back to life and grew back as strong plants.

So hope springs eternal in the human breast, not in the cynical way that the poet Alexander Pope meant it, but as the true expression of faith in life. The Gorse bush shows us how that can be.

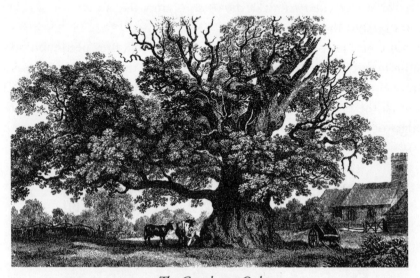

The Cowthorpe Oak

Oak

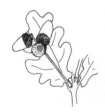

If Gorse people have given up on trying to regain their health then the Oaks are just the opposite:

> *Oak is for the type of people who, although they feel hopeless of any cure, still struggle and are irritated that they are ill.*[21]

It looks as though Bach saw these two as opposed ways of dealing with the same chronic problem; Gorse views the condition as hopeless while Oak struggles on despite the difficulty. From a diagnostic viewpoint this suggests a simple either/or choice. Faced with any longstanding life problem, see how the person behaves. The problem need not be a terminal illness, it could be physical or mental, a difficulty with work or a pathological relationship. The important distinction to be noticed is the kind of response made to a chronic condition.

The Oak people appear to be positive, making an attempt to keep on keeping on. 'They hate not being able to play their part in the game of life . . .' wrote Bach.[22] Yet this condition is damaging because Oak people ignore the warning signs of a breakdown in their health and need to limit their activity. This is an acquired behaviour, not the true type remedy or soul lesson. Indeed, appearing to struggle against the odds is a way to disguise the true problem; it is a kind of suppression, an unwillingness to face reality. As such, people in the Oak state are going nowhere even if they seem to be brave and purposeful. Theirs is a donkey determination and they need help to reappraise, reassess and reposition the life.

Oak trees are more written about than any others. Books list famous old trees and recount the folklore associated with them.[23] Such things are interesting in a scholarly sort of way but probably meant little to Bach: it is experience of the tree itself which leads to an understanding of the remedy state. For that we must meet actual specimens and observe the way that they grow. As with the other remedies, it is the life history which describes the gesture, even if the lore and language of tradition can help to make that description. If one word describes Oak it might be endurance. The Oak types and the Oak trees endure all that life brings, struggling without complaint.

This idea of endurance begins with the longevity of Oaks—many are said to be as much as a thousand years old. This puts an ancient Oak among the oldest living beings on earth. But it is not age alone which marks endurance; it is also submission to pain and difficulty, long-suffering patience and the will to continue to the limit of your strength. In this the Oak is the exact picture of endurance. Edmund Spenser, the English poet, wrote in *The Ruines of Rome*, 1591:

> ... *a huge oak, dry and dead,*
> *Still clad with reliques of trophies old,*
> *Lifting to heaven its aged, hoary head,*
> *Whose foot on earth hath got but feeble hold,*
> *And half disbowelled stands above the ground,*
> *With wreathed roots, and naked arms,*
> *And trunk all rotten and unsound.*[24]

He might have said that even a tree 'all rotten and unsound' puts out new leaves and flowers and fruits, providing shelter and food for birds, insects and animals. You can see such trees in the field, broken down and dying, yet still showing leaf upon a few small branches. Even at the end of its days the Oak tree struggles to live and provide sustenance for the other lives which depend upon it.

The tree begins with the seed, the acorn. In a 300-year lifetime a single Oak may produce as many as twenty-five million acorns, though fewer than a handful will develop into mature trees. Most acorns are eaten, almost as soon as they fall. In October rooks may settle in the branches and peck at the fruits as they ripen, chattering noisily as they snap the twigs. Later, come the spring, the same birds will gather these twigs for their nests. Of the acorns which fall to the ground, jays, squirrels, and mice all eat a share, or hide them as a store for the coming winter. Birds, pigs and deer will gather at certain trees looking for acorns, year after year. Only a few are overlooked and even those carefully planted in a nursery garden will be nosed out and eaten by hungry mice. The few left behind survive, germinate and grow. But their young shoots are attractive to mice and rabbits and are likely to be eaten during the next year or two. If they can survive that decimation, will they have sufficient growing space and light to develop? Probably not. But in woodland, once in a decade or so, a tree falls and leaves a hole in the canopy, so that the young tree may see the sky.

While we tend to see Oaks today as specimen trees in the middle of a field or in the line of a hedge, they are naturally woodland trees growing in the forests which used to cover lowland Britain, where the dynamic of growth and regeneration is notably different from trees in an open field or parkland. Of necessity, trees in a forest grow in the context of their companions. That is why Beech trees grow so straight and tall in woodland (page 223) as they race to get to the light. Perhaps that is why the Oak, to the contrary, developed its peculiar habit of dropping branches, often huge limbs, to allow light into the forest undergrowth.

For the first hundred years an Oak grows quickly if conditions are favourable. The first acorns appear after ten or twelve years, while the tree is still juvenile. But even before that, the immature Oak will begin to gather to it the various insects whose larvae eat the leaves, laying eggs on the roots, in the bark and buds. More pests attack Oaks than any other tree, though whether this is truly attack or attraction is questionable. L.J. Brimble in *Trees in Britain* noted that Oak has a peculiar attraction for insects and 'can count several hundred different species among its natural enemies'.[25] But are they really enemies? Evidence suggests that Oaks not only attract these 'predators' but carefully adapt their life cycle to provide for them. That, certainly, is in the nature of the Oak remedy state: Oak people seek the responsibilities that test their endurance. Thereby they avoid the real issue of facing their soul lesson. Dependable people, they attract to themselves those who need help and they will happily take on their burdens. 'They are discontented with themselves', said Bach, 'if illness interferes with their duties or helping others'.[26]

The Oak tree has a habit of producing a secondary growth of young leaves during summer—'the lammas growth' as it is called. Lammas Day is on the first of August and while every other tree has entered the stable period of summer the Oak uses its strength to produce new shoots and leaves. These are particularly attractive to certain caterpillars, hatching during August, which are unable to chew the older leaves from spring. These new leaves can actually be produced at any time of year if necessary. A.G. Tansley in *Oaks and Oakwoods*[27] noted that during the 1930s in the Forest of Dean the caterpillars of Oak Roller and Winter Moths 'very badly defoliated' the Oaks—but they survived by putting out new leaf.

Oaks have this facility for producing new growth from buds which have been dormant beneath the bark for many years. The 'epicormic shoots' are a reserve of life opportunity for the Oak which can be called upon if the main canopy of leaves is lost. This can occur if caterpillars eat the leaves or through the loss of branches (struck by lightening or broken in storms) or even through frost. Late frosts occasionally burn the young leaves and create a strange landscape of brown trees in spring. It does not occur often, since Oaks are one of the later trees to break bud. Other trees like hawthorn or birch are more frost resistant. But Oak leaves are soft and vulnerable just so as to be attractive to the caterpillars and larvae of moths and beetles.

Another aspect of the Oak is its facility for adaptation. Look at this first in terms of the remedy description. Bach said that these are people who have become adapted to their illness and carry on despite the handicap:

> *These people have physical diseases which tend to go on for years and, although they feel quite hopeless about themselves, they still go on trying and struggling.*[28]

This means that they have become subject to some invasive force, which causes physical problems, but the person will not give in to the difficulty. Yet Oak people become adapted to life with the problem, working hard, as if the problem were not there. In the tree we can see this illustrated in the way Oak deals with various parasites, such as gall wasps.

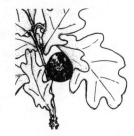

Gall wasps have individual and complex life cycles connected to specific parts of the tree. The well-known 'oak apples' are formed in response to eggs laid in the leaf bud. After hatching the females crawl down to the ground and pierce the young roots to lay eggs where a second generation of wasps (and galls) form. Some gall wasps utilize the leaves, others the male flowers producing 'currant galls' on the catkins. In each case the growth of the gall is in response to some stimulus produced by the wasp, the eggs or the larvae. It is a specific adaptation on the part of the tree, not fighting the wasp but accepting and getting along with it. Compare this with the Elm (page 192).

It is fashionable to look upon the pattern of growth as an expression of the selfish gene, to see any characteristic as being evolved to further the selfish prospects of the individual species. With Oaks such an idea does not square with reality; functionalism is given the lie by this tree which adapts its behaviour to help others rather than oppose them. Certainly the jays bury the acorns, just as do the squirrels and mice. In that they do a service to the Oak. But this illustrates co-operation and not a selfish cunning. The same is true of other relationships: the blue tit builds its nest in a hole in the Oak tree and then gathers the nearby insects to feed its young. The relationship between bird, food and nest is clear enough but the advantage does not accrue to the Oak, rather to life at large.

Examining the way Impatiens ensures efficient pollination in the flower (page 35), it was easy to speak of direction and will in the gesture of the plant. With Oaks we see an opposite process: an extravagant

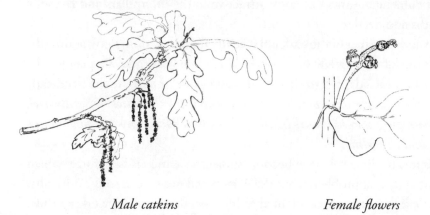

Male catkins   *Female flowers*

waste of pollen that is hard to understand. The Oaks rely upon wind pollination rather than any mechanical or insect-operated device. The male catkins generate prodigious volumes of pollen—several million pollen grains each—which are released into the air. Being very light, they remain airborne for days, making a kind of soup which washes

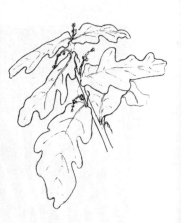

around the trees, slowly settling, but also travelling considerable distances on the wind. Some of the pollen lands upon as yet immature female flowers. These flowers are very simple structures, without petals or clear form other than the small red stigmas, like tiny lips (labia). Once the pollen has landed upon the stigmas the usual process of fertilization will lead to a swelling of the ovule and the production of the acorn. The part played by the billions of pollen grains (from Oaks, other trees and plants) which land upon the soil has not been considered, although it seems likely that there is a value to the process in the wider context of life on earth.

What emerges then, is a living eco-system where the tree is part of far wider life processes. This builds to a complex picture, a set of relationships which illustrate a pattern of life force that we call the Oak tree. Elements within the pattern are illustrative of the remedy state that Bach described for the Oak as one of the Four Helpers.

The form of an Oak tree depends upon the individual history—where is the tree in the journey from acorn to final decay? Each Oak has its own tale to tell and that is, in part, the reason for the old Oaks that we find named in books: Cowthorpe Oak, Gospel Oak, Majesty Oak, Major Oak, the list goes on. Each is famous for its age, its girth and more often than not the number of people who can stand within the tree. One such mighty tree, not the oldest nor the most decrepit, we call 'Bach's Oak'. It stands some thirty-six metres tall, with a girth of over seven metres, on the river bank near Crickhowell, just alongside the field where Bach made the Mimulus remedy in 1928 (page 51). Bach actually made the Oak remedy near Cromer at Felbrigg Camp but he cannot have failed to see this tree on his visits to Crickhowell a few years earlier. Bach's Oak has not yet lost any of its main limbs and has all the appearance of being totally strong and healthy. Yet walk around to the western side of the tree and you will see that it is completely hollow. On a number of occasions locals have put wire over the entrance to stop people climbing inside (nine adults can stand within) because youngsters have repeatedly set fire to the inside of the tree. One cannot say that the tree is unaffected yet it continues to grow as if nothing had happened. Of course, it is known that the central core of a tree is composed of dead wood; only the outer cambium layer next to the sapwood is truly living. Uniquely among the deciduous trees of Europe this Oak, *Quercus robur*, can endure 'half disbowelled'.

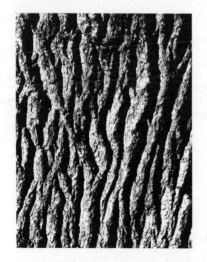

Oak bark

Patterning on bark shows that the living tissues of the tree are close to the surface. An image of the tree's energy can be seen from the lines and rhythms there. The Oak's bark is drawn with lines of tension; the surface cracking, splitting and furrowed as if under constant strain. Oak stands like an arm-spreading Atlas, shouldering the weight of the world, and that shows in the sweeping musculature of the tree and its bulging bark, networked with compressed force. Another picture of the energy system is drawn by the twigs and branches which criss-cross each other, changing direction in a confused and random way (almost like Scleranthus, page 120). Bach makes the point that 'the illnesses . . . are where much balance is lost, mental and physical'[29] and sufferers 'will go on trying one thing after another . . .'.[30] The twigs are brittle and snap off easily and this encourages the development of lateral shoots.* The clear purpose of the will appears confused by the multi-directional growth.

More could be said of the Oak. The hardness of the wood, (what Shakespeare called 'unwedgeable and knarled oak'[31]); the utility of the different parts of the tree; the bark for tanning; the acorns for pannage and even human food; the fungi and lichens that live on the rotten wood; the connection to the druids and their mistletoe mysteries; the story of King Charles; the builders who used Oak for the British navy and great

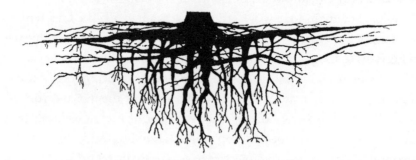

halls and castles; the huge network of the roots spreading out beneath the ground, like a second tree within the earth; the short trunk, long arms

---

* In springtime crows jump on to these twigs, breaking them off for use in nest building. The lateral buds then develop. These form the 'elbows' that were famously used in both boats and wood-frame buildings.

and horizontal limbs that make it look like a stocky weight-lifter; the brittle rigidity of the twigs and branches contrasting with the huge strength of the timber; the shape of the buds; the simple lobed form of the leaves; the acidity of the sap; it goes on and on . . . .

At the end of it all, look at the Oak tree and ask, what was it that Bach saw and felt in you which gave a clue to this remedy state? These are people, he said, 'who are struggling and fighting to get well . . . they will fight on . . . they are brave people, fighting against great difficulties'.[32] That is the Oak. It is the Oak tree and the Oak person: the gesture of the tree corresponds to the gesture of the emotional state. The emotional state corresponds to the tree. Those who take the remedy do not gain in strength and determination. They gain in understanding and that allows them to look afresh at the chronic life difficulty they face. They begin to see a new way to grow.

The third of the Four Helpers which Bach found in 1933 was either *Heather* or Rock Water. For both he travelled back to Wales. Weeks says that he found Heather 'near to the spot' where he had found Mimulus and Impatiens. This leads us to the Gryne Fawr valley, to Table Mountain above Crickhowell and the Sugar Loaf nearby. Rock Water was made at some forgotten well in the same area. It is frustrating to be so close and yet be uncertain exactly where he went. There are many mountain springs in the area and the whole region is ablaze with the flowers of Heather in August and September. He could have set off in almost any direction and come to both a Rock Water spring and Heather.

Heather

Both Bach and Weeks name Heather before Rock Water, so Heather first. We know Bach had the idea for Heather as a remedy when he was in Marlow in the springtime of 1933 (page 37). It was in the same breath, so to speak, as the discovery of Gorse. The golden yellow of Gorse and the purple of Heather are complementary colours and they flower at complementary seasons—Gorse in early spring, Heather in early autumn. Heather begins to flower in the first week of August, (the fifth of August in the Black Mountains according to a professional beekeeper—and

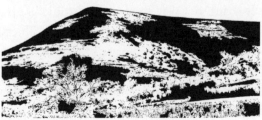

over a period of twenty years this has proved to be accurate, almost to the day). Bach makes the point that 'the Heather to choose is not the red bell-heather, but the beautiful slender small rose-pink variety such as grows on the Welsh or Scottish mountains'.[33] This is *Calluna vulgaris,* the common ling.

The first description of Heather is a longer text than that given to any other remedy; the account is rather vague. Bach must have been having a problem with it. It reads like a mishmash of Vervain and Chicory with the addition of some physiological pointers such as 'high colour', being 'well-built', excitable and energetic and prone to heart problems. Bach states and repeats the idea that these people want to influence others by petty, niggling interference, and that they want to create dependency. To see the sense of this we must remember what Heather is not. It is not a soul condition which carries with it one of the great lessons of life. Rather it is a way of treating with life as it has developed over a period of years.

> *This state of mind is so much part of their natures that is comes to be regarded as their character.*[34]

One wonders how such a state of mind comes about. A better delineation of the Heather remedy was needed and Bach provided it in the later editions of *The Twelve Healers.* At first he retained the references to a physiological picture: 'big, robust, well-made people, jovial and hearty'.[35] But his last description read:

> *Those who are always seeking the companionship of anyone who may be available, as they find it necessary to discuss their own affairs with others, no matter whom it may be. They are very unhappy if they have to be alone for any length of time.*[36]

Now it is clearer. These people have become lonely and they react by talking obsessively about themselves to anyone who will listen. From the earliest commentary upon this remedy, written by Victor Bullen in 1956, we learn that anyone may suffer from this at times.[37] There is the urge to talk about oneself, becoming unduly self-concerned, despite awareness of being boring. It is another way to react to chronic life problems. People talk obsessively about a divorce, a bereavement, an illness, an operation. Just as with Oak and Gorse, this happens, said Bach, because of lost hope, although sufferers may not be conscious of that as the cause.[38] When anxiety begins to replace normal, healthy optimism then some people may find themselves in the Heather state.

This thought is implicit in Bach's account of how he found the Heather remedy for a woman he knew. She was 'self-centred and utterly worldly' and he said 'What do you think is the most beautiful sight in the world? Have you ever seen anything that makes you think it possible that there is a God?' Her reply was 'Yes, the mountains covered with heather'.[39] She associated the wilderness landscape and the flowering Heather with the immanent Godhead. Bringing God into this may not simplify the matter! Or perhaps for some people it does. The sense of isolation which drives towards the Heather state is based upon an anxiety about meaning in life. Heather people become insecure and are secretly worried about life and death.

It is helpful to begin by accepting this idea. We might ask whether that person is capable of living alone. Without other people to chat to, with whom can the little worries and trivia of life be exchanged? If there are doubts that friends and partners really want to listen to one's concerns, what is to be done? As long as there is optimism and self-belief life can be managed. But when doubt sets in, loneliness can follow.

Eventually, Bach put Heather into the same group of remedies as Impatiens and Water Violet: the group for loneliness. Unlike Heather, the other two enjoy being alone. Heather needs to return to that same ease and acceptance of the self. The natural grouping of these three remedies can be seen in the way each plant is in retreat: Impatiens lives on the riverbank, Water Violet has actually taken to the water and Heather grows on mountain tops and wild heathlands, far from the busy streets of town. The romantic solitude of moorlands, open landscapes of mountains, untamed and unfenced, are sometimes too wide and wild for the town dweller's comfort. Left alone in the mountains, most of us feel our smallness and insignificance.

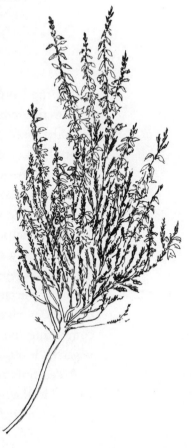

Each of the remedies looked at so far shows the gesture of the emotional state in the gesture of the plant. But with Heather little can be said in this context. Heather grows as a strong, dominant species, carpeting the ground. In sheltered gullies it grows as high as seventy-five centimetres but it is more usually a low shrubby plant. It lacks any clear structure, which might indicate

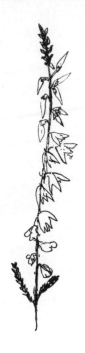

a lack of self-identity as with Cerato (page 115). The flowers cluster on stalks crowding so densely that the impression is of a massed colour rather than individual plants. Heather forms a specialized habitat, where each plant shelters its neighbour, so there is a closeness there. It builds into a miniature forest, excluding other species. This indicates the tendency of Heather people to sap the vitality of others, with their need for closeness and constant chatter. But it is a weak association. The flowers, once open, stay on the stalk for many months, slowly fading and drying out. They can even be found there the following spring as the new growth and flower buds form. Heather people are sometimes hard to get away from (Bach called them 'button-holers') and this attachment is like that of the flowers. But most of what can be usefully observed is related to the general environment, the landscape where Heather grows.

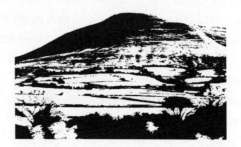

It is the landscape, the exposed, windswept moorland which really informs this remedy. Heather is as much an environmental essence, based upon the total geography of the place, as it is based upon the flower of the plant. If this is so, what does the land tell us of the remedy state? Heather grows in unfrequented places, where the soil is poor and there is no agricultural value to the land. A good field in the lowlands, by contrast, has been looked upon with particular intention by the owner for generations. The farmer imposes the thought form for the land use: grazing for cattle, grass for hay, a space for wheat or barley. No such intention is found on the moors where Heather grows; relatively it is a free space. As a result, the feeling of the land is different, less possessed, less directed. It is this sense of freedom which may be alien and generate loneliness; or else it can be comforting and create a sense for the unity of life. Either way, positive or negative, it plays into the experience of the Heather state.

A description of mountain scenery may add little to the image of where Heather grows. More relevant is a description of the experience of making a remedy there:

When we make a flower remedy, especially if it is a long way from home, there is not much else to do but sit and just be there. You sit and look at the sky, you look at the flowers, you sit and think and then you just sit. This morning it was so beautiful. The sky was intensely blue, the Heather vibrant pink-purple. The day was so warm and fine. Nobody else was there, no other people at any rate. There were a few wild ponies and the odd sheep, a couple of ravens 'cawing' at each other. Slowly, as I quietened myself, the quietness became immense—the silence stretched away over the great empty valleys below; the space filled with the warm, vibrant, living air.

The quiet joy of being there was so strong. Although it is hard to put into words, I felt that this is the remedy for unification. I felt a presence that is behind all individual things . . . like the spirit that is behind each species. There is the spirit that is behind the Heather or every other individual plant, animal or insect. Each plant knows how to be itself because it is connected to this spirit. The bees that were thronging the Heather flowers knew how to be themselves because of the spirit of 'bee-ness' that they are a part of. They fly up from the valley below, drawn by the scent of the Heather, gather the pollen and nectar from the millions of flowers and unfailingly navigate their way home. They know their purpose within this spirit and live it. But there are many, many other lives just as complex and purposeful. The spiders laying webs, the minute insects that crawl, buzz and hover, the gnats that hang like a mist suspended over a particular rock as if pointing a meaning to it. Then there are birds that curve and call in the air, the skylark thrilling high and clear. They come like the spirit of freedom that lives there wild and remote.

Many of us, I suppose, know this experience, the joy that we can have in such a place. But at the same time I saw that while the plants, the insects and the birds were each connected to their own spirit and knew their nature—I saw that human beings so often were not. It seemed that some people failed to contact this spirit in themselves and that was why they felt lost and confused. That was the message of the Heather. The negative state of the Heather remedy was this feeling of isolation, of loneliness, of being unable to endure the wild and open space of the soul, alone.

Then I saw that there really is a 'universal mind substance' that each of us can reach into and be a part of. That is the spirit that lies behind or rather within human beings. To reach to this spirit one had only to move

*towards it, rather than turning away. It carried all within it. It knew all,
saw all, and was all. To be a part of that unity was to be no longer alone.
It was the comfort and blessedness of communion, being one with all life,
separate but part of a united creation. It is a little like coming home, like
meeting your family, like knowing that you are not alone because you are
loved. Sitting up there with the Heather that morning I felt that I was no
longer a stranger in the land, no longer apart and isolated but one with
it all. I didn't want to leave. I sat there for three hours while the remedy
was making and they were like minutes, warm, rich and beautiful.*[40]

If the negative keywords for Heather are self-centered, self-concern
and self-obsessed then the positive keywords must point to a release, a
sense of unity, of being part of the whole without boundary or limit.
Most commentaries on Bach remedies have taken a negative view of
Heather and focused on the unpleasant symptoms of the lonely person.
But everything about the remedy points to a wider picture, a deeper
meaning and a more valuable application than even Bach wrote about in
his *Twelve Healers* description.

Rock Water

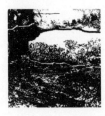

Rock Water is not a flower remedy in the strict sense of the phrase: it is
not made from flowers. Rock Water, said Bach, should be taken from any
well or spring 'which has been known to be a healing centre and which
is still left free in its natural state, unhampered by the shrines of man'.[41]
Later he modifies 'healing centre' to having had 'healing power'.[42] Water
from the spring is taken in a thin glass bowl and set down nearby so
that it may receive clear, uninterrupted sunshine. That's it, that's all. The
water is cold and condensation immediately forms on the outside glass.
After some time the condensation clears as the water in the bowl warms.
Later the familiar bubbles appear and the winking, spectral colours grow
stronger until the essence is made. Bach said this remedy only needed
about half an hour[43] although Nora Weeks speaks of three hours: she
erred on the side of caution.[44]

Rock Water is for idealists who 'have very strong opinions about
religion, or politics, or reform'.[45] They are ruled by theories, are disapproving, critical and strict 'and so lose much of the joy of life'.[46] They
want to lead by example but end up giving themselves and everybody else
a hard time. Was this Bach's perception of himself at this time? Certainly
much of his writing has a kind of passionate idealism and we might
suppose that he found the Rock Water remedy by the same process of

sympathetic resonance that led to Impatiens (pages 36–7); significantly, he mentions the severity of 'the inquisitor'[47] in relation to both.

Since there are no plants or trees involved, one cannot speak of the gesture of the flower reflecting the gesture of the person. Yet the basic presentation of a person in the Rock Water state shows the rigidity and obduracy of stone that contrasts with the softening, fluid movement of water. So the complementary gestures are illustrated immediately by the two elements involved. But the quality of this essence goes much further. To see it we must take in a wider perspective including a range of ideas, beliefs and history which surround the healing power of a sacred spring; consider the whole environment, both physical and metaphysical. It is for this reason that Rock Water is sometimes spoken of as the first 'environmental essence', although Heather shares in this as well.[48]

The only clue Bach gave to the environmental aspect of the Rock Water spring is his comment that it should have traditional healing qualities and that it needs to be 'unhampered' by any shrines of man's making: the shrine of nature is enough. Two thoughts come from this. Why should some springs or wells have been associated with healing and why might their quality be changed when they become built-up as a shrine or place of worship? There is a line of development in this, working backwards from the famous shrines, which become places of pilgrimage, to the simplest healing spring. Think of Lourdes, where the Virgin Mary is believed to have appeared to a girl in visions in 1858. Think of Saint Winifred's Well at Holywell in North Wales, or go back further to the Bethesda pool in Jerusalem. According to St John's Gospel, Bethesda pool was occasionally 'troubled by an angel' and of the waiting sick those who got first into the pool might be healed. Such springs may have a reputation built upon reality but they become places where people congregate, waiting and hoping for a miracle. All their thoughts create an atmosphere. Then the thoughts take on a concrete form in a shrine (Bethesda pool had five porticoes, *John* 5, 2) and also become structured into religion. The architecture of belief is built with priests, services, rituals and blessings. All of it is worthy enough, perhaps, but it creates a strong pattern of energy around the spring and water that flows from it; both become informed by the surrounding physical and metaphysical environment. Water, as we have seen (pages 61–7) is a medium that readily absorbs the thought forms and patterning to which it is exposed.

At the very least we can say that the water at Lourdes is charged and changed by the devotion and belief of the priests and pilgrims.

Belief in the sanctity of certain springs predated Christianity. The reported miracle at Bethesda pool linked Jesus to an older tradition and power. In pre-Christian cultures, we are told, there was a sense that the earth itself was holy and the land inhabited by divine presences. Wells and springs featured in ceremonies and religious observance. Nature worship is not well documented but the presence of weapons, jewellery and other archeological finds in springs may suggest votive offerings to the mother goddess (Gaia) or some other spirit which inhabited a particular locality. Caves and springs have been seen as an entrance to the underworld and so a portal to the mysteries of life and death. Alternatively caves were thought of as the womb of the mother goddess and springs as the issue from her body.[49] Francis Jones in the opening sentence of *The Holy Wells of Wales* makes the point:

> It cannot be stressed too often that everything relating to wells, whether in early form or in mangled survival, traces to one source—religion. There are in Wales wells which must have been sacred even in pre-Christian times, wells transformed from pagan to Christian usages, and wells that claim a purely Christian origin.[50]

The evidence for a cult of well worship, however, is sketchy, being based upon myths, legends, folk-tales, and obscure, half-remembered rituals. Little is known for certain about the pre-Christian well-worship in Britain. We can be more confident in the light of known history: the early Christians made definite efforts to adopt traditional pagan shrines, such as wells, for the new religion. They did so in obedience to the instructions of Pope Gregory I, who sent Augustine on a mission to convert England (597 AD), with a group of forty monks. Gregory told them to purify the pagan temples and to take them over for Christian worship. Subsequent directives tried to prevent 'heathen' worship at trees, wells, rivers and stones.[51] We can only guess how this was done. The process of converting pagans to Christianity called for people with absolute conviction, demonstrable virtue and courage, with the determination to convince others of their cause by living an exemplary life. The characteristics, most precisely, that Bach ascribed to the Rock Water person.

Rock Water, therefore, is linked to the tradition of sacred places in nature through pagan beliefs and to the missionaries and saints who converted Britain to Christianity. No doubt there was something of a struggle here between the asceticism of the monks and the more liberated fertility rites of the heathen. The early Christians wanted to demonstrate the correct way to live, to lead people to the new faith by example. But missionary zeal is an acquired state of mind, one that is not essential to the being. That is why Rock Water is one of the Seven Helpers. Bach wrote that Rock Water people 'hope to be examples which will appeal to others who may follow their ideas and be better as a result'.[52] But also, like the missionary, a Rock Water person wants so much to convert, 'any failure to make others follow their ideas brings them much unhappiness'.[53] In this Bach is perhaps siding against the saints and with the sinners. He said Rock Water people are excessively 'strict in their way of living'.[54] But the problem is one of balance. If the saint is too mental, ruled by theory and not by love, then there will be a problem. Asceticism can deaden the heart.

Christianity and the saints who gave their names to many of the healing springs modified the nature of the place, modifying the quality of the water by altering the pattern of thought in that area. Their ideas travelled across the land, carried by the water of streams and rivers—their thoughts and prayers sent out along the waterways. This was a part of the deliberately planned conversion of pagan Britain. The native belief in the divinity of wells and rivers was adapted and displaced while the medium was used to broadcast to the land. That is why so many churches were built upon springs and aligned with ancient sacred sites, the ley lines which Alfred Watkins observed in *The Old Straight Track*.[55] Such findings were confirmed by the water diviner Guy Underwood in his book, *The Pattern of the Past*.[56]

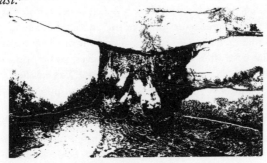

A Rock Water spring

Today it is hard to define what makes for a healing quality in any particular well. It is certainly more than the mineral traces dissolved in the water. There are some fifty named healing springs in Herefordshire alone.[57, 58] Frances Jones lists 370 healing wells in Wales,[59] although he notes that almost all saints' wells and those associated with churches and megaliths are also credited with healing powers. Most are good for eyes but others have a reputation for curing rheumatism, skin diseases, lameness and injuries. But it seems likely that 'every ancient spring was worshipped by our pagan forefathers, and there are traces of this in the medicinal virtues attributed to so many even at the present day'.[60] In other words, any account of a tradition of healing at a particular sacred spring is the residual memory of a far more extensive healing quality which was widely accepted in the past.*

It was the narrowing focus of Christianity which began to limit healing in holy wells to the physical body. In the old way, the spiritual health of a community was integrated with its physical health. Both were expressed in the health of the land, generally, and in the sacred trees and springs in particular. As the water flowed out into the valley it revitalized all life forms which lived there. The coming of Christianity, broadly speaking, changed this. Spiritual health was separated into the church and physical health became a measure of human suffering. Only water that was blessed in and by the church was holy water. It did not happen in a decade nor in a century, but slowly the sacred became profane. We have the residue of such things in the wishing well where people throw coins to raise funds for the local hospital.

---

* Robert Plot, in *The Natural History of Oxfordshire, 1677*, pages 48-50, makes the following observations: 'Beside these we have many other waters, not apparently (at least to any sense) of any *Mineral* virtue. . . . A very eminent one of these there is in the Parish of *Sandford*, not far from the *Great Tew*, which within the memory of many thereabout, hath done great cures upon putrid and fetid old sores, a long time before given over for incurable.... And thus (as I am informed by persons of unquestionable fidelity, that have often used them for their eyes, and in some other cases) do the waters of *St Crosses* in the suburbs of Oxford, whose Well was heretofore, and in some measure yet remains, so considerable for such like purposes, that the great resort of people to it has given occasion of change to the name of the Parish which to this very day we call now nothing but *Holy-well*. But of much greater Fame was the Well of *St. Edward*, without *St. Clements* at *Oxford*, now quite stop'd up; but as 'tis remembred by some of the antientest of the Parish, was in the field about a furlong S.S.West of the Church; this at least was believed to be so effectual in curing divers distempers, and thereupon held to be of so great sanctity, that here they made *vows,* and brought their *alms* and *offerings;* a custom, though common enough in those days, yet always forbidden by our *Anglican Councils,* under the name of *Wilveorthunga* more rightly translated *Well-worship.* . . .'

Whatever the original healing power of the wells, St Thomas, St Kevin and their brother monks conspicuously borrowed some of that power to further their healing ministry. But if every spring was sacred two or three thousand years ago we are dealing with a change in perception rather than any change in power or quality. Or rather, the two go together: the healing quality depends upon the way that we look upon the spring. The world is what we think it to be. As such, Bach was resonating the pattern of life force which surrounds a traditional healing well, with its history, myth and legend and all the thoughts and ideas that are and were associated with it. Part of this pattern has to include the very nature of water itself.

Water is essential for life in this world, being formed at the beginning. In a showcase on an upper gallery of the British Museum a collection of cylinder seals tell the story of the Babylonian version of *Genesis*. Apsu and Tiamat were the first beings. Apsu is called the Sweet Waters, Tiamat the Salt Waters. From their union existence began. In the beginning, says another genesis story, there was formless void, darkness and the deep. These are the conditions that Apsu and Tiamat embody, primeval chaos and the watery deep beneath the earth.

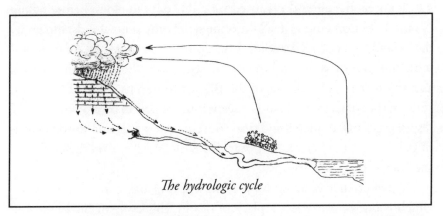

The hydrologic cycle

The movement between salt water and sweet water is still essential to the processes of life on Earth, as is the migration of water drawn from the ocean back up on to the land. The hydrologic cycle, a prosaic name for a most poetic process, is the cyclic movement of water around and through the biosphere. At every stage the salt and sweet are mingling, in blood, root, river and rain. Without pure water we cannot live, yet salt is the very stuff of life. It is the dynamic of such polarities which define genesis: light and dark, day and night, the visible and the invisible.

A Rock Water spring like St Thomas' well is a good place to wonder at such mysteries. From the hills of the border county of Herefordshire, sweet water begins its journey down to the sea. Water that flows out from such a source has come from the darkness and the deep. It is at the beginning, it is Apsu's. At every moment there is an individual birth for the water which leaps from the dark womb of the earth; out from the darkness into the day. The headlong fall of Apsu down from the hills to the plains and the coast is continuous, a constant flow of becoming.

The rivers of the world, small or great, flow out into the sea. The water from St Thomas' well flows into the River Monnow and out past Monmouth and Chepstow into the Severn Estuary. From here it is swept up into St George's Channel or out into the North Atlantic current towards the west of Ireland. Mixed now with the salt of Tiamat the water that was blessed with St Thomas' name has an unknown life in the oceans.

There is no rest in the sea. Always there is the rising tide, the swell and storm of waves, the drift of currents and the turbulence of life. Life, it is said, came from the sea. Agitation on the sea's surface allows some of the water to evaporate or be picked up by wind. Losing most of its salt, it enters the air and is carried for a few days in cloud before falling as rain, either on land or back into the sea. Some such clouds, blown by the prevailing South Westerlies form up over the northern Atlantic and settle over South Wales and the Brecon Beacons. The water falls to earth as rain on the open hilltops of the Black Mountains. Much of the rain runs off the surface of the land or seeps into the soil to be drawn up in the respiratory cycle of plants and trees. But some of it falls into the deep beds of ground water where it disappears from the life cycles on the surface of the planet. It returns to Apsu.

The water that is being born from a spring has come from a place which is out of existence, a place of death. This cycle of birth, life and death may not be attractive to the literal mind, but consider the deep places within the earth that are without light and life. The visible world is continuous existence, even into deep space; only the internal and the invisible part of the planet is really out of existence. When water has fallen upon the land and it disappears from sight it has begun a journey of transformation in the underworld.

Water may remain in a deep aquifer for hundreds of years: lying in the bedrock, creeping in the interstitial spaces, settling in caverns of silence.

Here there is static discharge. Ions are released in slow precipitates of chemistry; salts settling out in the darkness, like memories. In the holding quiet of the earth water waits, filtering out traces of the illumined world until it is polished to transparency.

St Thomas' Well is not on the maps. There are no signposts or tracks. Hidden away, it is placed between worlds, an Avalon of wonder. The water is icy cool, even in the hottest weather; the pool, shaded by trees and fenced from the farm animals, is a silent memory of the lake caverns far below. Sunlight falls, broken by the leaves to sparkle on the emerging water. Out of the rock crevice a steady and unfailing stream springs from the depth of the earth, from beyond our seeing and sensing. It is a place of renewal. Older than its Christian name, this well is a focus for releasing the potent forces of new life into the world.

So when we dip a glass bowl into the pool of this well or any other Rock Water spring we are in contact with the forces of the newborn. And just as a baby carries something of another reality, so this water has a memory of the underworld. If the land is healthy and the water pure, then the healing strength is there, naturally. By putting the bowl of water out in the sunlight we imprint upon it the clear light of life and the quality of the time and place, the environment around. The remedy then carries the imprint of a new beginning. This is the positive quality of Rock Water: to see all things anew and not through the prejudice of theory. It brings, said Bach, 'the understanding of allowing everyone to gain their own experience and find their own salvation'.[61]

Bach came down to Wales in August 1933 to make Rock Water and walking from the Abergavenny railway station on his way into town, he would have passed Holywell Lane. The lane is old but the town has changed. The Holy Well itself must lie under what is now a car park although this was meadowland in Bach's time. Jones says this well had the Welsh name *Ffynon y Garreg*[62]—The Rock Well. Was it here Bach made Rock Water? The name suggests that it is likely. The well was probably destroyed in the 1950s when the last section of Cybi brook (pronounced *kibby*), which once circled that part of the town's wall, was enclosed and buried in a culvert. Bradney, in *A History of Monmouthshire*, mentioned the Holy Well and how the original Benedictine Priory fell victim to the dissolution of the monasteries in the reign of Henry VIII.[63] Priory House was built on the same site in the eighteenth century but was demolished soon after the last war. There is also a small spring beside Holywell Road, as it now is, but this cannot be *Ffynon y Carreg* since it is the wrong side of the River Gavenny. In the 1930s there were open fields here, on the outskirts of town.

Rock Water is among the most important of Bach's remedies in that it pulls into focus many of the wider ideas which lie on the periphery of his discoveries. The remedy, he says, 'brings great peace and understanding . . . brings the realization of *being* and not *doing*, of being ourselves a reflection of Great Things…'.[64] It is not a popular remedy, few people elect to take it for themselves. And yet, it speaks to all of us who are trying to make a way in this life, trying to teach, demonstrate, learn, grow, support, parent, police—even those who are just trying to do their job properly. At one time Bach linked Rock Water to Vervain, Impatiens and Water Violet, three of the twelve type remedies, each of which could be said to have ambition to achieve something in life. The significant thought with Rock Water is that we should be a reflection of Great Things (Bach used capital letters to confirm the importance), meaning the great things which we carry as the aim for our life purpose; being a reflection 'and not attempting to put forward our own ideas'.[65] As one of the Helpers, Rock Water shows where we may get to on the path of life. With Gorse we have given up hope, with Oak we struggle on, with Heather we obsessively seek companionship, with Rock Water we take it all too seriously. Bach came to choose three more helper remedies, bringing the total to seven: with Vine there is a desire to exercise power, Olive people become exhausted and Wild Oat types lose their way.

10 · The Seven Helpers

BACH HAD BEEN SO KEEN to have his account of *The Twelve Healers & Four Helpers* published (by C. W. Daniel) that it had gone straight into print in the autumn of 1933. This superseded a version of *The Twelve Healers* printed privately in the spring, when he was in Marlow.[1] According to Weeks, he had already decided upon the three additional remedies which would bring the number of Helpers up to seven.[2] But these had to wait for the following year before they could be made and there is no mention of them in the first Daniel edition.

Bach did not prepare Vine and Olive himself; he asked people in Switzerland and Italy to send him the new mother tinctures.[3] These were proof, if such were needed, that anyone, anywhere, could make Dr Bach's remedies. Furthermore, they give the lie to any suggestion that Bach remedies must be prepared from the actual place or specimen originally found: nobody knows where these originals were made. Nor is it clear what lead him to choose them as remedies. It is possible that he saw specimens at the botanical gardens in Kew. There is a famous old grapevine at Hampton Court, dating from 1769; and many large houses had a vinery in the garden.

Vine & Olive

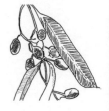

Olive and Vine are dissimilar emotional states but they are made from species which share the common experience of being cultivated by mankind since the beginning of recorded history. Noah, as the flood receded, sent out from the ark a dove which returned with an olive branch ('and lo, in her mouth a freshly plucked olive leaf', *Genesis* 8, 11). Noah was 601 years old when the ark came to rest near Mount Ararat, and after his long life and long voyage, he settled down. He 'was the first tiller of the soil'. He planted a vineyard. So olive trees and grapevines were closely identified with this second father of the human race. The domestication of the grapevine (*Vitis vinifera*) is thought to have begun in the Caucasus region, in the area between the Black Sea and the Caspian, while olives (*Olea europaea*) came from neighbouring Syria; both plants were selectively bred to produce more succulent and useful fruits. Their spread and cultivation through the Mediterranean and Middle

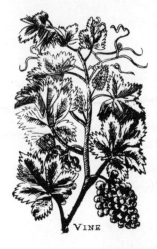

Vine

East is a thread linking the history and culture of this whole area.

After Rock Water, with its historical Christian connections, Bach was continuing a line of thought. Perhaps he was drawn towards plants which, quite specifically, had a long history of association with people; plants whose basic patterning had been modified by the demands of human cultivation. One quality of the Helper remedies, after all, is that they relate to the circumstances of adults who have grown sick as a result of their way of living. In the introduction to *The Seven Helpers* he reminds us that these remedies are for people who have been ill for a long time, for patients who do not 'improve when the right one of the Healers has been given'; they have moved away from their basic type.[4] The indication for Olive is deep exhaustion, the constant tiredness which grips you 'after much worry, illness, grief or some long struggle'.[5] Vine is for people who are 'critical and exacting'.[6] Both of these species, however, have lived in a chronic relationship with human beings and suffered at the hands of civilization. How is this? Look at the process of cultivation and it is easy enough to understand.

Left to grow in the wild, a young grapevine might be thirty or forty metres long; an old one might be hundreds of metres. Vines hang, rope-like, climbing over and through the branches of trees, trailing across the ground. But these wild vines bear no useful fruit, the grapes being small and full of seeds. So cultivated forms were bred to carry more favourable characteristics: plump, fleshy fruits which are full of juice and flavour. This is the story of domestication and plant breeding used for apples, wheat, maize: all the crops which have been developed for food.

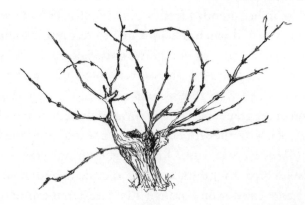

To grow grapes the plant must be approached with a defined purpose: getting from it what is wanted. Training is necessary. This is done by pruning and tying, forcing the growth into a chosen form. Whatever the age of the grapevine, it is always cut back to a stump. When the spring comes, a few shoots begin to grow. The farmer selects from these the ones he wants, maybe two or four that will be trained out along the wires or tied to a trellis.* Other shoots are removed. Vines grow fast and the tendrils reach out, exploring the opportunity to take hold of any support, to grow up towards the light. Out from the leaf nodes come secondary shoots, but these laterals must also be pinched out. The flowering stalk of the grapevine is a modified tendril and at an early stage a selection must be made: which will be allowed to grow into flowers and which will be cut away?

After flowering, as the fruits begin to develop, many of the clusters of immature grapes will be removed to force the plant's strength into the few remaining bunches. The leaves may be pulled from the branches to allow maximum sunlight to ripen the grapes. Even the fruit from the few late flowers at the base of the cluster may be removed so that the grapes ripen evenly and grow to the same size. The never-ending care and attention of viticulture means constant cutting and interference, limiting natural growth. When the fruit is ripe the grapes are removed, the vines cut back to the stump and all the new year's growth removed and burned. Nothing remains of all the effort. If a particular grapevine fails to produce a strong crop then the book advises that it should be rooted out. Domestic vines do not breed true to type from seed, so propagation is by cutting or grafting: more manipulation, selection and control. What a life!

Things are not very different for the olive tree. Wild olives are small with meagre flesh, so early growers selected and developed strains which gave more oil and weight to the fruit. At the outset this must have been a normal and natural process of preference for the improved variety. But, like grapevines, olives do not breed true to type from seed. So, to farm

---

* 'The safest pruning method is the Guyot, in which 2 shoots are grown upwards each year from a short stump. In winter, one is cut off to 4 ft and is bent down horizontally, and the other is cut back to 2 buds. This latter grows the two shoots for the following season, and should not bear fruit, while the long bearer bears fruit on all the shoots from its buds. These shoots are pruned back occasionally during the summer to about 6 in. above the bunches of fruit, and in winter this long bearer with all its shoots is cut right out at the base, and the 2 upright shoots used as in the previous year.' *The Royal Horticultural Society Dictionary of Gardening,* 1956, p. 2233.

olives, it is necessary to graft the chosen variety on to established root-stock. This means the tree's root is of one kind while the trunk, branches, leaves, flowers and fruit are of another. With grapes such grafting was also needed to establish strong, disease-resistant vines. With olives it was often done because wild olives (*Olea oleaster,* now named *O. Europaea, silvestris*) have deeper roots and are better able to resist drought.

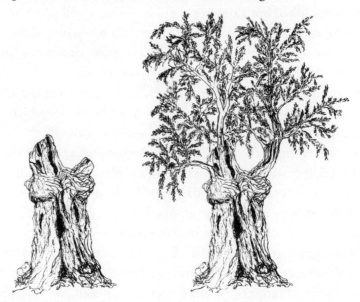

The life cycle of the olive tree begins with the graft on to an established young plant, which is, in itself, quite a shocking procedure. The 'scion', a short piece of twig from the selected tree, is inserted under the bark of the rootstock. If the graft takes then after a few years the join will not even show a scar. As it grows, the new tree must be pruned, keeping the centre open and the branches low for harvesting. Olives flower on the young, new wood of the previous year. The tree is kept in shape by cutting out older wood, providing a few main branches and then many slender young twigs: the reason for the characteristic 'leafy' form of the cultivated tree.

Olives flower in May and the fruits are generally harvested in the following February. Ways to pick the fruit vary but usually the branches are combed with a long rake or beaten with sticks. The fruit is gathered in nets or sheets laid out under the tree. A tree is said to continue productive life for at least a hundred years, although it may be older. Normally olive trees set fruit every second year (trees are often exhausted by a heavy crop), but if a tree fails through age, it must be replaced. Cutting it down to the ground forces new growth from the stool. There may be many

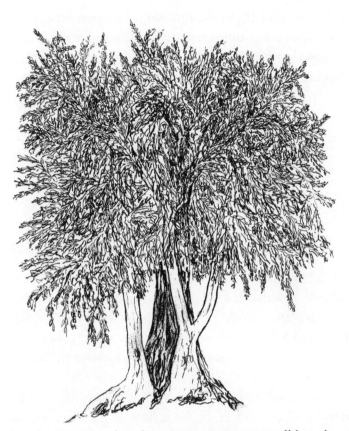

new shoots in the spring and in due course one or two will be selected as the 'new' tree—really the old tree growing again from the stump. Thus an olive tree is renewed, from the ground up. The younger limbs have a smoother, silvery bark; the old trunk is rasped, knobbled, cracked and broken. It's easy to tell new from old.

Both Olive and Vine show a pattern in cultivation which is chronically damaging to the species and to the land. But this is true of so much agriculture and should be no surprise. If we could identify with the grapevine, what might we feel? The depression and hopelessness of the Helper remedies; despair perhaps, and maybe a sense of fury and frustration. The Vine emotional state is said to involve a need to control, to dominate and enforce the will upon others—precisely what grapevines experience at the hands of man. With Olive, it is the constant cropping for thousands of years, the same trees in the same place, in the same soil even. No wonder the land is exhausted.

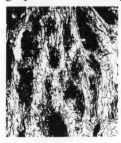

Old bark

It helps to recall Bach's thought that the Seven Helpers are not soul types but chronic emotional responses to life experience (page 145). What has happened to people who develop the Vine state? In their childhood they have found every impulse to self-expression ripped out or limited

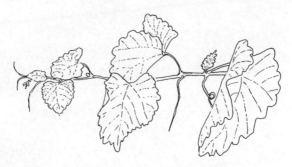

by their family. Each time they put out a new shoot it was cut or tied or trained into a particular form, maybe by a parent, or a sibling, a teacher, a bully at school or work. Whatever the individual story, the Vine types begin to learn that the only way to gain control is to follow that example and become in turn bullying, dominating, forceful adults. It is a learned approach to life.

Vine contained the basic disposition of the remedy state before all the interference of cultivation. In the gesture of the plant we can see a lack of sensitivity (smooth leaves without hairs) and a rather uncomplicated personality (the plain, simple leaf form). The plant suggests that these people lack a clear ego or identity—like Clematis (page 45) they lack the 'I' form of a strong, upright trunk—and perhaps that also accounts for the reactive need to dominate and control. Using the curling tendrils, Vines climb up and over others, gaining height by hanging on to them for support.

Charles Darwin conducted experiments with various climbing plants, including *Vitis Vinifera*. He observed how the growing shoot actually searches for a support and 'after a tendril has clasped any object with its extremity, it contracts spirally; but this does not occur when no object has been seized'.[7] This reflects the habit of the Vine person who only bullies those who can be seized upon. In its blind search, according to Darwin, the tendril can make an elliptical revolution every two-and-a-quarter hours. He made a significant distinction between the way vines climb, using tendrils, and how clematis climbs using the extending petiole of the leaf which wraps around adjacent stems. Clematis is much looser in

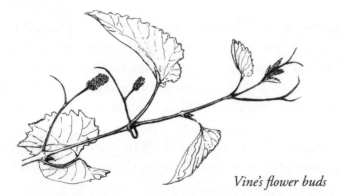

Vine's flower buds

its manner and gains stability by growing out through the branches of a tree; vines gain stability by taking a firm hold upon any support, spiralling around six or eight times, then thickening the sinews and pulling tight. The process is more powerful, although both plants achieve the same end: to get away from the earth and into the light.

Grapevines are made to grow in many different soils. But wild vines grow naturally where the soil is red, just as *Clematis vitalba* grows naturally on white chalk. This can be seen in the rust-red (blood-red) soil in many countries, in southern Spain for instance or in parts of Greece. The strength of the Vine remedy state owes much to the powerful soil in which the plants grow. The colour comes from iron, (iron sesquioxide, Fe_2O_3). The chemistry of this may be somewhat fanciful but it is possible to discern a symbolic relationship between on the one hand the white soil of Clematis, the tendency to go out of the body, anaemia and a lack of a proper respiration and, on the other, the iron in Vine, in haemoglobin and the oxygenation of the blood, in the red stalks of the wild Vine, in the fire and fury of the emotional state. Bach said of Vine patients that they are 'high coloured',[8] that is, red in the face; but they are also worldly, directed towards the physical and the material, 'certain of their own ability'.[9]

People in the Vine state, said Bach, are 'sure that they know what is right, both for themselves and for others . . . they wish for everything just in their own way'.[10] This is a widespread condition, surely, where an attempt is made to control the world around us (as widespread as grapes and wine, perhaps). This urge for dominance is observable in the vineyard where every other plant is eradicated and bare soil is measured out by the serried lines and symmetry of planting. Wild vines run riot, by comparison, in a fluid growth of freely-expressed form: let it be, let it explore the

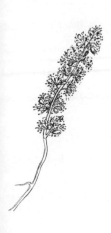

life opportunity, that is the message. Vine people 'give orders to those helping them'[11] and it is this domineering control which is damaging; where Rock Water is strict with self, Vine is strict with others. Like the Rock Water remedy, Vine essence softens and gentles the heart; we can sense this in the softness of the flowers and the sweetness of their scent.

Vine flowers have no petals and this also shows a lack of emotional sensitivity (page 49). There is a lack of empathy towards other people and how they feel. When the buds open, the cap (calyptra) is pushed off

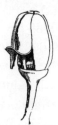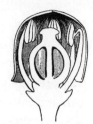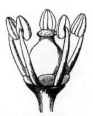

An opening vine flower

by the developing stamens beneath. Again, the gesture is one of force and pressure rather than the gentle receptive unfolding of other flowers. Yet the flowers lead to fruits which are sweet and full of juice, carrying a generosity in a dry land. The positive side of the Vine remedy is based upon a need to give, just as Olive gives, giving until exhausted. And, if as the Gospels say 'each tree is known by its fruit',[12] then grapes are renowned for their flavour and usefulness. Vine, therefore, is a story of almost violent contrasts.

In chapter five of *Heal Thyself*, Bach wrote about the relationship of parent and child. He was concerned (probably as a result of personal experience) that family should not be a battleground of conflicting wills.

> *For very many their greatest battle will be in their own home, where before gaining their liberty to win victories in the world they will have to free themselves from the adverse domination and control of some very near relative.*[13]

It is in the family that Vine behaviour will be learned and reinforced and in the family that gentleness, love and freedom can shape the future life. The Vine remedy has the potential to break the powerful legacy of dominance and control so often handed down from generation to generation.

Where Vine types are 'high coloured', Olive people 'are pale, worn-out and exhausted'; perhaps after a long struggle with illness, grief or some worry.[14] The condition is more than tiredness, rather it is complete depletion. We recognize it readily enough in others, reading signs of pathological exhaustion in the eyes, the face, in body language; the dogged attempt to keep going despite the loss of pleasure and appetite for life. Bach said that 'in some, the skin is very dry and may be wrinkled'; like the dry and wrinkled bark of the olive tree.[15]

In the Mediterranean, wild vines grow in the cooler shade of any small valley or seasonal watercourse but olives grow on the open hillside. Here they are exposed to the full force of the sun. It is this burning dryness which the olive trees can withstand, indeed they love the intensity of light and crave the warmth of the sun. To obtain moisture in a dry land the olive tree has an enormous wide-spreading root structure extending far beyond the canopy of the tree. That's why olives are set well apart within a grove. Wide spacing also allows maximum light to reach all parts of the tree. The leaf is narrow, a slender ovate form, dark above and pale grey beneath: the dark absorbs light and heat while the white-grey reflects. The two tones allow the olive tree to regulate the amount of light absorbed and moderate the effects of temperature. Curved stalks rotate the leaves so that in high summer many move to face into the stem. This gives a shimmering effect of light and dark. As the leaves alternately absorb and reflect light there is a dynamo movement of building energy within the tree. Stand or sit beneath an olive tree on a hot summer day and you will feel the refreshing coolness of the shade but you may also enjoy the benefits of the stored energy which pulses with vitality within the tree.

Olive trees have provided useful products for mankind since the beginning of recorded history: as food; as oil for cooking, preserving, lighting and cosmetics; as medicine; and as a wood for building and ornamentation. All this has given the olive a central place within society. Consequently there are strong traditions surrounding olives and their cultivation. In his *Encyclopaedia of Bible Plants*,[16] F. Nigel Hepper combines an account of the plant's life history with references found in the Old and New Testament. He suggests that Job may have had the olive in mind when he lamented the short life for 'man that is born of woman' and compared it to a tree:

*For there is hope for a tree, if it be cut down, that it will sprout again,
and that its shoots will not cease. Though its roots grow old in the earth
and its stump die in the ground, yet at the scent of water it will bud and
put forth branches like a young plant.*[17]

There is also the reference in Psalm 128 which calls for a blessing from
the Lord:

*Your wife will be like a fruitful vine within your house; your children
will be like olive shoots around your table.*[18]

Both quotations allude to the capacity of Olive for regeneration, sending
up young shoots (children) from the table of the cut stump. In the New
Testament there are significant references to the Mount of Olives and
the Garden of Gethsemane (meaning oil press),[19] where, while Jesus
prayed, his disciples fell asleep.[20] In Luke's Gospel,[21] Jesus, risen from the
dead, walks with his disciples as far as Bethany, just beyond the Mount
of Olives, before his Ascension. The olive tree links the experiences of
exhaustion, life, apparent death and regeneration.

Those who wrote the scriptures made accurate observations of the
plants in their land. In *Job* (15, 33) there is a reference to the way that the
abundant flowers of the olive soon drop, and in *Deuteronomy* (28, 40) we
read that the small olives may also fall from the tree—both indicative of
the fact that the trees produce more than they can sustain. This suggests
that like the Oak (pages 151–2), Olive is proliferous, even if the effort
does not reach fruition. The energy of the tree is given outwards to the
land around, like a light. We see this clearly when it comes to making the
mother essence. The creamy-yellow pollen of the flowers colours spring
water almost immediately so that it glows golden in the sunshine. The
essence makes rapidly as the energy is quickly released.

A book on olive oil makes the comment: 'Imagine a thousand years
of continuous cultivation and not an ounce of innovation'.[22] Olive trees
have been enslaved, servants of a system of agriculture which has not
changed over the centuries. It is a system caring little for the balance of
nature, only for what may be taken out from the land. Yet the Olive continues to give, uncomplaining, and still anoints a barren earth. It does so,
as do all plants, by converting sunlight into energy. This can be utilized
as oil but more particularly as a flower essence.

Noah's dove, which returned with an olive leaf, stands as the emblem
of peace—a truce between God and man. We might see it as forgiveness.
But of all the trees and flowers, Olive is forbearing, tolerant and continues

giving of energy, long after another species would have given up. Bach says that, in the Olive state, people 'feel they have no more strength to make any effort'.[23] The Olive remedy finds the resources for renewal. Where does this come from? From the light.

Wild Oat, the last of the Seven Helpers, 'is a remedy that may be needed by anyone'.[24] This is an important distinction. Up until now Bach had differentiated according to the individual emotional state or mental outlook of the person—Gorse for the hopeless, Clematis for the dreamy—and here, with the nineteenth remedy in his new range, he settled upon something more general and universal. Wild Oat, he says, is an all-purpose remedy to use 'in cases which do not respond to other herbs [essences] or when it seems difficult to decide which to give . . .'.[25] For those at a loss to make a choice among either the Twelve Healers or the other six Helpers then 'in all such cases try the remedy Wild Oat'; it will guide our further choice.[26]

Wild Oat

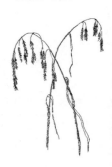

At the time, Bach probably did not realize he was half way through the discovery of his thirty-eight flower remedies; indeed, he may have thought himself at the end.[27] Then Wild Oat would have tidied up any loose ends within the new system of healing. But Wild Oat is pivotal among the 38 as the only remedy which can help to orientate towards a true direction. At one point Dr Bach grouped the remedies in formation and put Wild Oat in pole position (page 280). Another time he set all the remedies in a circle but placed Wild Oat at the centre. If the different remedies discovered up until that time helped people to understand their soul lessons or overcome chronic problems, then Wild Oat was there to help, like a compass, to rediscover the true path in life. Or, like a map it helps to show where we are.

Wild Oat is found throughout Britain and in many parts of Europe. Reference books speak of it as frequent or common. Yet it is almost unrecognized, being only a humble Brome grass: *Bromus ramosus* (or *B. Asper* as it was). Bach must have seen it many times as he walked the lanes of southern England. It is pre-eminently a plant of roadside and track, of hedges, banks and woodland verges. It grew originally, perhaps, inside woodland, persisting after trees had been felled, left behind in the cleared ground, a marker species. Margaret Plues in her *British Grasses* (1867) noted that it grew in 'nearly every hedgerow, especially such as border woods and shady lanes'[28]—it is as common as . . . grass. She liked Bach's Wild Oat and called it 'lordly . . . the tall stature, large panicle bending gracefully, and long branches drooping slightly in flower, and arching more and more as the ripening seed adds weight to the long spikelets . . .'.[29] Other writers note with regret that it is a tall, coarse grass and not recommended for agricultural purposes.[30]

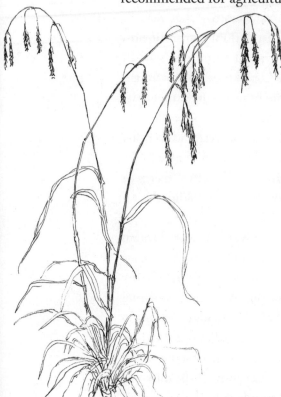

It is the unusual height of *Bromus ramosus*, up to two metres, which first draws our attention. It gains height, as we might climb a tree to see where we are. But it stands as a fragile and delicate grass, moved by the slightest breeze, with none of the strength of a tree. Since it grows in shade, sheltering amongst other plants, it needs height to get into the light and gain space. But it appears rather as a plant seeking to orientate itself, facing about. The slender, tubular stems extend upwards like an aerial, the nodding heads bend over as if watching and sensing. The stems are held in a sheath which opens out into a narrow ribbon-like leaf that carelessly falls back upon itself. The sheath is covered in hairs which add to the appearance of sensitivity and make the stems shine, silvery, like antennae.

Unusually, Bach gave an indication for the duration of treatment when using Wild Oat: 'try this for at least a week' and 'if the patient does well, continue with it so long as they improve before changing to another remedy'.[31] It is as if the person needs retuning, needing to resonate with the Wild Oat for 'at least a week' in order to orientate and realize the best path to take—renewing contact with ground control, so as to remember the correct route to follow.

The primary gesture of the Wild Oat is questing, growing upright and upwards. But the strong 'I' form of Impatiens and Vervain is missing as the vertical movement falters and the head bends over and looks back towards the earth. Bach describes this human gesture:

> *Those who have ambitions to do something of prominence in life, who wish to have much experience, and to enjoy all that which is possible for them, to take life to the full.* [But:] *their difficulty is to determine what occupation to follow . . .*[32]

Their ambitions falter. They want to do something, having the ambition to make a clear vertical movement, to make a mark in the world, but they lack the firmness of purpose and the sustained will to follow through. 'They have no calling,' said Bach, as if to reinforce this idea of an outside message, 'no calling which appeals to them above all others'.[33]

So they fall back within the mundane labyrinth of life, knowing perhaps that they might fly but lacking the initiative of a Daedalus* and the will to develop such soul qualities as are required. How might it be to see our soul's greatness beckon and not know how to move out from the shadows and into the clear light of the sun? It must lead to disappointment, 'delay and dissatisfaction'. The word 'delay' leads again to the thought of a journey: the soul's journey, the journey through life, the journey upon the path of our calling. At various times in a life we all stand at the crossroads and wonder which path to take; Wild Oat is for those who remain there, irresolute and undecided.

Bromus ramosus likes moist ground and will not normally grow in open spaces exposed to the full force of the sun: never on the hilltop or in the thin dry soil of downland where Rock Rose or Gentian are found. Other grasses grow there but not *B. ramosus*. In the sunlight a clear and strong will is needed for survival. This is not the wild oat (*Avena fatua*) seen in cornfields, a weed of cultivation. Bach just borrowed the name. His Oat prefers the dappled shade of ambivalence, the excuse of uncertainty being given as a reason to avoid action. So different to the assertive Vine people 'certain of their own abilities'. Even the flowers are constructed so as to avoid direct light.

Wild Oat flowers towards the end of July, coming late in the season. Two glumes hinge open to reveal yellow stamens (the male, pollen-producing parts) and the white feathery stigmas (the female). These all hang down from the spikelet so that the pollen dusts over the stigmas. But the glumes rarely open fully to expose them since this requires the warmth of strong sunlight. When they do open it is only for a few hours, then, after pollination, the flowering is over. As a result, Wild Oat is a remedy which can be difficult to make, the combination of weather and full flowering being elusive. Pollination often takes place while the

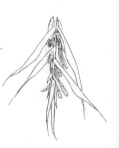

---

* Daedalus, an inventive Athenian, is said to have constructed the Labyrinth in Crete for King Minos, who then imprisoned him. With his son Icarus he contrived to escape by making wings of feathers and wax. Daedalus flew to Sicily. Icarus went too close to the sun, however: the wax melted and he fell back into the sea.

glumes are only partially open—self-pollination. This points to the Wild Oat problem of self-preoccupation and the lack of involvement in life. Cross-pollination (page 126) indicates a more developed soul potential which can lead to change.

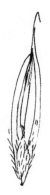

Seeds form within the shelter of the glumes and are only released at the end of summer. They appear as narrow shards weighted at one end by the kernel which remains attached to the 'lemma', a sort of sail (like the flight of a dart or arrow) which guides the seed in the wind. As the seeds fall they turn back towards the earth and spear themselves into the land (like Clematis, page 46). Each seed has short bristly hairs which act as barbs, forcing it into the earth or at least forcing it into the seclusion of the vegetation below. Thus the seeds find a protected place for rapid germination. Wild Oat is an opportunist wriggling into the shelter others create. Chancellor says of Wild Oat people: 'they have the tendency towards drifting into uncongenial environments and occupations and this only increases their sense of frustration'.[34] The behaviour of the seed suggests that there is a perverse intention here, as though the Wild Oat person seeks out difficulty just to show the impossible nature of fate.

Nora Weeks' account of what Bach had in mind with Wild Oat focused on the need we have for 'a definite purpose in life'.[35] People are often bored, she said, or lack any real interest in their lives. They do uncongenial work, devoid of creativity, and this saps strength leading, inevitably, to ill health. In truth, Bach put it more strongly (as can be read in *Collected Writings,* see particularly *Free Thyself* Chapter 6, pages 97-98) and emphasized the need for every individual to recognize and respond to their life purpose. This is the calling of the soul to fulfil its potential and so to develop those innate qualities each one of us possesses in order to become true human beings. Our challenge, says Bach, is 'that we may realize our Divinity . . . for through that Divine Power all things are possible to us'.[36] If the terminology (Divine Power) is an obstruction then substitute 'the power to dream' for what we dream, that we may become.

11 · The First of the Second Nineteen

BACH LEFT CROMER IN MARCH 1934 and the following month moved to the Oxfordshire village of Sotwell in the Thames Valley. Here he remained for the next two and a half years until his death. During 1934 he made one new remedy: Wild Oat. Nora Weeks suggested that it was a year of consolidation[1] with 'long quiet days spent working in the garden'. He made visits to London to see patients but, as far as we can tell, he settled down. He made furniture (both for *Mount Vernon* where Nora Weeks lived and Mary Tabor's house, *The Wellsprings*) and wrote *The Twelve Healers & Seven Helpers,* which came out in July. No doubt he spent time walking, as he got to know the area. This was the calm before the storm.

During the five months from March to July in 1935, Dr Bach found nineteen new remedies: an average of one every week or so. (The first nineteen had taken six years.) The process was exhausting, of that there is no doubt, since before finding a new remedy he experienced the intensity of each emotional condition the remedy would help. Once started, he was on a roller-coaster ride of feelings and mental states, impelled to find a plant which would ease the onrush of symptoms. Weeks tells us that during the winter he had begun feeling restless and sensed this indicated he was to make a new set of discoveries.[2] But it is characteristic of the Second Nineteen that they were not planned out in advance as the others had been. They were forged in the fire of immediate experience, rather than theory.

Aspen, Elm and Cherry Plum all flower around the same time, in late February or March. Weeks said that Cherry Plum was the first to be found. She recalled that Bach had been in great pain for some days with a sinus inflammation.[3] As often happens with sinusitis this was combined with intense and persistent headaches. However, the physical trauma was not to be the basis for the remedy. It was the feeling he had in relation to the pain: a fear that he might lose control and be driven out of his mind. In view of Bach's medical history, his earlier neuralgia and experience of

Cherry Plum

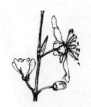

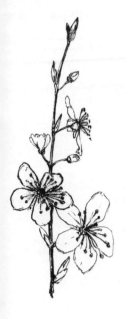

constant pain (page 38), it would seem that the emotional state was the novelty here. This was not the tension pain of the Impatiens type but a reactive mental strain: the feeling that he was losing ground in some battle for the mind. Look closely at his choice of words to describe the Cherry Plum remedy and this makes sense:

> *Fear of the mind being over-strained, of reason giving way, of doing fearful and dreaded things, not wished and known wrong, yet there comes the thought and impulse to do them.*[4]

What 'dreaded thing' was he referring to? What might he have felt driven towards, knowing it to be wrong? Whence came the impulse and the thought to behave in this way? Elsewhere he spoke of impulses 'that come upon us', impulses 'to do things we should not in the ordinary way think about or for one moment consider'.[5] Perhaps for each of us the dreaded action is different: suicide, murder, cruelty, perversion, whatever dark shadow fills the mind when the light of conscience is obscured. We each know where the threshold lies which we should not and would not normally cross. This is not a great madness but a small personal battle for sanity and control. Cherry Plum, said Bach, 'drives away all the wrong ideas and gives the sufferer mental strength and confidence'.[6]

This is very much a remedy of light and dark and if we look at the tree in flower in early spring, that is what we see: the intense white blossoms clustered on the black branches, with only the bright beginnings of green leaf buds. Cherry Plum, *Prunus cerasifera*, is the first white blossom of the year, coming before pear, cherry or other fruits, earlier than the blackthorn sloe. It is a slender, small tree with slightly drooping branches, of no great physical strength, even weak in appearance.

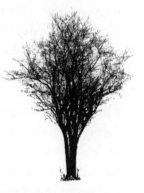

There are often several stems in the trunk, as though several trees are growing together, like multiple 'I' forms. The single upright trunk of Oak or Elm (page 191) betokens, by contrast, a clear and strong individuality. It is expressly the problem of Cherry Plum that this individual integrity has been breached. The same thing can be seen in the bark, which is smooth and speckled without clear energetic structure lines. Like the Aspen (pages 195–6) the emotional structure is open. But the strength of the gesture is to be found in the brilliant and exuberant flowering, not in the structure of the trunk and branches. The scent is strong and heady

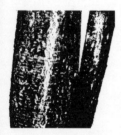

and reinforces this experience. Like Olive, this tree is alight with the blaze of the spirit. It shines into the darker recesses of the mind, clearing and ordering mental confusion.

Cherry Plum is a somewhat unstable species. Many authorities seem uncertain as to how to classify it and so omit it from the listing of British trees. Miles Hadfield notes that 'in nature the cherry plum varies greatly; in those districts in which it is believed to be centred, it is said to be difficult to find two trees showing quite the same combination of characteristics'.[7] This parallels the instability of the emotional state. Although the flowers are almost certain to be pollinated (this can be observed as the greeny centres blush pink), fruit formation is sparse, totally absent in many years. This lack of seed production suggests a poor adaptation to the material world. Plants like Scleranthus and Impatiens, by contrast, are prolific in both production and germination of seeds. They represent emotional states where the individual is better adjusted towards life on earth. We might compare Cerato which does not readily set seed or germinate except in controlled conditions, and it also shares Cherry Plum's susceptibility to interference and the tendency to be misled. The cherries are sweet and juicy when they do form, though the colour may vary from yellow, through orange to plum red: there is no consistent standard. With the Cherry Plum state there is a pressure from the non-physical world that distorts normal boundaries, breaking through the controls which would otherwise bring certainty in the process of life. We are right to be afraid.

Although the cherry stones germinate easily, the plant has a natural tendency to sucker, sending up new stems from the root. For this reason it is used for grafting more profitable stock (plums) and is often planted as a hedge. There was a Cherry Plum hedge which Dr Bach was said to have planted at *The Wellsprings*, in Sotwell. This habit of suckering shows the other aspect of Cherry Plum: the need to stabilize the mentality by involvement in the practical material world, where roots draw strength from the earth. So the white light of the flowers draws down the mental clarity, but the future for the plant lies in the root's regeneration within the earth. This will be a key to understanding the Second Nineteen: Cherry Plum, Elm and Aspen all throw up suckers from the root and in each case the trees fail to propagate as successfully through germination of the seeds.

Demented with the pain of sinusitis, then, Bach went out to look for help. Finding Cherry Plum in flower, the same process of resonance that he had used with the earlier remedies (page 36) came into play. He resonated the agony and fear and the flowers responded with 'mental strength and confidence'. Weeks said that he prepared a remedy using the flowers and felt better immediately. The following day the whole episode was over. He made the remedy by the boiling method (pages 199–203) not using the thin glass bowls of his previous preparations. But the nature of the remedy was the same in that the qualities of the Cherry Plum brought him back to himself. In *Ye Suffer From Yourselves* he had written that:

> *The action of these remedies is to raise our vibrations and open up our channels for the reception of our Spiritual Self, to flood our natures with the particular virtue we need.... They cure, not by attacking disease, but by flooding our bodies with the beautiful vibrations of our Higher Nature, in the presence of which disease melts as snow in the sunshine.*[8]

Cherry Plum is like sunshine and snow, like the bright light of the Alps. Over many years it has been noticed that there are always a few days of brilliant sunshine towards the end of February, no matter how wet and dull the winter. It heralds the coming spring. This is the quality of light that shines in the blossom of the Cherry Plum.

Elm

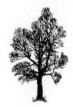

Having found the Cherry Plum remedy, Dr Bach must have taken some time to reflect and consider his position. After all, he had written and published accounts of his discoveries on several occasions and here he was, apparently, about to start all over again. What might he have felt and thought about it? In some respects a look at his life indicates that it was enjoyable discovering these new remedies. It is occasionally pointed out that making Bach mother essences today is a pleasant and rather enviable occupation. But it carries with it responsibilities and certain anxieties, even if, unlike Bach, the remedy maker benefits from knowing what to do next. For him it must have been a double difficulty. So if the message came to him that a new sequence of nineteen remedies might be in the offing (as a message had come to him at least once before), his first thought may have been 'oh no!' rather than 'what jolly fun!'. Another nineteen remedies, he may have wondered, wasn't that too much responsibility, too much for one man to bear? And then, of course, there he was, already in the second of the new mental states. At least that is how he described the remedy later on:

*At times there may be periods of depression when they feel that the task
they have undertaken is too difficult, and not within the power of a
human being.*[9]

At the time he probably looked at it all and felt overwhelmed. He was
one of

*. . . Those who are doing good work, are following the calling of their
life and who hope to do something of importance, and this often for the
benefit of humanity.*[10]

And yet, what he was set to do he clearly felt was beyond his strength
and power. He may have decided to take a walk. Reaching for his hat and
coat, and calling his dog, Lulu, he stepped out into the fresh March air.
And as he went across the fields he looked up at the flowering Elm trees.
These tall people, so strong and capable, were covered in a soft pink of
flowers which answered the doubt and depression: all was well.

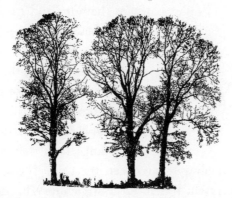

Bach's Elm is *Ulmus procera*, the Common or English Elm. In the 1930s
it was one of the commonest trees of the midland counties of Britain.
Druce, in his *Flora of Berkshire*, 1897, called it 'abundant, and one of the
conspicuous features of our valley scenery',[11] although it is probably not
a native. Being 'conspicuous', it was a tree which Bach must have known
well enough. But it was the flowering of the tree, at that moment, which
caught his eye. Again there was a resonance between the mental state and
the flower, an equivalence which Bach experienced directly because of his
awareness of his own emotional circumstances.

The first impression of *Ulmus procera* is the massive column of wood
(*procera* means tall), the huge pillar of a trunk, often more than thirty
metres high when fully grown and with a girth of five metres or so. It
is an erect tree with a few large upward spreading arms carrying a great
density of smaller branches. When in bloom there is a contrast between

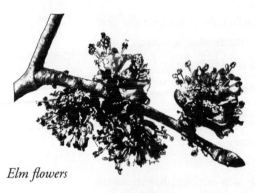

Elm flowers

the strong trunk and the flowers. One writer comments 'when the flowers are fully out in March, the whole tree glows warmly in the sunlight'.[12] This warmth acts to lift the mood with gentle strength and determination.

The flowers are complex. It is the male part of the flower which gives most of the pink colour, as the taller anthers are red until they open and shed their pollen, when they quickly blacken. This pollen is windblown, and the rate of pollination is very high. Where the flowers cluster on the end of each twig seeds form, each inside a thin, papery vessel (samara) like a flat disk. These fruits, which ripen a few weeks after flowering, are green at first giving the false

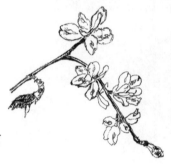

Seeds forming

impression that the tree has burst into leaf. Later, as they dry and turn brown it looks as though these 'leaves' are dying, just at the time that the true leaves are opening. Not least significant among this contrary information is the fact that not one among these perfectly-formed seeds will germinate. The English Elm is effectively sterile.

This strange fact, that the seed will not germinate, cannot always have been the case. The species must have adapted from others which were fertile originally. What does this say about the Elm remedy state? To understand it we need to consider something of the history of the species and how it manages to survive. There are several closely-related species of elm in Britain although it often needs a specialist to distinguish them.* The situation is complicated by the fact that

---

* Several books give a detailed account of the English Elm and its parentage. The best may be Alan Mitchell's *Trees of Britain* (Collins 1996). Very briefly these are the points at issue. It is assumed that seeds are killed off by the cold March conditions in Britain and that this points to a Mediterranean ancestry. So the English Elm was probably brought from southern France (or Spain) by pre-Iron Age tribes, possibly for religious reasons. Unfortunately, nowhere in Europe can we find any wild populations of *Ulmus procera* and it is unlikely that the originals would have died without trace in a mere few thousand years. It may be that this is a species so unstable that it changes according to location. If so the adaptation of plant forms, thought to be extremely slow and steady, may actually be extremely unstable and rapid under certain circumstances. This is, interestingly, the conclusion made by Jonathon Weiner in *The Beak of the Finch*, concerning the time taken for evolutionary change by Darwin's Finches in the Galapagos Islands.

many English Elms were planted in the eighteenth century for both their landscape value and utility as hedgerow trees for field enclosure. The enclosure of common land (from about 1700 to 1850) required a dense, fast-growing tree which could be laid as a hedge to contain stock. These trees were grown on from suckers and were therefore clones. John Evelyn, in *Silva, or A discourse of Forest Trees* (1664), described the process of digging a trench twenty metres away from a mature Elm* and how, by cutting the roots there, it is possible to force new shoots to spring up.[13] These are suitable for planting on as trees. There is a suggestion from Hadfield that similar young shoots may have been imported from France. He says 'the British elms are a puzzling collection, the status of them is not properly understood'.[14]

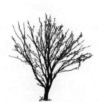

Ulmus glabra   *Ulmus procera*

Bach's Elm, nevertheless, is distinct from other elms. The outline and structure of the tree is significant: while *Ulmus procera* is upright, like a column, *U. glabra* is more fan-shaped in form. So, while the flowers look the same, the quality of the remedy state makes Bach's Elm (*U. procera*) the choice because of the strength of the 'I' form. This clear, upright gesture shows self-determination and will: the Elm state concerns those people who are strongly motivated by their soul purpose and know what they are doing in the world. Yet this species has come to a point in its evolution where it can only propagate itself by suckering, sending roots through the earth like blind moles. The comments made about Cherry Plum apply here, although the condition is made more extreme by the total lack of seed propagation. A person in the Elm state (and not for this reason alone) suffers as though blind, unable to see a future. The seed represents the future in every species; here that future is beyond reach.

---

* Elms can reproduce from the root in this way as much as forty-five metres from the parent tree (see H. N. Ridley *The Dispersal of Plants Throughout the World*, p. 660).

To make this point more clearly, look again at Impatiens (pages 33 ff.) with its certainty and headlong rush to achieve its aim. Impatiens seeds are ninety-nine per cent viable. Then consider Cerato (page 116) whose seeds fail almost entirely and whose soul lesson concerns a deep uncertainty about what future to take. Elm, in this particular respect, is like Cerato: suddenly uncertain.

To assist with differential diagnosis compare the Oak tree and the Elm; it will illustrate the differences between remedies. Both states are for strong people who are normally effective in the world: both trees are large and expansive with hard, durable timber, although the gesture of the Oak is less vertical, more spreading and receptive. The furrowed bark of both trees has a similar picture of strength and energy in the network of force lines. The distinct differences lie in the roots, the leaves, the

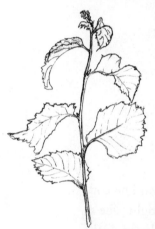

flowers and the seeds. The Oak person struggles on, keeping going while the Elm falters and becomes depressed. The Oak continues to work for the future, producing seeds, even in old age. By propagating through the roots the Elm shows a different approach and therefore is likely to bring about transformation in the material world. Oaks are more prosaic and more predictable—this is reflected in the smooth and simple leaf of the Oak. Elm's leaves are small, rough and hairy with a sharply toothed margin. The hairs contain a mild irritant (like stinging nettles) which stimulates the life force. Elm flowers are prominent, opening before the leaves; the reverse is true of the Oak's.

Another aspect of Elm's gesture is shown in the problems encountered with Dutch Elm Disease. First identified in 1919, it arrived in Britain in 1927 and first peaked in 1935, the same year that Bach chose the remedy.[15] The disease is caused by a fungus, which is spread by a small flying beetle. In the 1970s a new strain of this fungus appeared, far more virulent than the first, and this progressively destroyed all the remaining mature *Ulmus procera* in the country. True, a few hybrids or closely related species survived and the disease has not attacked Wych Elm (*U. glabra*) to the same extent. By 1990 it seemed that the English Elm was finished. But not so. While the disease continues there are many trees which have grown again, from the roots of course, and there are now thirty-year-old Elms flowering once more.

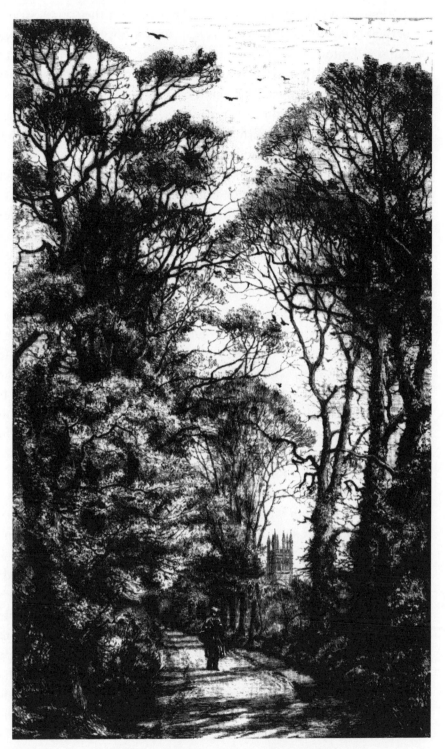

The old elms at Magdalen College, Oxford

These young trees continue to die, however, and they stand, stripped of their bark, alongside others which appear healthy. Dutch Elm Disease can travel through the roots, since a stand of trees will be linked together underground. These trees may come into leaf in spring but by summer the leaves yellow and die. It is a cycle of chronic infection, an illness that may never be thrown off. What may be needed is the space and time to get ahead of the problem: maybe Elm can do it with some additional stimulus, but it will need additional strength.

It has been suggested[16] that Elm stands half way between man and nature, that it is a species not really wild but linked to man and the land. This fits with its use for hedges on farmland and to create a picturesque landscape. It has been cultivated and tamed. It grows by roads and tracks where people walk, not as a forest tree. It has become dependent upon us, for we are now the architects of the landscape. Elm has no seeds to venture out alone. As such, the tree mediates between nature and direct cultivation. In terms of the remedy, the Elm type of person is seen as well-adapted to human life, successfully following in the scheme of society; doctors, judges, priests or teachers are often cited as potentially Elm.[17] Such people may have developed beyond simple competition for survival, living more altruistically. But uncertainty, like a virus, secretly undermines their position—supposing they are wrong? In some respects this is an interference pattern, such as Cherry Plum experiences. Here it is a sense of inadequacy, worming a way into the mind as self-doubt. Like Cherry Plum it is the massed flowers of Elm which show the power of the spirit. Elm reconnects us to the source of our true strength when we have become too rooted in the material world. No matter how important the responsibility we must learn to offer it up.

Gilpin, writing in 1791, said of the Elm 'no tree is better adapted to receive grand masses of light'.[18] A reminder that all plants and trees have the same, simple, self-evident purpose: to receive light. But it is pertinent to ask just what that light really is. As we shall see, these Second Nineteen remedies are directly concerned with bringing light into the world (page 241). If Elms do this more effectively than others it is because they have the life potential to bring about changes in human society. What does Bach say? 'Those who are doing good work, . . . following their calling, . . . something of importance . . . for the benefit of humanity'. The Elm tree is their succour and support.

Close on the heels of the flowering Elms comes the Aspen. It flowers *Aspen*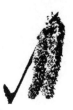
late February to mid-March, depending on year and location. As with
so many of the Second Nineteen, there is no record of how Bach came
to choose Aspen, other than Week's comment that he experienced the
emotional state of each new remedy in turn and that this guided him
to the appropriate tree or plant which carried, as it were, the antidote.[19]
So Bach was being spooked by the invisible world—he wrote of 'vague
unexplainable fears' that 'may haunt by night or day'.[20] In the four-line
description he repeats the word 'vague' and states in three different ways
that these fears have no rational explanation. Those who have experienced
such a fear easily recognize the condition; a fear that 'something terrible
is going to happen', although we cannot tell what.[21]

Bach's experience in finding the previous remedies suggests that
he was developing as a psychic. This carried a risk of being available
to interference, as we have seen with Cherry Plum. Another risk in
being open to the subtle world is feeling the full force of a destructive
power which sometimes lurks, unseen, beyond the physical senses. This
negativity is frightening, even terrifying, although it may be difficult
to describe to others. They will say that we are imagining it! Yet Bach
described how this fear might make a person tremble or sweat 'from the
abject fear of something unknown'.[22]

If this Aspen fear is so subtle and yet so intense, what will be the
gesture of the tree equivalent to it? With Elm, strong, capable people
who are successfully dealing with the material world are helped by a tree
which is tall, deeply-rooted and long-lived, with hard, durable wood.
Aspen is almost exactly the reverse. It is a slight and slender tree, lacking clear shape and structure with a delicate, open form. It has a shorter
life (maybe sixty years) and never attains any substantial size, growing
to about fifteen metres or so. While Elms grow in parks and farmland,
Aspen is much more adventurous. Being a pioneer it grows up to the
boundaries of climate in the north. It is often the first tree to appear in
open ground. As a species Aspen is easily overlooked, for while it is a
pretty tree its appearance is nondescript. In textbooks it often gets only
the briefest mention in comparison to other more significant poplars.
Aspen struggles to maintain a place in the world.

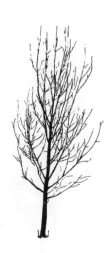

Details of the tree's gesture, describing the emotional state, are clear
to see. First there are the leaves which tremble and flutter in the slightest
breeze. The Latin name *Populus tremula* and the French name *Tremble*

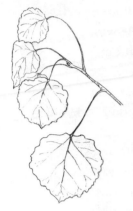

both recognize this. Aspen, then, is said to be for that trembling fear; it is a literal picture. This shaking movement of the leaves is most pronounced and invariably observed. Lauder (1834) said of Aspen 'there is a superstitious notion among the vulgar, that the tremulous motion of its leaves was occasioned by its having been the wood of which our Saviour's cross was made'.[23] Johns notes the same belief and makes the comment: 'This peculiarity obtained for the Aspen the unenviable distinction of being selected as the poetical emblem of restlessness, inconstancy and fear'.[24] There is no rational basis for the idea that the tree trembles because of the Crucifixion. Johns is rather pedantic in dismissing the notion as superstition, which of course it is. But his appeal to reason with an account of *how* it is the flattened stalk which causes the leaf to flutter does not explain *why* it does so. It is usual to point to some competitive advantage for the plant in its form and behaviour. But there is no credible case here for evolutionary benefit. What the 'poetical emblem of restlessness' tells us is that the tree is a picture of trembling fear, just as Oak is a picture of strength and endurance. Both trees have been written into folklore in the attempt to explain the gesture and form of their growth.[25]

The image of the trembling leaf is reinforced by the quivering tension felt in the trunk of the Aspen tree. This is a perceptible shaking; it can be sensed if you stand with your back to the tree. Aspen is the remedy for people shaking or trembling in a similar way, either mentally or physically. For the most part the trunk is silvery smooth, though it begins to become furrowed with age. The clean surface of the bark is a sheaf of protection, though it is marked in places by strange black diamonds, drawn like stuttering runes on the trunk. The flowers tell us little more, although their soft grey hairs speak of an etheric sensitivity, hidden and mysterious. Male 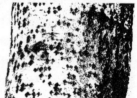 and female flowers grow on separate trees as pendulous catkins looking rather alike, at least at first glance. Significantly, both types of flower grow outwards from the bud and then downwards towards the earth. While Agrimony (page 96) or Vervain (page 105) flower along a vertical stem growing away from earth, pointing to the sky, Aspen does the opposite. To escape from this fear of the unknown and unseen, a person in the Aspen state needs to be pointed towards physical reality, just as someone waking from a nightmare reconnects to ordinary dimensions of life in this world.

When the seedpods of the female swell and break open, a white fluff containing seeds is carried far away from the parent tree on the wind. These seeds can germinate within a day if they fall on damp earth. Aspens crave light and will generally only grow on the fringe of woodland, lurking on the edge of the tree community. The roots are shallow, with 'the root-branches running almost horizontally';[26] an observation also made by Johns.[27] This indicates superficial contact with the material world: trees

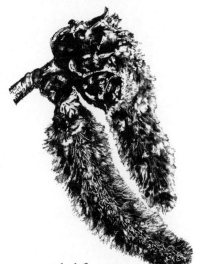

with deep-diving roots represent a stronger involvement with life at a physical level. Like the Elm and the Cherry Plum, the Aspen sends up suckers from the root: a sign of the hidden forces at work.

There is little evidence of the positive aspect of the Aspen state. The growing strength of the Aspen as it nears the earth can be seen: the trunk begins to furrow at ground level, showing a stronger network of energy. But this is not a clear emblem of the strength which overcomes fear. It might be indicated in the golden-yellow leaves of autumn, which fall to earth early but are slow to rot. However, when the essence is made by the boiling method (page 199) the scent of balsam is strong, sweet and aromatic. The mother tincture is plum-coloured, or light claret. It shows a gentle warmth and fire which penetrates the grey mists of early spring, driving away the occult penetration, bringing peace.

Bach commented of Aspen that 'sufferers often are afraid to tell their troubles to others'.[28] This silent apprehension, a kind of quiet anonymity, is apparent in the tree. Yet of all Bach's remedies, the Aspen most clearly proclaims its trembling fear. It is among the easiest to see and understand of the plant gestures. The signature of the tremulous leaf has been noted by poets since Chaucer, but Bach was the first to make the connection between this and the healing potential of the flowers. He saw how the qualities of Aspen inform the tree and how they resonate the positive expression of strength and protection, protection from a fear of the supernatural.

12 · The Boiling Method

THESE NEW REMEDIES were prepared using a new method. While the First Nineteen had all used 'The Sunshine Method', Bach now introduced 'The Boiling Method'.[1] It is hard to fathom why he did this —he left no written explanation. Certainly the weather in February and March, when he went to make Cherry Plum, Elm and Aspen, was likely to have been an immediate problem. Bach needed to make the essences at once as he was struggling with the discomfort of the emotional state. Waiting for clear, sunny weather could have meant an indefinite delay in these early months of the year. In addition, as Nora observed, 'the sun in early spring has not the strength it gains later . . .'.[2] But there has never been a satisfying explanation as to why Bach chose to *boil* the flowers, nor why he continued to use the boiling method on into the summer, when he found others in the series of the Second Nineteen.

In *The Twelve Healers*, the description of the process is terse:

The specimens, as about to be described, were boiled for half an hour in clean pure water.

The fluid strained off, poured into bottles until half filled, and then, when cold, brandy added as before to fill up and preserve.[3]

It comes down to that simple process: boil for half an hour. As with the sun method (pages 59 ff.) it is important to select the site, to ensure that the flowers are freshly opened and at the peak of flowering. A bright day is the best choice, but the weather needs to be good rather than perfect. As before, there are things to do before setting out, such as collecting fresh spring water and preparing all the necessary utensils.

The flowers are picked with about fifteen centimetres of twig, flowers, buds and leaves so that they fit within a twenty-centimetre saucepan. A white enamel pan is best. Secateurs may be needed. Flowers are gathered from several different trees where possible, so as to three-quarters fill the pan. With the lid on, take it to the cooking stove—maybe a portable gas burner or the stove at home, if nearby. Gas is a better source of heat than electricity or solid fuel; it is more direct and does not carry any electro-magnetic charge.

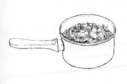

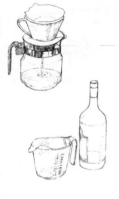

A measured two pints (1.1 litres) of fresh spring water is poured into the saucepan. With the lid off, the water is brought to the boil and then simmered for thirty minutes. Then, replace the lid and put the saucepan outside to cool. The liquid is later filtered and, as with the sun method, an equal volume of brandy is added to that portion of the essence to be saved. This mother tincture will be stored in a dark-glass bottle, labelled and kept in a cool, safe place. All the utensils need to be carefully cleaned and boiled before they are used again.

There is something rather shocking about this boiling. It is a more physical process, with less of the delicacy and fineness of the 'thin glass bowl' and the ethereal, dancing light of the sun method. To stand and watch as the flowers wilt and then brown in the heating water is to witness some kind of disintegration. The colour and life go out from the flowers, forced out rather than released, taken rather more than given. As the liquid comes to the boil it quickly takes colour from the plant material. And, as steam rises, there is a constant agitation of small droplets which fizzle on the surface of the water, bouncing, it seems, into the air. This appears to be the reverse of the air bubbles that form within the bowl in the sun method.

The rising steam carries a scent of the essence: with Cherry Plum it is almonds, with Chestnut Bud a spicy, sugary smell, with Star of Bethlehem it is fresh and sweet like a pleasant cooked cabbage; Willow is the same. The Star essence, when it has cooled, also has a strong, tangy taste with a golden, greeny-yellow colour, brilliant. Pine tastes like old timber, fousty and dry; Holly can be an intense, bright green (from the leaves); Elm makes a thick, syrupy liquid which is slow to filter; Walnut is dark amber, impenetrable; Sweet Chestnut and Hornbeam both have a sharp taste which is strong and stimulating. Red Chestnut makes a deep plum-coloured essence. Each has a specific character in taste, colour and smell.

Significantly, only those remedies selected by Bach utilize the boiling method. Essence makers who have followed after him, whether in California, Australia, or elsewhere in Britain and Europe, have all worked with the sun method. Perhaps Bach would have used the sun if it had been available. The various attempts to explain the enigma of 'the boilers' seem to make this assumption. Weeks, as cited above, suggested that the early spring sun was not strong enough to make an essence. And yet Bach had made Gorse by the sun method in April. Furthermore, she does not explain why he continued to use the boiling method in May, June and July of the year when, surely, there would have been sun enough. Could it be that 1935 was particularly cloudy with few suitable days? Records show that during May and June there was average bright sunshine and it was exceptionally fine weather in July.* So poor weather does not explain matters. It is sometimes said that the Second Nineteen were trees and woody shrubs; being tougher they needed to be boiled. But even this is a partial truth since several are delicate, fleshy plants such as Star of Bethlehem and Mustard, or the soft flowers of Red Chestnut and Wild Rose.

Is there any significant difference between the sun and the boiling methods? Some people have made a boiling remedy (like Star of Bethlehem) using the sun and consider the resulting essence to be every bit as satisfactory. Although both methods use the same spring water and similar flowers, there is a clear departure in the quality of the fire element which actually does the making. Both are using the energy of the sun to bring about a transformation in the making of the remedy. The difference is that sunlight comes from outside our planetary system while fossil fuels come from within the earth. Having been through a number of processes of transformation, photosynthesis being the first, the sun's energy has been changed when it becomes the fire used for cooking. Light from the sun has been metamorphosed into fire in the form of the three other elements: earth, water and air—making coal, oil and gas. It is this quality of transformation that becomes characteristic of the boiling remedies.

Bach says of the Second Nineteen:

There is no doubt that these new remedies act on a different plane to the old. They are more spiritualized and help us to develop that inner great self in all of us which has the power to overcome all fears, all difficulties, all worries, all disease.[4]

---

* The National Meteorological Archive offers a comparison of the hours of sunshine during 1935 with the average for fifty-five years. Records made at the Radcliffe Observatory in Oxford, ten miles from Sotwell, show that April was more cloudy than average but that July was exceptional:

April	127.3 (average 147.4)
May	188.5 (average 190.7)
June	196.2 (average 195.2)
July	274.3 (average 192.3)
August	200.0 (average 176.2)
September	144.7 (average 140.7)

What does he mean by 'more spiritualized'? The remedies are not a quick or easy path to spiritual enlightenment. But working with these emotional states is doing the real work which leads to spiritual development. Overcoming life difficulty leads to the evolution of soul qualities. In other words it is the work done to transform suffering into learning, pain into insight, disease into health which leads to spiritual growth. Learning comes through the experience of difficulty; no knowledge comes from ease. We become transformed by going through the fire. And it is just this relationship which makes the boilers distinct. They are remedy states people experience as a result of difficult life-involvements; they arise in reaction to life problems. And being prepared by the boiling method, they have this common theme of pressure, intensity and, indeed, pain.

It is for this reason that 'suffering' is often associated with these later remedies. Bach had 'great suffering to bear' according to Weeks and the word is used frequently to convey the difficulty he worked through.[5] But making this a slightly Christian virtue (He suffered for our sins) is to miss the point. The suffering is the process of transformation and the remedies serve to help us find a way in it, before removing it from our path.

> *Disease is the result of wrong thinking and wrongdoing, and ceases when the act and thought are put in order. When the lesson of pain and suffering and distress is learnt, there is no further purpose in its presence, and it automatically disappears.*[6]

So it is the failure to learn the lesson which leads to the suffering. Suffering also comes from resistance, when struggling to sustain a situation against the weight of what happens in life. It is actually the root meaning of the word: Latin *suffere*, to sustain, which comes from *sub* in the sense of 'up from underneath', and *ferre* to carry [Chambers]. So the sense is of carrying up from underneath. This is just what the fire does in the boiling method, thus confirming the image of upward growth in the evolution of the soul.

This carrying up from underneath is important. The energy of the sun is given and received, falling from above. The fire that comes from within the earth burns beneath the essence. It carries the energy upwards on the return journey. This parallels the journey of the individual who incarnates on earth and grows back along the path of soul evolution. *The Twelve Healers* described the qualities of twelve types of descending soul. The boiling remedies describe the pathway of the ascending soul and the varying experience of life-lessons which attend the return.

So the boiling method brings more to the preparation of the mother essence than a convenient alternative to the sun's rays. The process is different. Just as the flowers collapse and disintegrate in boiling water, so old patterns are broken down as change enters our life. Water and fire act together to soften and dissolve; gentle and fierce. Resistance to change causes suffering and that suffering is like a cooking for the soul.

13 · Holding Back from Involvement in Life

THE THOUGHT THAT PEOPLE SUFFER in order to learn, or rather that failure to learn brings suffering, may have been uppermost in Bach's mind as he approached the next of the remedies: Chestnut Bud. This one, he said, is about making full use of observation and experience to 'learn the lessons of daily life'.[1] Some people only need to have an experience once and they learn from it what they need to know and build that into their life patterning. Others find they need to repeat the experience, often several times, before it becomes effectively a part of them. Bach speaks of these lessons in terms of 'error' and 'fault', so we may suppose that he has quite specific experiences in mind.

Chestnut Bud

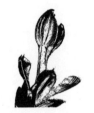

What kind of thing, then, was Bach thinking about at this time with Chestnut Bud; what were these lessons? Where might the feeling arise that he was failing to learn from experience? He may have been concerned with his work, or his relationships, or, thirdly, progress with his personal life purpose. We can only guess. But considering what his situation may have been does give a context for the meaning of Chestnut Bud. At this time Bach was living at *Wellsprings,* in Sotwell, with Mary Tabor. Nora Weeks lived at *Mount Vernon,* possibly with Victor Bullen for company.* His group of close friends also included the Wheelers. It is likely that some entanglement in their relationships led Bach to think, with regret, of either his or their failure to learn from past experience. We often say of other people that they head straight into the same kind of situation as they have just left, be it employment, a love affair or just a dream. Chestnut Bud applies to such experiences as soul guidance

---

* In her book *To Thine Own Self Be True*, Mary Tabor sketches an impression of how matters may have been between them as a group. The hero of the tale is Davidsson, a thinly-disguised version of Bach; there is 'the lady of the flowers' who lives alone in the 'corner house, standing up above the road'. Notes on the wrapper of the book say 'This book is the outcome of the author having seen the personal example of Dr Edward Bach, one time Harley Street Specialist, who carried the principle into living effect'. The principle is 'follow your own desire'. Published in 1938, by C. W. Daniel, there is an indication here of another side of Bach's work as a teacher.

to understanding, helping people to learn what is really happening. Like an able counsellor, the remedy shows how patterns of behaviour are repeated and the consequences of that.

In Dr Bach's work, the discovery of new remedies, there was also the risk of making 'the same error on different occasions'. He was involved in a complex process of learning and teaching, listening and talking simultaneously. With these boiling remedies he had to study himself and his emotional responses most closely and yet still allow guidance and intuition to speak to him. If he had felt depressed and overwhelmed with Elm and frightened with Aspen and Cherry Plum, it may be that at this point he lost track of what he was being shown. A Chestnut Bud situation is like the game of *Snakes and Ladders:* one can fall back into old ways of thinking and acting, slip away from knowledge and experience achieved through hard work. Bach said, life is 'for the purpose of gaining all the knowledge and experience which can be obtained through earthly existence . . .'.[2] But at times we fail to see that. If experience is repeated without gaining knowledge, it must be repeated yet again. Was Bach being shown something that he failed, at first, to see?

Error, fault and failing are words which appear frequently in Bach's writing. 'Our whole object is to realise our faults . . . Disease is entirely and only due to faults within . . . The only cure is to correct our faults . . .'[3] So look carefully at Chestnut Bud as the remedy which most definitely helps in the recognition of error. Recognizing these personal failings is the most important task for life on earth:

> An understanding of where we are making an error (which is so often not realized by us) and an earnest endeavour to correct the fault will lead not only to a life of joy and peace, but also to health.[4]

This brings us to the third context for Bach of Chestnut Bud: the progress he was making in his personal life purpose. He had an operation for cancer in 1917[5] and *sarcoma* was given as joint cause of death (with cardiac failure) on his death certificate in 1936. His whole adult life was a struggle with 'the real cause and cure of disease'.[6] Maybe as the Chestnut leaves were unfolding, Edward Bach had to re-examine his personal understanding of his own health and how it related to his soul's purpose. Perhaps the spectre of a dragon long slain rose again to frighten him. No small issue this, but then the boiling remedies are not dealing with small matters. When considering how Bach saw the relationship between body and soul, it helps to read his 'fundamental truths' in *Heal Thyself*:

Thirdly, we must realize that the short passage on this earth, which we know as life, is but a moment in the course of our evolution, as one day at school is to a life, and although we can for the present only see and comprehend that one day, our intuition tells us that birth was infinitely far from our beginning and death infinitely far from our ending. Our Souls, which are really we, are immortal, and the bodies of which we are conscious are temporary, merely as horses we ride to go a journey, or instruments we use to do a piece of work.[7]

So, to him, any bodily illness was of little account. But that is precisely the context of faith and knowledge which is hard to achieve and easy to fall away from. The life lesson may need to be shown more than once before it is understood.

The Chestnut Bud remedy is prepared, not from flowers but from the opening buds of the Horse Chestnut tree, *Aesculus hippocastanum*. This is one of the first big trees to break into leaf. While there are aspects of the tree's gesture which are relevant (like the broken pattern in the bark, see White Chestnut page 253), it is specifically the stage of bud-burst which characterizes this essence. The Chestnut, then, is emblematic of all trees in every spring. Each bud has formed in the previous season; we can even see the scar of the last leaf. Within the closed bud lies all the potential for new growth and development—miniature leaves, stems and flowers lie closely folded inside.

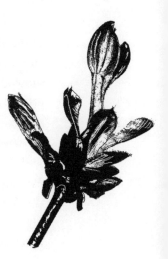

As the bud opens and the shoot explores its unique pathway into space, into the life of the tree within the year, it unfolds individually within a set pattern of potential. Each bud is from the same blueprint but expresses a single and unique form. It is like the individual person exploring the potentials within a life. In every life there are opportunities ('it contains the lessons and experiences necessary at the moment of our evolution . . .')[8] and the only question is whether the opportunity to learn is taken. That is where the Chestnut Bud remedy comes in. Those who fail to learn and grow into their potential 'do not take full advantage of observation and experience . . .'.[9]

Why is this remedy made from leaf buds and not from flowers? Because spring leaves are so expressive of a new season, of new beginnings and new growth. They develop moment by moment before our eyes. But leaves are also the organ of respiration. They absorb light and air to create, through photosynthesis, the energy which sustains life on earth. This physical activity parallels the way experience and observation lead to learning and sustain the life of the soul. Respiration works at many levels. Living efficiently means taking in life experience and building from it soul qualities. That is, saying 'yes' to the lessons of life.

Chestnut Bud is often described as a remedy for children, either slow learners or for the foolish person who does not make supposed progress in life. Young buds may equal young people. But anyone can become stuck in life and need help. And this way of freeing up learning for the soul means a person may usefully take Chestnut Bud even on the day before death. Most of life, after all, is spent repeating the pattern of the past.

Larch

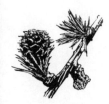

Next came Larch. This remedy helps those 'who feel they will never be a success';[10] people whose confidence in themselves is low. This is a natural sequal to the Chestnut Bud experience in that, even if the lesson to learn can be seen, it may still be felt that failure will follow. It may be clear enough what must be done to fulfil the life purpose, but such people hang back because 'they do not consider themselves as good or capable as those around them'.[11] For Bach it seems again to point to self-questioning and self-doubt. The challenge is there but not the will to succeed. We know that Bach did succeed; yet Larch was one of the stages of difficulty to deter and delay him. That is characteristic of the boiling method remedies: they represent difficulties overcome on the pathway of life.

The Larch condition is not inherent, not something we are born with, not integral to the soul. It grows up as a response to trauma, a response to a particular setback. After an accident there may be a loss of confidence. Larch is there for those who have engaged with life, taken a knock and subsequently feel defeated. Larch calls for the attempt to be made, even at the risk of failure. Bach described this situation by saying that these are people who 'do not venture or make a strong enough attempt to succeed'.[12] We all know this, surely. It is not only Scots who are brought up on the story of Robert the Bruce and the persistent spider which kept rebuilding its web. It was an Irish poet, Thomas More, who wrote:

> There was a little man, and he had a little soul,
>   And he said, 'Little Soul, let us try, try, try'.

And an Englishman, William Edward Hickson, who wrote:

> If at first you don't succeed
>   Try, try, again.

Larch is the 'try again' remedy.

Observations on other of Bach's plants suggest that the form of the Larch tree should be either very forward and confident or else tentative and hesitant. In fact it is both. The Larch is another immigrant species to the UK; *Larix decidua* was probably not introduced until about 1620. If it was here at an earlier date it was very scarce. The reason why it was introduced and then grown so extensively is its strength and adaptability. It can grow in quite rugged and adverse conditions. The great plantings of Larch by the Fourth Duke of Athol in the eighteenth century (said by some to have grown twenty-seven million trees on 15,000 acres of barren land) were a recognition that it was strong enough to grow on the rocky and hilly ground of Scotland. Seeds and seedling trees were originally brought from Italy, where Larch thrives in the Alps and the Apennines, and more recently from Germany. The new forests were economically viable because Larch is a particularly durable and useful timber for ship-building, poles and pit props. It grows fast and straight, with a single trunk and few branches. Yet, despite this forwardness and apparent strength, the Larch is sensitive to pollution and prone to fatal diseases, just like the Elm (page 192). This is probably due to monoculture and over-planting in unsuitable conditions. But it is nonetheless indicative of an inherent weakness in the species.

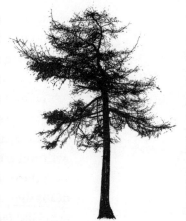

Larch seed forms within the shelter of a cone (Larch is a conifer, like pine or fir) and has a small wing which will carry it some distance on the wind. Like Clematis, Wild Oat, and Hornbeam, the Larch seed illustrates a tendency to drift in life: there is a temporary dissociation from any involvement in the material world. When the seed lands, germination is uncertain but seedlings may root in the cleft of stones or in some small ledge where others cannot succeed. This habit contrasts with other species which require altogether easier conditions and more fertile soil in which to grow. Like Mimulus (page 52) Larch braves difficulty. In Evelyn's *Silva* (1786, Hunter edition) there is a footnote concerning Larch:

> . . . *it is remarked that those trees which have been planted in the worst soils and the most exposed situations, have thriven the best, which is a great encouragement. Some trees cannot bear too great a luxuriancy . . .*[13]

There is a story that the first Larches planted in Scotland were imported with some orange trees. The Larches failed when put into the hothouse with the oranges but, when thrown on to the rubbish heap, given up for dead, they quickly revived and grew into strong trees.[14] Larch seedlings are easily set back ('being rather prone to damping off and sun scorch')[15] so that discouragement can set in early. Equally Larch cannot survive in waterlogged ground, preferring to use an extensive root system to search for moisture. As with Scleranthus (page 120), this indicates a need for deepening involvement with the material world.

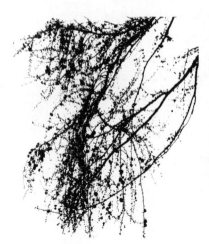

Larch starts out as a typical conifer with a small vertical shoot breaking into six to eight thin, needle leaves which radiate like the spokes of a wheel. For the first four years it is an evergreen. Thereafter the young tree becomes deciduous, the leaves turning yellow, then brown and finally dropping to the ground. This behaviour is unique among British trees. It emphasizes the point that Larch begins life in a normal way, like other conifers, and then, suddenly, changes. The way the leaves brown, yet remain on the tree through the autumn and early winter, has prompted the observation that every year Larches give the impression they are dying. The poet William Wordsworth, who took a strong dislike to the Larch for some reason, wrote:

> ...*in winter, it is still more lamentably distinguished from every other deciduous tree of the forest; for they seem only to sleep, but the Larch appears absolutely dead.*[16]

In practical terms this may be a strategy for survival, allowing the tree to grow in the mountains up to 1,500 metres in the Alps and up to 550 metres) in Scotland. But the poetical image of a tree giving up on life is a more pleasing explanation. Compare the unremitting struggle of the Oak (page 151), which never stops trying, with the apparent inclination of the Larch to give up at every opportunity.

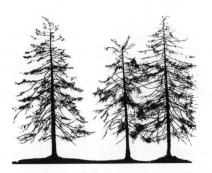

In several respects the form of the Larch tree may be regarded as the inverse of Impatiens. The Impatiens person is sure of himself, reflected in a clear and powerful geometry within the structure of the plant. Larch is lacking just that confidence and this is reflected in the slender, drooping branches which hang from the trunk like loose-slung cables reaching out towards the earth; at the tip they turn upwards, as if trying, at the last, to lift their line. Indeed, the young side shoots begin by growing upwards at an angle but slowly bend under their own weight. This downward swooping gesture may help to shed snow which otherwise could weigh down the branches and snap them off. But it strongly expresses the Larch remedy state which collapses without resistance, not asserting the will. This is seen in the growing tip of the tree which seems to lose the impetus of going upwards, and curves over, flattening out at the top.* It seems the effort of vertical growth cannot be sustained.

Yet the Larch does, eventually, build a powerful, columnar trunk. It is a fast-growing tree, reaching a height of twenty-five to thirty metres in fifty years. It then only increases in girth, living 200 years in some cases. The timber is resinous (trees used to be tapped for turpentine) and is resistant to both fire and water. So, in the end, it has a strength and stature which speak of the positive quality of the remedy. When the tree is young the bark is scratchy and irregular, flaking like dried skin. As the trunk expands the bark seems unable to grow at the same speed, so that cracks appear. Sticky sap oozes from the crevices like a weeping eczema. This is milky-white and strongly aromatic. It is as if growth is painful

---

* This flattening-out is seen in *Larix decidua* but not necessarily in the hybrids grown commercially. *Larix* x *eurolepsis*, Dunkeld Larch, is a cross between *L. decidua* and the Japanese Larch *L. kaempferi*. It has a more upright stance producing straighter timber. It is the more natural and curving *L. decidua* which is used for making the remedy.

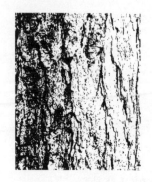

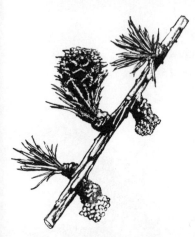

Male and female Larch flowers

for the tree. The painful and traumatic experience which lies behind the shaken confidence of the Larch state, perhaps? When it is older the bark develops vertical fissures, though these lack the strongly networked structure of Elm, Oak or Sweet Chestnut.

Larch flowers in April, with spring. Males and females appear together on the same branch. The males are smaller with yellow, rounded pollen-producing sacs; they point downwards from the underside of the branches. The females are purple-red, sitting upright on the top of the twigs. The flowers do not open from a bud, but, like all conifers they are gymnosperms (meaning 'naked seeds') so they grow with an exposed ovule which is waiting for pollen to fall.* Each ovule is protected by a small bract. After pollination this continues to grow and will, in time, help to form the cone. Positioned as they are it is certain that pollen will fall from the males on to the females. Pollination is inevitable; it cannot fail. Every flower makes a cone; these remain attached to the branches for several years waiting for windy, dry weather which will shake the seeds free. So Larch has a history, a long story of the past to tell: the several generations of the cones are evidence of continuity.

Larch is a pioneer species: it grows on the frontier where conditions are hostile; in cold, wet, poor soils. Only a tree with great determination can make it. So a strategy has developed which allows it to wait for favourable conditions. But not only self-propagation is planned for. Because Larch is deciduous, dropping its leaves each year, it slowly builds a nourishing loam on the ground. It is a tree that helps to build soil; this is said to be because it puts in calcium.[17] Most conifers poison the earth with acidity.

---

* There are two major divisions among plants: gymnosperms and angiosperms. The distinction is made in the structure of the reproductive organs of the female flower. Gymnosperms do not have an enclosed ovary—pollen falls directly on to the naked ovule—there is no need for the stigma and style found in angiosperms. Gymnosperms are the older group in evolutionary terms; they were the dominant vegetation 300 million years ago, in the Carboniferous Period. Today there are still examples of such 'primitive' species as *Ginkgo*, and among the conifers there are the ancient Redwoods of California, *Sequoia sempervivens*: one of the largest and oldest life forms on earth. Angiosperms do not appear in the fossil record until about 100 million years ago although they soon became the dominant plant form in many parts of the world.

Larch has leaves which rot more quickly and is 'by far the best improver of heath or moor pasturage known in this country'.[18] This is success for the tree and then success for the land use thereafter. When a tendency to expect failure is overcome, determination and success follow, making a strong contribution to the evolving consciousness of life on earth.

Hornbeam

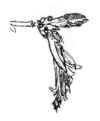

There is a third remedy which fits into this little group concerning people who are holding back from involvement in life: Hornbeam. Bach did not note the order of discovery, nor did Weeks, but Hornbeam flowers at the same time as Larch and has certain qualities in common. While Larch stands back through lack of confidence, Hornbeam stands back through lack of determination and strength. It is 'for those who do not feel they have sufficient strength, mentally or physically, to carry the burden of life placed upon them . . .'.[19] Once again Bach is feeling burdened. This time the burden is not responsibility, as it was with Elm but the weight of work, the slog of it, the feeling that too great an effort is required. The shift in emphasis is really quite subtle between these early boiling remedies. It can be explained clearly enough, however, by visualizing Bach at this time and allowing ourselves to resonate with his state of mind. He knows how to do his present work (Chestnut Bud), he has regained the personal confidence to attempt it (Larch) yet he cannot quite shake himself into action, he still cannot, as it were, get out of bed. Why? Because 'some part of the mind or body needs to be strengthened before they can easily fulfil their work'.[20] Note the use of 'easily'. It can be done but it is such a great effort.

Hornbeam, *Carpinus betulus* is a deciduous hardwood. In the textbooks it is invariably called inconspicuous, little known and with few distinguishing characteristics. This may often be true, but when the tree is in flower it is sensational, a magnificent display of force, vitality and colour. Clarke Nuttall has it nicely described when he writes: 'Suddenly the tree is clothed, as it were with a dripping green-gold garment'.[21] This cloak of gold lamé shimmers in the sunlight, a dazzling burst of energy. The brightness of the flowering is akin to Olive and it follows therefore that Hornbeam is for a kind of tiredness or lassitude. It does not happen every spring and the flowers are often subdued or even missing altogether. But every

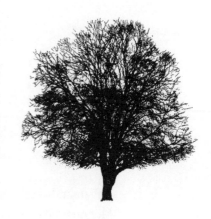

few years (after hot summers it is said) the tree puts on a display which is truly memorable. And then our curiosity is aroused to enquire what strange and exotic species can that be.

Hornbeam grows naturally in the south east of England and not at all in the north; perhaps it is only the weaker southern temperament that calls for Hornbeam's support. The ancient forests to the north east of London were mostly Hornbeam. Here it was coppiced for firewood in previous centuries and was especially prized for its heat and bright flame. The wood takes fire easily. Burning equals transformation of energy; a person in the Hornbeam state needs to transform energy, to galvanize the will into action. The timber is extremely hard. Gerard said '. . . for in time it waxeth so hard, that the toughness and hardness of it may be rather compared with horn than unto wood; and therefore it was called hornbeam or hardbeam'.[22] The hard, white wood was used in the days before iron and steel for the moving parts of machinery, like the cogs used in a water or wind mill, by wheelwrights, for ploughs and other farm implements. But there is no tree lore associated with the Hornbeam,[23] it has just this beauty in flower and utility in the timber.

The trunk is smooth, a dull grey-brown but shot through with vertical, silvery lines which waver like light. The picture is one of electrical energy shimmering in the bark. The trunk is rarely circular and has a corrugated or fluted appearance, like braided muscle fibres which bulge beneath a smooth skin. It begins to branch quite low down and each bough branches out in turn. so that the tree has an elegant, forked form;

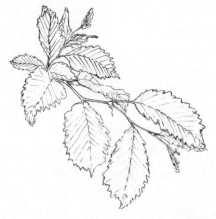

the main boughs are quickly lost in the smaller branches. These twigs are slender and covered by a density of leaf growth. The leaves have a notched edge and are strongly ribbed, an indication of strength and a kind of

irritability, like Impatiens (page 43); not that Hornbeam is
an irritable emotional state, rather that some irritability and
excitement would help to get things moving. The leaves
often stay attached through the winter, making Hornbeam
useful as a hedge.

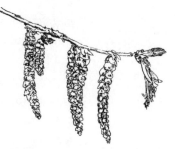

Male catkins and female flower

Hornbeam grows readily in any soil: 'no soil, however
wet or dry, comes amiss to it; and undiscouraged by the
most ruthless pollarding, it at once starts to grow again'.[24]
This shows the powerful intent to get on with life. The life
force in Hornbeam is so strong that when two branches
touch or cross one another they often grow together and
fuse as one.* Hornbeam is a picture of braided strength.

Male and female flowers are found on the same tree. The
male catkin is showy and appears a little before the leaves
are fully open. The females are very inconspicuous, looking
like unfolding leaf-buds pointing downwards at the end of
the twigs. When pollinated, small red styles protrude. The
seed is a nut which is carried by a three-winged bract which
acts as a sail. It flies like a helicopter and may be blown up
to a hundred metres from the tree before coming to rest.[25]
As with Clematis (page 46), the fruits stay on the tree well
into the winter. There is a parallel here in the need for the

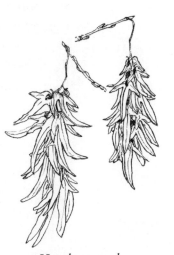

Hornbeam seeds

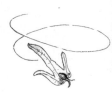

Hornbeam person to get down into life, to get deeply involved with the
world. The wing of the seed is emblematic of the tendency to remain
detached from the earth; downward-pointing flowers, of the need to
engage in physical reality.

Hornbeam is one of those remedies which must be taken to fully
appreciate the quality of the emotional state. Then the difference can
be felt. People become so habituated to the Hornbeam feeling that 'the
affairs of everyday seem too much for them to accomplish . . .'.[26] Lethargy
slowly creeps up. The sudden flowering of the Hornbeam, like the remedy, brings a sudden access of strength and determination. The gears

---

* Hunter's notes in John Evelyn's *Silva* record that in Germany (in 1786) Hornbeam
was planted so 'as that every two plants may be brought to intersect each other in the
form of a St Andrew's cross. In that part where the two plants cross each other, he
[the farmer] scrapes off the bark, and binds them closely together with straw. In consequence of this operation, the two plants consolidate in a sort of indissoluble knot,
and push from thence horizontal, slanting shoots, which form a living palisado, or
chevaux de frise; so that such a protection may be called a rural fortification. These

engage (like the cogs of the mill of the mind) and become active and purposeful once more.

Here, then, are three more remedies made from trees. They share a common feature in that each emotional state has a characteristic reluctance to full involvement in life. Chestnut Bud lives but does not register the significance of what is experienced; this is a mental withdrawal from learning the lessons of life. Larch withdraws from actively participating and so misses the opportunity to learn from involvement, remaining a bystander. Hornbeam, needing to activate the dynamo of wilful engagement in living, uses mental weariness as an excuse for holding back. When these three lessons are learned and integrated into life then the individual soul actively participates in making use of experience to progress and grow.

---

hedges, being pruned annually, and with discretion, will, in a few years, render the fence impenetrable in every part. It is not uncommon in Germany to see the side of high roads thus guarded for many miles together and it were to be wished that this example was followed in some places of this kingdom. I am the more inclined to recommend such hedges, as the Hornbeam is not delicate in point of soil, but will even thrive on land seemingly barren. When properly pruned, it will put out strong lateral shoots within three inches of the ground, by which means it makes an impenetrable fence against cattle. It is also of quick growth; a thing of great consequence in the improvement of waste land.' Evelyn, Sir John, *Silva, or A discourse of Forest Trees and the Propagation of Timber in His Majesty's Dominions'*, with notes by A. Hunter (second Hunter edition) 1786, p. 141.

14 · Finding Fault with the World Around Us

NORA WEEKS, writing about Edward Bach's experience of the new remedies at this time, said that 'for some days before the discovery of each one he suffered himself from the state of mind for which that particular remedy was required'.[1] So, having got over his weariness with the help of Hornbeam, he next encountered the bitterness and resentment of Willow. 'It's not fair' is the thought which characterizes this state of mind. What was it that Bach found unfair? Perhaps his ill health, perhaps the rejection of his ideas by the medical establishment, perhaps just the difficulties he experienced in discovering the remedies, we do not know. But Willow he described as being:

Willow

> *For those who have suffered adversity or misfortune and find these difficult to accept, without complaint or resentment, as they judge life much by the success which it brings.*[2]

This resentment he felt to 'an intensified degree' so that he might then be drawn towards the plant or tree which could counteract it.[3] Just what it felt like for Bach is clear from the description:

> *They feel that they have not deserved so great a trial, that it was unjust, and they become embittered.*[4]

All the boiling remedies describe our responses to the trials of life: that is exactly what they are about. When faced with trauma or misfortune one person will wonder if they have the courage or will to carry on, another feels deep sadness, anger or despair. People who get caught up in the Willow state have more than a fair share of difficulties, or so they feel, and complain of injustice. They respond, said Bach, with 'less interest and less activity in those things of life which they had previously enjoyed'.[5] So they punish themselves. Their energy slows down and turns inward, concentrating like gall to a poison which permeates life so that, inevitably, matters get worse. Willow needs to learn to say 'yes' to life and to work with renewed energy to overcome adversity, no matter how difficult the problem.

There are many types of willow; Bach chose *Salix alba*, subspecies *vitellina* or *Salix vitellina*. The vitellina willow is different because the

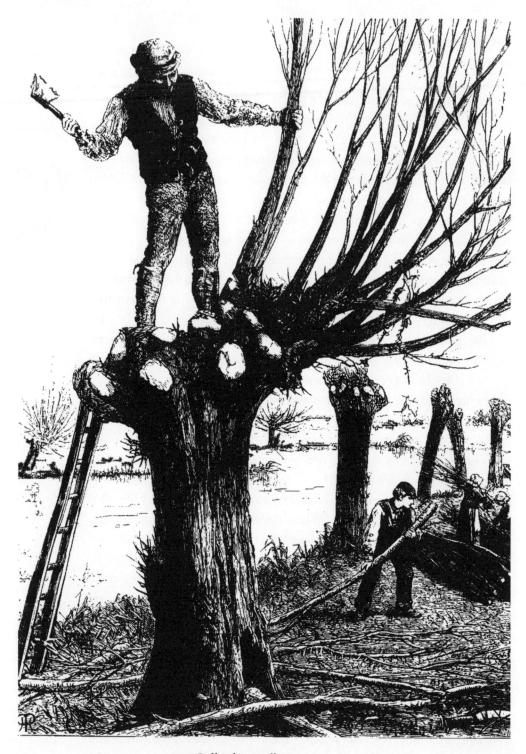

Pollarding willow

twigs are a bright egg-yolk yellow (Latin *vitellus*, egg yolk) rather than brown. In other respects *S. vitellina* is like *S. alba*, a tall open tree with narrow lanceolate leaves which are shiny green above and downy olive-grey beneath. The whiter underleaf gives the name 'white' willow. These leaves flutter in the breeze, hence Tennyson's couplet:

> *Willows whiten, aspen quiver,*
> *Little breezes dusk and shiver.* [*The Lady of Shallott*]

Willows are often found along the riverbank in damp, low-lying ground. Left to grow they can achieve twenty metres. But more often (especially in years gone by) they are pollarded. Pollarding involves cutting the growing crown out of a tree, reducing the trunk to three metres. This stimulates regrowth in Willow just as it does in Olive (page 175). This was done regularly every few years to harvest a crop of poles for building, fence making and so on; it also supplied a source of firewood. 'It is the sweetest of all our English fuel', remarked Evelyn regarding the scented smoke. He devoted several pages to the willow in his *Silva*, listing forty or more other good uses for the wood including 'plattens for clogs' and 'rafters for hovels'. Willow grows rapidly, up to three metres in a year in ideally wet conditions: 'it groweth incredibly fast, it being a byeword in this country, that the profit by willows will buy the owner a horse before that by other trees will pay for his saddle'.[6]

So, with money to be made from commercial planting and pollarding of willows the tree had been pressed into service. Like Vine (page 173) it is the very strength and vitality of the species which invites exploitation. And how does the Willow feel about it? Resentful perhaps? Willow's response is to grow back with such vigour that it actually becomes an emblem for the affirmation of life. Ezekiel, the Old Testament visionary, described God's renewal of the Covenant with Israel by saying 'He set it like a willow twig and it sprouted . . .'.[7] Break off a twig or cut off a branch and set it in the earth and it will strike roots and grow; Willow is so responsive to life opportunity. Most trees will not grow from such 'sets' or cuttings and none with such willingness. Logs cut in the winter and stored will sprout leaves in the spring as if they are still part of the tree. Willow is so alive that it will regrow if it is cut down to ground level.

And yet, Willow has also been a traditional symbol for sadness and lamentation:

By the waters of Babylon, there we sat down and wept,
when we remembered Zion.

On the willows there we hung up our lyres. [*Psalm 137*]

The Israelites had not deserved such misfortunes (or had they?). 'From that time the willow appears never again to have been associated with feelings of gladness. . . . It was a tree of evil omen, and was employed to make torches carried at funerals.'[8] Maybe the Rev. C. A. Johns missed a point here. The link between Willow and funerals is in the symbol of rebirth after burial in the earth.* This is what happens to the Willow tree; bury a branch and see. The lamentation of the Israelites exiled in Egypt can also be seen as symbolic of the exile that the soul experiences in the physical world. The resentment of the Willow person is based upon a rejection of life as much as on a sense of unfairness. If this appears to be wandering too far into the realms of theology and metaphysical speculation, bear in mind the vital concept that, in the Willow state, the individual has lost belief in the fairness of life. Ezekiel made the point that God (and life) would deal justly with the individual. Willow people deny that reality.

There are other, more tangible pointers which illustrate the gesture of the Willow state in the tree. Bach implied that Willow people are concerned with their success in the material world. The way the tree roots deeply into the earth shows this. It has a massive fibrous root system which searches everywhere for water. It is well known that willow roots can block house drains. But this affinity for water shows how Willow people feed upon the emotional drama of complaint and blame. There is an intensity of feeling in all the water plants. Willows grow by rivers and in marshy land. It was this characteristic which gave rise to the idea that it contained help for rheumatics and the aches and pains associated with damp places. In 1763 the Rev. Edmund Stone experimented with willow

---

* Jacqueline Memory Paterson in *Tree Wisdom* [Thorsons 1996] connects Willow to the legendary Greek Orpheus and his journey into the Underworld searching for his dead wife Eurydice (he wore a Willow wreath and took his lyre), to Circe, Hecate and others. She develops the theme of pagan ritual and magical uses, seeing Willow as the witches' tree, a tree of divination, psychism, water, the moon and the night. Much of this comes from material found in Robert Graves' *White Goddess* [Faber 1961]. All such ideas can be woven within the tapestry of the Willow state. However, with Bach's *Salix vitellina* it is the strength of the golden sun that makes for the change from bitterness to renewal, the sweetness of the tree which, like the music of Orpheus, can charm both the ferryman Charon and the dog Cerberus.

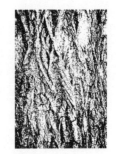

bark (*S. alba*) thinking the bitterness was reminiscent of Peruvian bark (cinchona), used in preparation of quinine, a treatment for malaria. He claimed some fifty people with rheumatic disorders were helped by willow bark. But his report to the Royal Society was ignored. Perhaps the problem was that 'pious folk belief held that God planted cures where diseases originated'.[9] It was a case of an infant science dismissing the traditional Doctrine of Signatures.* But later research showed that the *salicin* found in Willow was related to our present-day manufactured aspirin, so he was probably right.

The seeds of the Willow are like masses of fine cotton wool floating on the wind: a contrast with the root's desire to become immersed in the physical world. Only if they land on damp soil will they germinate and then, almost immediately. So the cycle of growing in damp conditions is repeated. Chancellor, in *Handbook of the Bach Flower Remedies*,[10] describes Willow people as wet blankets, spreading gloom and despair. They are sulky, 'believe their prayers are unanswered and their efforts unrewarded…they take without giving'. They would not admit to being happy even if they were happy. This is in contrast to the vitality and lust for life seen in the seed, in the networked strength of the bark, in the lanceolate leaf with its serrated edge (see Impatiens page 43), and in the

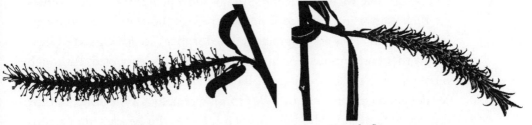

Male flowers   *Female flowers*

greeny-yellow of the flowers with their sweet scent and nectar (see Holly page 240). When in the negative state Willow people become emotionally congested and inflexible. The positive is illustrated in the flexibility of the twigs which bend without breaking (this is what makes this Willow useful for basket-making), in the easy dancing movement of the leaves

---

* The Doctrine of Signatures, a medieval medical theory, held that the physical appearance of plants indicated the diseases that they would remedy. Thus the bulbous roots of the Lesser Celandine (*Ranunculus ficaria*) were the signature for haemorrhoids; the spotted leaves of Lungwort (*Sticta pulmonaria*) made them suitable for lung complaints.

and branches when the wind blows. A strong wind shows how responsive Willow can be as it allows itself to be shaped by outside forces.

Most of all, however, the contrast between resentment and joy can be seen in the colour of the twigs. Willow stands at the first motivation of a love of life: without that things appear unjust, unkind, depressingly difficult and unfair. This love of life is in the golden, egg-yolk-yellow of the winter wood. In early spring, on a bright, clear day, look at the Willow against a brilliant blue sky: a halo of purple and gold can be seen. This is the positive quality of Willow, shining with life force and strength. It is often thought that the Willow condition is like a lower form of life. But these are people who are qualified and capable, although experiencing a great challenge. Only those who are able to carry much are given the greater load. Accepting that load without complaint, transforming the bitterness into sweet acceptance, makes a real contribution to the evolution of the soul consciousness of life on earth.

Beech

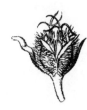

The complaint about life's circumstances is continued by the next remedy: Beech. This is for intolerance, criticism, fault finding. 'For those who feel the need to see more good and beauty in all that surrounds them'.[11] Typically, Bach softens the description. But the point is made clearly that this is another remedy for those who look out into the world and do not like what they see. As with Willow people who blame others for their misfortunes so Beech people criticize the world around for its imperfections. They are judgmental. Life for them could be good enough if only they concentrated less upon what needs to be corrected. 'Although much appears to be wrong', said Bach, they need 'to have the ability to see the good growing within'.[12] But this is a remedy for the critic, not the criticized. However valid the criticism may be, the Beech state narrows and restricts joy in life and so narrows and restricts vitality, leading inevitably to ill health.

To find a remedy for this Beech state of mind, Bach needed to be clear about what such people really feel; what leads them to those circumstances? Beech people are not exactly dominant, but they develop an urge to suppress the freedom of other people's self-expression. Again, this is not a soul type but a condition which builds up over time owing to a reactive dislike for something—expressed as 'life does not do what I want so I will criticize everything and everybody to show how wrong it all is'. This finds expression in setting straight the natural tumult of experience, seeking exactness, order and discipline; in the narrow standard of getting it perfect; in a pernickety, fussy attention to cleanliness and detail. All of this expression looks at the external form because the person is internally discontented.

At the end of the year, when Bach had found the last of the Second Nineteen remedies, he organized all thirty-eight into seven groups. Beech he put into the group for *Over-Care for Welfare of Others*, along with Chicory, Vervain, Vine and Rockwater. All five remedies share the same dissatisfaction with the external circumstances of life and a feeling of superiority towards others. In each case this outlook deflects attention from the real problem: the individuals themselves. The problem for the Beech person is a lack of self-worth. Those who do not value themselves find it hard to value and honour others. Katz and Kaminski in *Flower Essence Repertory* make this point that Beech suffers from

> *...an inner sense of inferiority and hypersensitivity which is projected on to others. Very often such persons grew up in an environment of criticism and harsh expectation and so they inwardly feel very vulnerable and insecure. However, they learn to cope by condemning others instead of healing themselves.*[13]

It may be that Bach had himself grown up with criticism and harsh expectation—his father wanted him to join the family business—so perhaps this was a familiar state of mind.[14] We may imagine him recognizing the problem and once more resorting to his walking meditation in search of the flower, tree or place that would ease the harsh thoughts and bring him back to being:

> *Tolerant, lenient and understanding of the different ways each individual and all things are working to their own final perfection.*[15]

The Wittenham Clumps are a mile and a half north-east of the village of Sotwell. Here a famous group of hilltop Beeches stand guarding an old Iron Age fort. A few miles further away, across the River Thames to the east, there are the Beech woods of the Chiltern Hills. In either direction Bach would have come into the characteristic Beech woodland, said by some to be like entering a cathedral, such is the silent calm and peace. To experience fully the tranquillity of the Beech tree, stand in a Beech wood. Here the tall, smooth trunks rise like slender pillars to the vaulting leaf canopy. Shafts of light, green from the translucent young leaves, shine into the shaded aisles, which are carpeted with dry brown leaf litter of earlier years. So complete is the high roof's delicate tracery of branches that other plants are starved of light. At the woodland edge, brambles, hollies and hazels may survive, but even here the low sweeping branches of the Beech trees close out the sun.

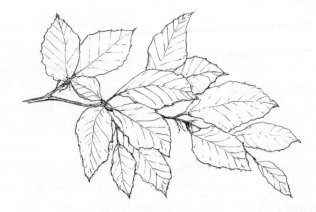

In the Beech remedy state a person becomes isolated, lonely and cut off from others. Criticism and intolerance push people away. It is the same with Beech trees. Edward Step remarks 'it is a powerful competitor with other trees, and if left to fight their own battles unaided, the Beech will be the conqueror'.[16] Evelyn also noted this and commented that in a mixed wood of Oak and Beech, the Beech will dominate and ultimately take over completely. Beech is said to have 'an evil reputation of symbolising selfish ambition, the ambition of a forest prince in the rivalry of the monarch oak'.[17] The good old English Oak, always popular. Boulger goes on to say 'the well-drained soil in which [Beech] delights is by it drained yet more thoroughly; so that it has a marked power of holding the ground against other species . . .'.[18] Or, as Mitchell says, 'Beech can grow up under any species but none can grow up under Beech'.[19]

What does this tell us of both the Beech people and the Beech species? Each of the remedies in the Second Nineteen illustrates one of the ways of grappling with the world. Here, personal insecurity leads to other people being pushed away with criticism, just as Beech trees prevent other species from entering into their growing space. This dominance, like that of Impatiens (page 43), suggests a kind of vulnerability—Beech cannot tolerate competition and the rough play of life and so closes out all other species. Although they appear strong and confident, Beech people are sensitive and vulnerable (shown by the soft hairs that protect the opening leaves). The Beech tree has a superficial hold upon the land: the roots spread outwards over the ground (often above the ground) and rarely penetrate to any depth. In a gale a Beech tree may be upturned, and

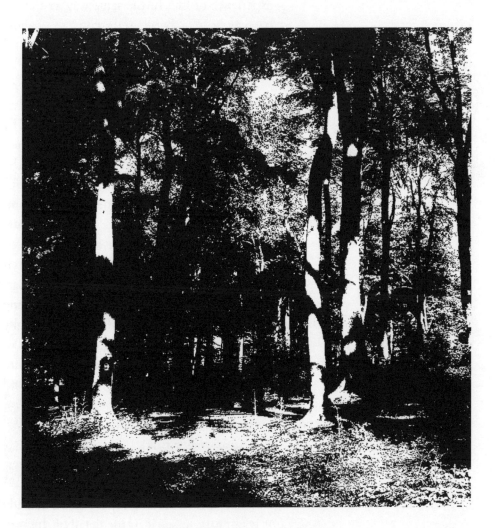

Shafts of sunlight in a Beechwood

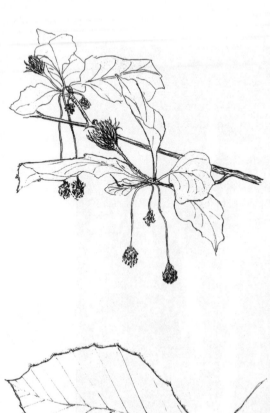

its great, flat plate of roots torn from the earth. It is an uncomfortable picture of a tree which is physically successful yet with a shallow experience of life. In the same way, criticisms by people in a Beech state concern shallow or superficial matters: this is not a profound condition.

Beech flowers do not tell us a great deal more. Male and female flowers appear on the same tree. The males hang like dangling ear-rings. The females appear at the growing tip of the branch like a little nest of wiry spikes, unfriendly. The Beech forms a nut inside a barbed casing. This is nourishing, though nothing like as useful as the acorn. Therefore, we might suppose, there is a value to life in the Beech condition, and some good comes from criticism. But it is not of great value in the scheme of things.

The leaves are beautifully pleated, opening like a perfect parasol or fan, geometrically balanced; further evidence of the push to perfection. The leaf buds are long and thin, like an accusing, pointing finger. The bark of the tree is smooth, showing only the occasional wrinkle like a slipping stocking. If we are looking for the positive, 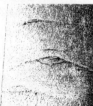 tolerant, understanding aspect of the remedy it is not easy to see it in the detail of the tree. Rather, Beech pushes us to the extreme of experience so that we react from the negative to the positive, like the light and dark within the Beech wood.

15 · What Has Got Into You?

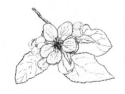

FOLLOWING CLOSELY UPON BEECH comes Crab Apple. Here the finger-pointing and judgemental attitude of Beech is turned back upon us, not in order to question something fundamental but as we worry about seemingly superficial aspects of our health. In the Crab Apple state 'often it is something of apparently little importance,' said Bach.[1] People have a feeling 'as if they had something not quite clean about themselves'.[2] There is a sense that something is wrong and, searching for an explanation, people fix upon a trivial concern, like the small skin blemish which is most easily seen. The condition of the skin is an expression of overall health—skin disease is regarded as analogous with disease of other organs and bodily functions—so it stands to reason that a small spot on the nose is a token of wider internal disorder.[3] But it can be difficult to know what signals what problem. So a sense of proportion can be lost here. That is one aspect of Crab Apple.

Secondly, concern about these superficial problems may become a fixation. Bach commented that some people suffer from a 'more serious disease which is almost disregarded compared to the one thing on which they concentrate . . . which seems so essential to them that it should be cured'.[4] A third factor in the remedy description is a kind of despondency which Bach said can go with Crab Apple, if treatment fails. Furthermore, he spoke of this as 'the remedy of cleansing'—this is a complex remedy which describes several conditions simultaneously:

> *Being a cleanser, this remedy purifies wounds if the patient has reason to believe that some poison has entered which must be drawn out.*[5]

So Crab Apple also operates directly at a physical/medical level. More than any other of the remedies, perhaps. But this cleansing may be needed at a more subtle level, not just for the physical body. Non-physical toxins may have entered into us: emotional poisons, ideas which shadow the clarity of the mind, experiences with a residual sense of being contaminated, infected or defiled. Then Crab Apple helps by bringing cleansing purity of light into the darkening places where the wounds are.

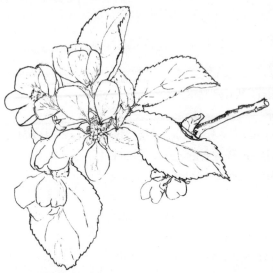

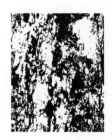

The Crab Apple remedy is prepared from the flowers of the wild apple tree, *Malus sylvestris*. As with Cherry Plum (page 186) these blossoms are a blaze of sweetness and light. That is what makes the essence, the purity of the light, the tender softness of the petals with their pink glow of vitality, opening to the golden heart of the stamens, a soft purifying fire. That is it.

The tree is small and variable in form with a knarled and crooked trunk and a head of dense, interlacing branches. It is shallow rooted, just like Beech (page 224), which denotes the superficiality, and a tendency to be blown over by the wind or pulled over by the attraction of water lines.* The bark is furrowed, irregular, wrinkled and liable to flake—a sign of the diffused and erratic energy in the skin. Noticeably, the bark is frequently covered with moss and lichens. Crab Apple is the chief habitat for mistletoe (*Viscum album*) a parasite which draws nourishment from the sapwood by rooting in through the bark, like a cancer. Bach's own cancer has already been noted. Does this point back to his 'more serious disease which is almost disregarded compared to the one thing on which they concentrate'? The fruit is, of course, the crab itself, green, sharp to taste and a poor eating apple compared to the fat, juicy flesh of domestic ones. But the wild crab is stronger. The little apples will last right through the winter without rotting. The apple is the emblem of health, cleansing and purity, as well as knowledge. The seeds are the small pips found in the core, inside the five-pointed star which forms from the five-petalled flower; a symbol of time and eternity. Yet there is little material here to explain Bach's choice of Crab Apple as a remedy. His selection was informed by what countered the mood of that moment: an empirical experience.

Crab Apple is one of the most popular of the Bach flower remedies (page 284). Someone unwell feels infected, invaded, as if some poison or foreign entity has taken over the body and corrupted the normal

* Water diviner Guy Underwood considered that trees in an orchard could show the path of water or line of earth force as the trees lean over in the direction of the energy flow. See Guy Underwood *The Pattern of the Past*, Museum Press, 1968.

programme of living. A virus does this and so does a cancer. In Bach's writings the words clean, cleanliness, cleanse, pure and purify occur repeatedly as he describes first the need for intestinal cleanliness and its relation to diet,[6] then the cleaning power of his nosodes,[7] 'the spiritual power that cleanses mind and body, and heals',[8] and later the use of clean, pure water for the remedies and 'the clean pure beautiful agents of Nature'.[9] It is not that Bach was obsessed by cleanliness, rather that he realized illness of any kind calls for purification. Crab Apple is the remedy of purification. Purification can range from the simplest act of washing our hands before eating to the most complex rituals of isolation, sacrifice and initiation.* The white apple blossom is the purifying light which acts within the Crab Apple remedy.

If Crab Apple involves the sense that 'some poison has entered which must be drawn out',[10] it is easy to see how it related to Bach's state of health at the time. His friend Nora was clearly appalled by what she saw him going through and described how he needed superhuman courage to survive.[11] His body was 'completely covered' with a rash during the hottest part of the summer. During the year his hair had fallen out, he had leg ulcers and failing eyesight. At one point, she tells us, he was haemorrhaging, presumably bleeding from the bowel, and this only stopped when he found the next remedy. Not a pretty tale. Furthermore, according to Nora,[12] his sensitivity at this time had grown to the point where he was aware of the illness of a patient before they arrived at the house for a consultation. On occasion, he even experienced the symptoms of their illness in his own body a couple of hours before their arrival. This kind of openness to metaphysical experiences—the resonance of the disease and suffering of others—was an extension of the resonance of mental states Bach had experienced when searching for remedies. But it is not healthy and may indicate too great an openness and susceptibility to outside influences.

Out of these experiences, Bach contrived a description of the next remedy state: Walnut. Like Crab Apple, this contains the idea that something has entered the person which is causing damage and distortion. Having cleared the poison out of the system, Walnut is there to close the door and make sure that it does not return. 'This remedy,' he said, 'gives constancy and protection from outside influences'.[13] Outside influences

Walnut

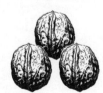

---

* A concise introduction to this subject is available in *The Encyclopaedia Britannica*, fifteenth edition, 1993, Volume 26, pp. 910 ff.

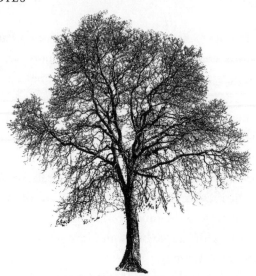

abound—advertising, electro-magnetic signals, peer pressure or psychic attack. The intent here was to protect the person and so maintain control of the soul's purpose. Bach's purpose at this time was to find these new remedies. So the prompt for Walnut was that something was interfering in his work.

> *For those who have definite ideals and ambitions in life and are fulfilling them, but on rare occasions are tempted to be led away from their own ideas, aims and work by the enthusiasm, convictions or strong opinions of others.*[14]

Dr Bach himself can be recognized in the phrasing 'definite ideals and ambitions in life'—it carries an echo of the Elm description, 'doing good work and following their calling in life'.[15] The temptation to be led away from his own ideas must have come from some specific experience. It is as though he came under the influence of a Vervain type (page 105), someone convinced they knew better. But it could equally be that he was experiencing a more subtle form of psychic interference—ideas being put into his mind which subverted his own mental processes. The action of the Walnut remedy rebuilt the integrity of Bach's thinking so that he was once again clear about his path and direction.*

The link between Walnut and the mind is generally made because the nut itself looks like a brain. Not a new thought, but one expressed clearly by William Cole in 1657:

---

* One of the arrangements which Bach gave to the 38 remedies put Walnut opposite to Wild Oat—suggesting that Walnut had a function in giving or maintaining the direction of the life (p. 280).

Wall-nuts have the perfect Signature of the Head: the outer husk or green covering, representing the Pericranium or outward skin of the skull whereupon the hair groweth.... The kernel hath the very figure of the Brain and therefore it is very profitable for the Brain . . .[16]

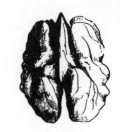

The same thought was expressed in poetry by Abraham Cowley, at about the same time:

Nor can this head-like nut, shaped like the brain
Within, be said by chance that form to gain,
Or Caryon called by learned Greeks in vain;*
For membranes soft as silk her kernel bind,
Whereof the inmost is of tenderest kind,
Like those which on the brain of man we find.
All which are in a seam-joined shell enclosed,
Which of this brain the skull might be supposed.[17]

According to the Doctrine of Signatures† the form of the nut pointed to its value as a medicine for the brain. These days the idea would not be taken literally. But it is not the physical medication that is sought, rather the idea that lies behind the form: what Walnut represents.

The English walnut tree, *Juglans regia,* is not a native but has probably been grown in Britain since the time of the Romans. It came originally from Persia (the modern Iran) and northern India. It was always grown more extensively on the Continent and its Latin name gives it prominence: *regia* as in regal and *Juglans* as for 'Jovis glans' or Jupiter's nut. In the Golden Age mortals might eat acorns, apparently, while the gods ate walnuts.[18] The tree is also linked to the Greek goddess Artemis[19] (Roman, Diana), who 'is goddess of the wild, virgin nature, all the inviolable places where humans dare not enter'.[20] She is a goddess of the wilderness. Baring and Cashford in *The Myth of the Goddess* make the revealing comment that 'there was a purity, an uncompromising autonomy about Artemis that related the uncharted empty spaces in nature to the solitude required by every human being to discover a single identity'.[21] This has a strong echo of the Walnut state. Artemis is also the virgin huntress, the ruler of childbirth, unmarried girls and transition to motherhood. At weddings in Rome, young boys scrambled after walnuts thrown by the bride-groom 'as a sign that he had laid aside childish amusements',[22] according to some authorities.[23] But it was more likely that this was a ritual gift

---

* Greek 'kara' = head, so Caryon.

† See footnote on p. 221.

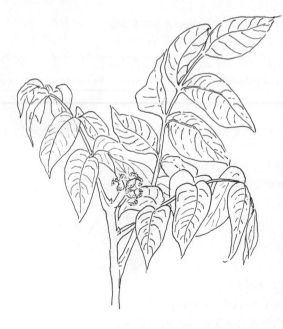

to propitiate the goddess for the loss of one of her maidens. So in classical tradition at least, Walnut is linked to rites of passage and the developmental stages in human society.

Such ideas derived directly from what people observed of nature and the character of the Walnut tree. The female flowers have a striking resemblance to the womb: hence the connection with Artemis. The male flower is a large pendulous catkin, like the penis. So the signature here is rather explicit and walnuts have therefore been regarded as a 'symbol of fecundity'.[24] To make the Walnut mother essence for a Bach remedy only the female flowers are used[25] which leans away from the sexual allusion and looks more to the image of the womb as a protected environment, a place for growth, development and the coming into being for a new life. Bach picked up on this connection to new life in his further comments:

> Walnut is the Remedy of advancing stages, teething, puberty, change of life. For the big decisions made during life such as change of religion, change of occupation, change of country. The Remedy for those who have decided to take a great step forward in life, to break old conventions, to leave old limits and restrictions and start on a new way.[26]

Every new life and every stage on the path of life can be a 'great step forward' and needs protection. At times of change the structure of our energy patterns is loosened to accommodate the new situation; without that loosening people cannot change. But this leaves them more open to interference and the intrusion of distorting forces which may throw them off course. Walnut then acts as a shield, a defensive barrier within which it is safe to assemble the new pattern of identity.

The female flowers grow in the axil of the leaves, often two or three together. They appear as a swollen, green bud, flask-shaped, with two small feathery horns or curving green tongues which grow out from the ovary. These are the stigmas awaiting windblown pollen from the male catkins. When pollinated they blush, coral-pink. This subtle colour change takes place with several flowers (for instance White Chestnut and

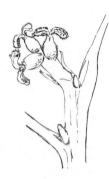

Female Walnut flowers

Cherry Plum, pages 252 and 187). It is a chemical messenger signalling the internal transition. The green fruit swells and internally membranes separate out the different parts which become the kernel of the nut, its skin, the hard shell and the fleshy outer layer. While the nut is forming the inside is like a clear jelly within a wrinkled white skin.

The outer flesh looks like a large unripe plum, 'only the pleasant, alluring flesh of the plum is here represented by a thick, green rind beset with bitter tannin glands which repel with acerbity all attempt to interfere with it'.[27] No bird, insect or animal will penetrate this 'epicarp', so the young are allowed to grow, protected. When the fruit is ripe it will usually fall with the epicarp intact. This covers the hardened shell of the nut within, which in turn is protecting the now tasty kernel. Crows do find ways to break in but more accessible fruit is usually available. Squirrels bury the fruit whole, allowing the bitter outer coat to decay in the ground.[28] Humans harvest walnuts. Juices in the husk stain the hands of those who pickle them and this juice used to be extracted to make a dye. Dr Bach himself used Walnut stain on the furniture he made for *Mount Vernon* and *Wellspring*s, the two houses in Sotwell. Such a dye penetrates the wood and permanently changes its appearance.

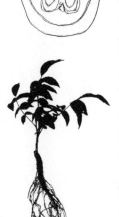

When the nut germinates it quickly puts down one thickened root, like a slim carrot, with many smaller fibrous roots attached. This swollen taproot is characteristic and explains why it is difficult to transplant walnuts trees after they are one or two years old. The seedling tree remains attached to the old shell for some time, continuing to take nourishment from the kernel of the nut. There is a tenacity here, holding to the past while yet growing strongly with a deep-diving intent to anchor in the physical world. With other plants, like Chicory (page 102), the deep root is indicative of an association with the past. With Walnut the link to the past is understood differently, earning the remedy the name of 'the link breaker',[29] or 'spell breaker'.[30]

When the spring leaves first open they are purple-bronze in colour, powdered with gold spots. They look very exotic. The colouring results from the presence of tannins and volatile oils, which have a strong and characteristic odour. This deters all animals which might otherwise eat the fresh young shoots: Mrs Grieve notes that 'no insect will touch the leaves'.[31] This smell is rather like that of Impatiens (page 43), another plant which keeps animals away to avoid molestation. It is said Walnut roots contain the same chemical, and that it poisons other plants. The Walnut remedy takes from all this a quality of isolation and deterrence. In summer the leaves are still scented and oils vaporize in the warm sun. Although they are tougher and less attractive to eat they maintain a shield against predators. By then they have formed a dense shade acting as a barrier to other species. Parkinson remarks: '. . . by reason of his great spreading armes it taketh up a great deale of roome, his shadow reaching farre, so that scarcely any thing can well grow near it.'[32] This antagonism contrasts with the Oak (page 154) which is so receptive and responsive to other species. Walnut offers isolation where an individual may develop alone without the influence of outside forces.

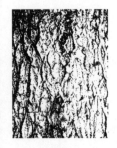

When young, Walnut bark is smooth and green, almost like Beech (page 226). But as the tree ages a pattern of shallow fissures develops giving the appearance of flat ribboning which curves up the trunk and branches. There is no great significance in this but it shows how the Walnut tree changes with age. Bark protects a tree, and when smooth it suggests a sealed coating of energy which has little exchange with outside forces. Older bark shows how the structure has developed—in this case with a more open network of energy which still protects and strengthens the tree.

Walnuts were usually planted deliberately to harvest the nuts; at least, that used to be the case. Writing in 1946, A. L. Howard laments that 'less and less interest has been taken either in the trees or their fruit, and only in a very few cases is any care and attention practised today';[33] far truer now than then. Trees can still be seen in country areas like Herefordshire. They stand sentinel, by a farm gate or in the hedge behind a cottage, a welcome sight when it is known how helpful their protective influence can be. Like Elms (page 194) they represent a link between man and the land. Evelyn wrote of the traditional husbandry in France and Germany, where it was the invariable practice to replant and replace old, decayed walnut trees. No young farmer might marry until he had planted his quota of these trees.[34] Today it might be difficult to find ten young men, married or not, who have tasted a home-pickled walnut this year, let alone planted a walnut tree. Such is the demise of our rural economy.

Holly   It is significant that Dr Bach put both Walnut and Holly under a heading *Over-Sensitive to Influences and Ideas* (page 281); they are next to each other in the text of *The Twelve Healers & Other Remedies*;[35] they flower at the same time. We must assume that, no matter what threatened

Edward Bach at this time, the preparation of the Walnut remedy served to protect him, making him less sensitive to outside influences and ideas. But what if the influences were no longer external but had come from within? The next remedy would need to deal with the effects of such an invasion: Holly. This is the remedy 'for those who are sometimes attacked . . .'.[36] That is how the description begins. Suppose the attack had got past the guards and a negative pattern of interference had actually taken up residence?

The Holly state is very serious, for it describes all kinds of strongly negative emotions which not only burn within a person but express themselves in destructive, even violent behaviour. It is for 'jealousy, envy, revenge, suspicion, the different forms of vexation'.[37] Vexation is a nicely old-fashioned word, but here it does not mean a trifling ill humour but a kind of agitation, intensely malicious. More particularly, it means the experience of being shaken by violent feelings (Latin *vexare*, to shake). Everyone knows what it feels like to be shaken by our own anger or to be shaken by the anger of others. This might well be the most important of the Thirty-eight Bach remedies, since it is for hatred and rage.[38] But Bach put it another way, saying it was a protection 'from everything that is not Universal Love'.[39] He was attempting to avoid the negative characterization of emotions which grow larger the more they are concentrated on. Anger is not wrong in itself, but the lack of love can cause problems. Hatred results from the absence of love; the two are mutually exclusive. Holly is for any persistent negative emotion which violates the sanctity of life.

To understand why Dr Bach chose Holly as a remedy, it is necessary to understand what happens when a person gets jealous or in a rage.* Contemporary neuroscience reckons that 'emotions are complicated collections of chemical and neural responses' leading to 'circumstances advantageous to the organism'.[40] Yet while there may be occasions when anger is useful and appropriate it is essentially a negative reaction to life circumstances. It is not a 'part of homeostatic regulation',[41] bringing balance to the organism or 'survival-oriented behaviour'[42]—at least as far as Bach remedies are concerned. Anger is a reaction to the invasion of an

---

* Shakespeare illustrated the process in *Othello* (1604). Othello and Desdemona are in love. Whispered interference by the wicked Iago poisons and corrupts Othello's mind so that he becomes consumed with jealousy. The result is the tragic collapse of his love leading to murder and suicide.

individual's sense of self; this may mean a breach of integrity, of standards of behaviour, a reaction to the power of something far stronger, a threat to the sense of self-control. Invaded (by physical or non-physical interference) a person may react with outrage. To that extent it is a natural and appropriate response. But the problem arises when outrage becomes habitual. Someone who is habitually angry must experience an habitual stimulus. The invasion or attack which breaches the sense of self has so broken down the natural defences that a part of the being is taken over, it has become occupied territory. Anger then is the reaction to a foreign pattern of activity *within* the boundaries of the self. Far from indicating that homeostasis is at work, it indicates that homeostasis has failed. This is an important concept, since invasive diseases like cancer may be related to anger and the Holly condition.

Holly, *Ilex aquefolium*, is well known for its prickly, evergreen leaves and red berries making it so attractive in winter. It is generally a small tree, slow growing and, unusually, tolerant of shade. While it also grows in the open, this habit of sheltering beneath other trees explains much about Holly and why it was chosen for the remedy. Johns says, 'the Divine Power which fixed its rate of growth ordained at the same time that it should thrive under the shade of its lofty companions. Hence we frequently see it deepening the gloom of a forest, where it is rarely visited by even a few straggling sunbeams . . .'.[43] A tree or plant which grows in the shade requires a dark green leaf to absorb as much light as is available.* This must be significant. Holly needs light; the Holly remedy brings the light of love into the darkness of negativity.

The leaves have an average of fifteen prickles each,[44] arranged both sides of a strong central spine. These prickles force leaves, which would otherwise be flat, to angle into repeatedly changing curves. Each leaf is then set so that maximum light is received whichever direction it comes from. At the same time, any unabsorbed light is reflected by the shiny, waxy surface. It bounces back into the thick of the bush so that other leaves may absorb it in turn. The foliage is very dense, with branches growing in all directions, so the structure of the tree is often hard to

---

*Anthony Huxley in *Plant and Planet*, Allen Lane, 1974, p. 216, says: 'In Britain the common holly is regarded as perfectly hardy ; in the eastern United States a thriving plant will be treated with awe, because it nearly always succumbs to the scorching caused by reflected sunlight off the long-lasting snow.' The very capacity to absorb light becomes harmful when subject to excess.

detect. There may be several small trunks with smooth white-grey bark, which has the effect of bringing light into the middle of the tree, just where it is darkest. Young shoots grow vertically from the base of the tree, their bark green for photosynthesis. All this presents a strongly black and white appearance.

Much is made of the fact that Holly has these prickly leaves: it is said to be a form of protection to deter grazing cattle or deer.[45] But if it is a defensive measure, why does Holly have smooth-edged leaves at the top and outer edges of older trees? Because cattle cannot reach so high? (No giraffes in Europe.) That may be true, but the leaves at the top of a full-grown tree have all the light they need—that is why they have fewer prickles and the leaves are flat. Because some commentators force the issue of defensive or competitive behaviour among plants and animals, Holly is seen as hostile, with the leaves evolving a spiky form. As with the Holly remedy state it is important not to concentrate solely on the negative (anger, jealousy, hatred or greed) but to look for the positive stance, the light in the darkness.

The spiny form of the Holly leaf acts to interlock one branch or shoot with another and thereby one tree with another. This forms a supportive matrix (as with the Gorse, page 148) which helps younger trees to resist movement by the wind. A careful reading of Darwin shows that he was well aware that spines, prickles and hooks serve to assist in plant growth rather than plant defence.[46] Holly trees cannot tolerate movement at their roots (anger shakes the root of our security). When exposed to wind a juvenile, solitary tree will often die back with silvery, dead wood among the bright green new shoots. So this habit of linking arms, as it were, brings support and strength to the group: one reason why Holly is such a good hedging plant.

There is a natural tendency for Hollies to grow together. The seeds are often passed by roosting birds after they have eaten the berries. Each berry has three or four seeds so they are 'planted' in groups. Holly is one of the few trees, therefore, to grow in the understorey of beech woods where pigeons may settle for the night.[47] The small seedling Holly has a long tapering root and in the first years the leaves are at their most curved, contorting themselves in an attempt to find both light and support. Growing in leaf-litter or thin grass at the foot of a full-grown tree or within a hedge, the young Holly will encounter difficulty because of the lack of light and moisture. Only great determination will win through. But Holly can sustain itself, even growing in among the roots of a full-sized oak tree. This shows more of the positive determination which enables the Holly state to be overcome.

The spines on the leaves (*aquifolium* means needle-leaves) are a sharp reminder of the need to reawaken love within. While the negative energy of the Holly state is turned outwards—we are angry with someone rather than with ourselves, we are jealous or envious of others—it is necessary to internalize and find the cause of the problem. The sharp prick of Holly's needle-leaves is painful but stimulates the life force, just as it does with Gorse (page 147). Gorse provides a kick into action. With Holly it is a stab to the heart, homœopathic one might say.

Extraordinary as it may seem, Holly trees were once pollarded (see Willow, pages 218–9) and the branches taken for fodder. They needed to be crushed in a chaff-cutter, but like Gorse, they were nourishing for stock. Where stands of Holly grew for such a purpose they were called 'hollins'. 'One well-defined group is in the Olchon valley in Hereford-shire, where the gnarled pollards stand in a landscape of Celtic fields and ancient stones'.[48] In this area the Holly thrives and it is here that I have most often made the mother essence for the remedy. These trees may form a simple 'hollin' or perhaps a sacred grove. There is something very unusual about the place. There are no pre-Christian records which might explain the history. But it is likely that agrarian, pagan rituals were enacted which involved Holly as the winter king.[49] This is remembered in the *Holly-Tree Carol*:

> Of all the trees that are in the wood,
> The holly bears the crown.

Such a folk memory was recorded in *The Romance of Sir Gawain and the Green Knight*. To quote Robert Graves: 'The Green Knight is an immortal giant whose club is a holly-bush. He and Sir Gawain, who appears in the Irish version as Cuchulain, a typical Hercules, make a compact to behead one another at alternate New Years—meaning midsummer and midwinter'.[50] Sir Gawain represents the sacrificed oak king. This is complex mythology but it was adopted and adapted by early Christians[51] much as was the worship of wells and springs (see Rockwater, page 165).*

---

*'The use of the holly and the ivy was taken over by the Christian church, just as many other features and elements of heathen worship were taken over from time to time on the time-tested principle that it is easier to absorb popular customs than to eradicate them by condemnation' — Moldenke, H. N. & A. L., *Plants of the Bible*, Chronica

Jesus then became the sacrificed god-king; His crown of thorns, a holly wreath; the four-petalled white flowers a symbol of His purity and the cross; the red berries the drops of His blood. The English name Holly then becomes holy.

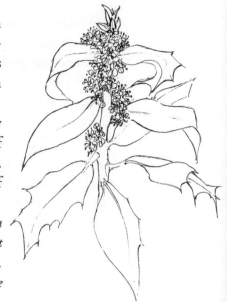

How much does this play into the Holly remedy and perception of the Holly state from Bach's point of view? He was often overtly Christian in his writing. Of Beech he said that at its best it was an example of perfect tolerance:

> It was Christ allowing the soldiers to place the crown of thorns on His head, to pierce His hands and feet with nails without His having one harsh thought. Instead He pleaded on their behalf, 'Father forgive them for they know not what they do.[52]

Holly in flower

This would actually be better applied to Holly. Perfect tolerance is the acceptance of the world's anger and contempt, welcoming in negativity but overcoming it with love. Holly has become the tree of Christ's love, the tree for Christmas.[53] We bring Holly branches into our homes (but only for the days until Twelfth Night) in memory of the renewal which comes after the darkest day of the winter solstice and the renewal of the light of the world. It is still considered to be bad luck to cut down a Holly and when mechanical flails trim the hedges in Herefordshire, Holly trees are always left to grow—often the odd Oak as well.

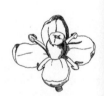

Female flower

The Holly remedy is made from the flowers by the boiling method. Weeks said we can use the female and/or the male flowers.[54] These grow on different trees (the reason why not every Holly bears a berry). The two types of flower are rather similar in construction and appearance: clusters of white around the neck of the twigs, contrasting with the dark leaves. The obvious difference is the female ovary which appears as a small green dome surmounted by four stigmas in the form of a disk. The female flower also has false (vestigial) stamens which are not

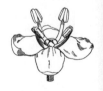

Male flower

Botanica; 1952, p. III. The Roman festival of Saturnalia, described by Pliny as a time when people exchanged wreaths and presents, is quoted as an antecedent for the use of holly at Christmas. But the wreaths were of holly oak, *Quercus coccifera*, a different species. It is an evergreen and has a leaf somewhat like *Ilex aquifolium*. John Parkinson, in his 1640 *Herbal*, repeats Pliny's comment that holly was a safeguard against witches and lightening. Popular folk belief then confused the two trees but borrowed freely of the associations to support the notion that holly had special powers as a tree.

effective in pollination, just as the males have a vestigial ovary. Apparently this is a tree still differentiating its male and female qualities. The female flower buds develop during spring, leading straight to flowering in May, while the male buds develop during the previous summer. It is almost as though it would flower twice in the one year. Similarly, for an unknown reason, berries sometimes remain on the tree, neglected by birds, not just through the winter but on into the following summer. Flower buds in the autumn, with berries at the same time as the blossom, suggests a sustained and perennial energy within the tree, again like Gorse. Love, like hope, springs eternal; it is always there in potential. Holly is sweet-scented and its flowers produce abundant nectar, whose sweetness brings a throng of bees.

One other point about Holly concerns colour: of the leaves, the bark and the berries. Red and green are complementary colours. An easy way to see this is to use a table lamp with a green shade. It will cast a green shadow on to the wall, but place your hand so that the green light falls on it and a red shadow will appear. Conversely, a green shadow will be cast by red light. The complementary colour is stimulated as the light shines into darkness. This effect applies to shadows falling within all green-leafed trees. But the red of the holly berry is beautifully equivalent to the dark green of the leaves. The young shoots, which are green, turn to silver-grey and when mature carry a shading of red. Now, the colour of anger is red, there is no doubt, just as green is the colour of envy or jealousy. These are colours seen in the aura. But equally red is for animation and green for balance and harmony. So Holly as a remedy acts on the point of choice. The energy can be negative or positive according to the intention of the individual; this follows the direction of the soul. If an individual's freedom has been usurped by an outside pattern of activity it will be more difficult for the choice to be made and sustained. We will meet the negativity and be confused as to the process involved.

The Holly remedy, said Bach, may be given when other remedies fail to have the desired effect, or if the prescriber feels too many different remedies are indicated. This is one of the so-called 'catalysts' which Bach recommended—Holly for the active and intense person, while Wild Oat is for the weak and despondent type.[55] Holly was chosen because of this quality of light and dark, positive and negative. Like Beech it prompts the individual to stand forward, to step into the light. Here all may be clearly revealed and seen for what it is.

16 · The Coming of the Light

IT IS APPARENT THAT DR BACH'S FLOWER REMEDIES are centrally concerned with bringing light to the light body. Cherry Plum is about light; Crab Apple is about light; Holly is about light. Many of the flower remedy plants can only be described effectively in terms of a pattern of light. While allopathic medicine looks for chemical action, and homœopathy turns on like curing like, flower essence therapy talks of vibration, resonance or pattern of energy. But these things—pattern, resonance or energy—end up describing the essential qualities of light.

We know that light is only a narrow band in the electro-magnetic spectrum. Visible light lies in the middle of the wider range of waves, from x-rays, through ultraviolet to infrared, microwave and radio waves. Only when they reach our planetary system and meet physical matter, first in the atmosphere and then on land, do these waves illuminate an object. Light does not exist in outer space. Light waves which do not contact a physical body pass by, travelling on into the darkness of space: the moon appears in a dark night sky. Other electromagnetic frequencies are just as invisible and unrecognized, unless there is a suitable receiver for the signal. Radio waves are all around, but we are ignorant of their content until we 'tune in' to the appropriate waveband and then hear the broadcast. In the same way, physical bodies are the aerials or satellite dishes to pick up the electromagnetic waves in the visible spectrum: light.

No great surprise in this. Green plants have physical bodies and their most essential function is to receive and utilize electromagnetic waves in the visible spectrum (light). Through the process of photosynthesis green plants are able to collect radiant energy from the sun and give it physical form. Light energy is thus transformed into chemical energy. The key to this process is chlorophyll* which allows air, water and minerals to

---

* Chlorophyll has a similarity to haemoglobin both in structure and function. Haemoglobin, found in the blood of mammals, is the carrier transporting oxygen and carbon dioxide for respiration. People breathe eight or ten times a minute when the body is at rest. Plants have a longer cycle with a full breath in and out once every twenty-four hours. During that time we might draw 8,000 breaths. It follows that a

be transformed into sugars and the material of plant life. These sugars, in varying forms, are the building blocks of the food chain as roots and leaves, fruit and seeds are eaten by humans and animals. So photosynthesis, by transforming the light of the sun, is the fundamental process which sustains life on earth.

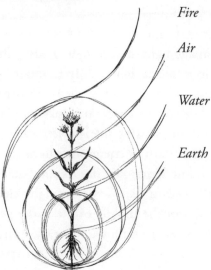

Fire

Air

Water

Earth

Bach spoke of how the sun method (page 61) involved the four elements—earth, air, fire and water.[1] This thought has wider application in the context of plant life. The fire element is the light which brings energy from the sun. Air is represented by oxygen and carbon dioxide, the gases of photosynthesis. Water is also part of the chemical equation, but principally the medium circulating sugars within the leaves, stems and root of the plant. Earth is in the plant root, just as the root is in the earth. These four elements are equivalent to the four parts of the plant. Earth for the root; water for the stem; air for the leaf; fire for the flower. They all interrelate, but the lower is drawn upwards by the higher. Water draws minerals from the earth; transpiration from the leaves draws water up the stem and into the air; the heat of the sun initiates photochemical reactions, releasing oxygen into the atmosphere. The effect of light falling upon earth is to raise each element within a living form to participate in the element above. Light-sensitive organisms grow towards the sun;

---

human metabolic rate is far higher than that of plants. Nonetheless there is a complementary symmetry in the respiration of plants and people: in the oxygen/carbon dioxide cycles, in the red and green of haemoglobin and chlorophyll, in the conversion of heat and light to sugars and these sugars into movement and heat.

there is an ascending energy. Conversely, the energy in light is transferred through air and water into energy within the physical world, in the earth element. There is a double movement: light enters the earth through photosynthesis resulting in an upward growth in plants.

The form of the plant determines the qualities of light brought down into the earth. Differently coloured flowers absorb and reflect different parts of the visible spectrum. Blue reflects blue but absorbs all other parts of the colour range; white flowers reflect almost all visible light while black absorbs. Photosynthesis generates in different plants varying forms of sugar, starch and carbohydrate. And if the form of the plant absorbs different energy patterns then the growth of the plant expresses different patterns of ascending energy. This is apparent in the gesture of the plant, be it structured like Impatiens or more random in growth, like Clematis or Cerato. Plants with a strong geometrical structure radiate patterns of energy which order and structure the environment. In this way plant life has an additional meaning and purpose. Like the light in outer space, this radiant pattern of energy may be invisible but it becomes manifest when attention is focused on the plant. The satellite dish or receiver in this case is human consciousness. The physical plant can be utilized as food for the physical body. The energy form of a plant can be used as food for the light body.

Such an idea supposes that we have a light body, that there is more to us than the physical body. Hard to prove to the sceptic. But this thought certainly was written into everything Bach said about life, health and disease. A person does not need to be clairvoyant to 'see' the light body of a plant. It is something which can be tested empirically by anyone who cares to spend a little time. Of course, time is important since the metabolic rate of plants is so much slower. If one plant breath takes twenty-four hours it may be necessary to sit for ten or fifteen minutes before the pattern of life force in a tree begins to permeate awareness. But in time it becomes clear that each plant gives out energy as well as absorbing the light energy of the sun.

Plants use this ascending energy in general growth but focus it more particularly into the flower. Here, where the fire element is expressed, a transformation takes place leading to new life through fertilization and seed production. The broadcast energy in the flower is at its most excited and radiant: blossoming, shining with light. The intensity of the pattern is greatest as the flower opens, ready for pollination. Scent, colour and design signal this moment to insects making a pathway to the nectar and pollen. It is at this moment that flowers are picked to make an essence—combining the sun's light with the fire element of the flower. The broadcast pattern of light energy is then released in the spring water. The flower essence becomes a vehicle for preserving and transferring this light resonance to another person in another place.

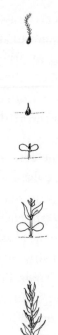

If the flower is at the apex of ascending energy in the plant then the root is at the base of descending light. In the root starch is stored: a supply of energy for the next year's growth. Similarly seeds fall back to earth, pellets of energy and life potential. But there is a further descent where the light energy fixed in the physical form of plants decays and becomes transformed again. It can become coal, oil and gas—fire, or the potential for fire, in solid, liquid or gaseous form. This is the fire used for the boiling method.*

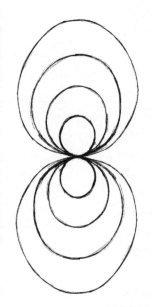

The fire is thus transformed—from light, through the sugars of photosynthesis, to the hydro-carbon compounds of fossil fuel. Fossil fuels are then burned releasing light, heat, gases and water into the atmosphere. A similar path of transformation can be seen in the hydrological cycle as water carried in the air falls as rain, enters the earth and settles in aquifers underground. It is then reborn to the light in a spring or source. This cycle parallels the cycle of physical birth, life and death of human beings on earth. Like spring water, they are born and live on the surface of the earth, in the light. After death the physical body returns to darkness, to the elements of which it was made. Return to darkness or return to light?

This may be wandering into the realms of metaphysical speculation. Yet these observations are not invented but based upon what can be seen in the world around. This process of

---

* That fire of this kind is associated with the Bach remedies made by the boiling method has a curious but significant parallel in the legend of Prometheus. Prometheus stole fire from the gods. As a punishment Zeus created Pandora. She took the lid off a great jar she carried (Pandora's Box) and released into the world all kinds of misery. The problems caused by these difficulties are like the life problems the boiling remedies help to overcome. In another tale, Prometheus is punished by Zeus by having his liver

observation led Charles Darwin to conclude there was an evolution in species accounting for the changes in type, whether plant or animal. His theories form the basis for contemporary 'scientific' explanations for human life: the descent of man. As far as they go these make sense and explain the adaptation of physical form to a changing environment. The problem is that no account is taken of the evolution of consciousness. Neo-Darwinian theories about life suppose an evolution based only upon physical or material form: the earth element alone. Include the idea of consciousness at the beginning of creation and it is easy to suppose a parallel evolution of both physical and non-physical forms: matter and spirit.

Light is invariably the emblem of spirit: divine light, the light of love, the light of creation. Physical light, so vital in photosynthesis, matches the light of the spirit. These two inform the populations of the world, plants and people. It is obvious when this light of the spirit shines strongly in a person, or if it shines at all. It can be seen when that same light shines in nature, more than the common light of day (see overleaf). It is this light which potentizes the mother essence in the making of a Bach remedy. It is the qualities of this light which can be described by reference to the form and gesture of a remedy plant.

The Universe is God rendered objective; at its birth it is God reborn; at its close it is God more highly evolved. So with man; his body is himself externalized, an objective manifestation of his internal nature; he is the expression of himself, the materialization of the qualities of his consciousness.[2]

With these words at the end of *Heal Thyself*, Bach expressed his sense for evolution of life and consciousness. The thought can be expressed another way. People are born with particular qualities—physical, emotional, mental and spiritual. These can be equated to each of the four elements earth, water, air and fire. They are the qualities given for life. These qualities are set to the test of reality on earth and there is the opportunity to evolve greater capacities such as for love and learning; the great soul lessons which Bach described.[3] Through this process, life on earth evolves. That which is learnt in life burns as soul flame certainties, soul flame qualities. These are carried with us as we enter another level of reality, the next dimension.

---

pecked out by an eagle. A gruesome picture. But the liver is traditionally the organ of emotions, so there is a further link between fire and emotional trauma.

≈ ≈ ≈ ≈ ≈ ≈

The same William Wordsworth who thought so little of the Larch tree (page 210) was eloquent about light and how our eyes acclimatize to mundane reality:

> *Our birth is but a sleep and a forgetting:*
> *The soul that rises with us, our life's Star,*
> *Hath had elsewhere its setting,*
> *And cometh from afar:*
> *Not in entire forgetfulness,*
> *And not in utter nakedness,*
> *But trailing clouds of glory do we come*
> *From God, who is our home:*
> *Heaven lies about us in our infancy!*
> *Shades of the prison-house begin to close*
> *Upon the growing Boy,*
> *But he beholds the light, and whence it flows,*
> *He sees it in his joy;*
> *The Youth, who daily further from the east*
> *Must travel, still is Nature's priest,*
> *And by the vision splendid*
> *Is on his way attended;*
> *At length the Man perceives it die away,*
> *And fade into the common light of day.*

Wordsworth found but a painful inspiration in nature to bring him back towards the light:

> *To me the meanest flower that blows can give*
> *Thoughts that do often lie too deep for tears.*

(From *Ode: Intimations of Immortality from Recollections of Early Childhood*, written 1802–4, first published 1807)

17 · Making the Pattern, Breaking the Pattern

LEONARDO DA VINCI, great genius of the Italian Renaissance, was particularly interested in botany. He made careful studies of plants, which he used in his paintings. They were often symbolic, allowing the painting to be understood at several different levels.* A small four-petalled flower (from the genus *Crucifer*) held by the infant Jesus, pointed to knowledge of His coming crucifixion: the plant chosen to foreshadow the future. The geometry of flowers and their patterns of growth and form were also used by artists and architects to express the divine impulses of balance and harmony within creation. This found its clearest and most brilliant expression in the Gothic cathedrals, especially in the rose window, with its twelve-fold geometry and dazzling colour.

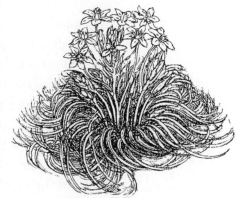

Leonardo's Star of Bethlehem

One of Leonardo's drawings shows the small flowers of the Star of Bethlehem. These have a perfect geometry, just like the cathedral window. Six pointed petals surround six stamens, which form a coronet around the six-celled ovary with its single style (interestingly 6+6+6+1=19, like the Second Nineteen remedies). The flowers express a formal design, yet Leonardo has drawn leaves as a wild, swirling vortex of lines. They are like spiralling water. Surprisingly, for Leonardo was usually accurate in his depiction of plants,[1] this is not as the leaves are found in nature. When young, the leaves are straight like small spears; by the time the flowers open, they have begun to die back and collapse. Why would Leonardo choose to exaggerate the picture of Star of Bethlehem in this way? What might be the symbolism? It might be that he has drawn the inner character (the soul quality, if you will) of the plant. This combines

---

* 'Leonardo knew the iconography of plants in a painting would convey specific historical meanings to the viewer. Often painters scattered plants about their canvases as allegorical decoration.' William A. Emboden, *Leonardo da Vinci on Plants and Gardens,* Christopher Helm; 1987, p. 105.

static geometry with the generative movement of life force. The dynamic movement of the leaves could represent the turbulent experience of life which supports the pure, crystalline form of the flowers; spirit born into the material world.

Star of Bethlehem

The beautiful white flowers of the Star of Bethlehem (*Ornithogalum umbellatum*) were chosen by Bach as a remedy for shock and distress:

> *The shock of serious news, the loss of some one dear, the fright following an accident, and such like.*
>
> *For those who for a time refuse to be consoled this remedy brings comfort.*[2]

It is not difficult to imagine that Bach would have occasion to need such a remedy, although there is no record of any particular event which prompted its discovery. Nor is it known whether it came before or after Walnut and Holly in the sequence. It flowers from late April through to early June, reaching a peak in mid-May.

A vital ingredient in Bach's five-flower rescue combination, Star of Bethlehem is one of the most significant remedies in the whole Bach system. The action of the remedy brings balance and calm to those caught up in the swirling whirlpool of life trauma—just such a picture as Leonardo drew. The geometry of the flowers helps to reassemble the structure of life when it has been tumbled and broken by shock.

The six-pointed star of this plant is unique among Bach's flowers. The others are mostly five-petalled, like the rose family (Crab Apple and Wild Rose) or four-petalled (like Mustard and Holly). To see the significance of this, take a piece of paper and a pair of compasses; then draw a circle. This circle is one. It is a perfect construction, a line without beginning or end, a symbol of unity.

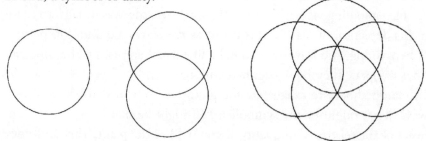

Place the point of the compasses anywhere on the circumference of the circle, and, using exactly the same setting (radius), draw another circle. The second circle passes precisely through the centre of the first. One leads to both two and three: there are now two circles and the

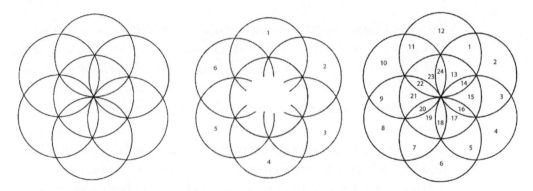

overlap—that which joins them. Where the second circle crosses the line of the first there are two more points on which a circle may be drawn. Continue in this way and, if the setting of the compasses is maintained, six circles fit precisely around the first.

Again this is a perfect construction, just like the single circle at the beginning. It has moved from 1 to 2 to 3 to 6 and 7. Many ideas have been based on this simple drawing: it may explain why there are seven days in a week, six to work and the seventh day of rest. The number of sections in the drawing add up to both 12 and 24. This gives the months of the year and the hours of the day: divisions of time and space.

If, as well as a pair of compasses a straight edge or ruler is also used, by bisecting the original circle it is possible to construct many other geometrical forms. Connect the points 12 – 9 then 5 – 2 and a cross is drawn. Connect 1 – 2 – 3 – 4 – 5 – 6 and there is a hexagon; 12 – 10 – 8 – 12 then 11 – 9 – 7 – 11 and there is a Star of David; many more patterns can be created.

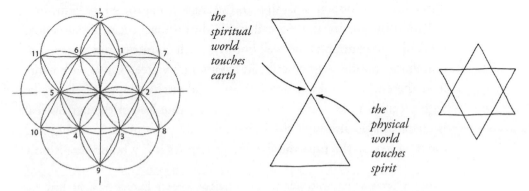

The Star of David is composed of two triangles, sometimes used to represent the coming together of heaven and earth: one pointing down for the spiritual world, one pointing up for the physical world. It is the balance of forces represented by the triangles which leads to harmony and health. That is the positive state for Star of Bethlehem: order and balance. All of this geometry can be seen in the star form of the flowers.*

For those who experience trauma there is a dislocation between the physical and subtle body—the geometry is distorted. This may happen as a result of physical accidents (broken bones, wounds, bruising, a fall) or as a result of some psychological trauma ('serious news, the loss of someone dear, the fright following an accident').[3] In both cases there is disruption in the normal flow of energy and information. The remedy acts to repair this by realigning the matrix of subtle and physical links in living forms.

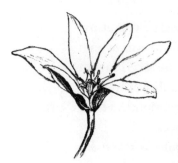

There is another way to interpret the quality and gesture of Star of Bethlehem. The flowers shine with light, lying like a carpet of stars among the grass. They are particularly sensitive to sunshine and only open on warm, clear days (like Gentian, page 130). The buds unfold afresh each morning. One local name for Star is 'eleven o'clock lady' (the French call it *dame d'onze heures*). The flower may last up to three weeks before the petals tire of this daily movement and collapse. On the back of the petals is a broad green stripe which camouflages the flowers when closed. Opening in the sun, they bring a sudden sparkle of light to the meadow grass. Looking more closely into individual flowers reveals six points of yellow pollen as the stamens surround a golden jewel in the heart of the star, warming and strengthening the white light.

Parkinson, writing in 1629, called this 'the ordinary starre of Bethlehem [which] is so common, and well knowne in all countries and places, that it is almost needlesse to describe it, having many green leaves with white lines therein, and a few white flowers set about the toppe of the stalke with greenish lines down the backe'.[4] The white line in the narrow leaf is characteristic although the leaves are only prominent in spring and often wither by the time the flowers appear. As it is a bulb there is only

---

* The medieval masons who built the cathedrals of Western Europe thought there was particular meaning in these geometrical constructions. The area where two circles overlap was called the *vesica piscis* (fish bladder) and it has a constant proportion of 15:26 which was used as a scale throughout Gothic architecture and Renaissance painting. It is the basis of much sacred geometry.

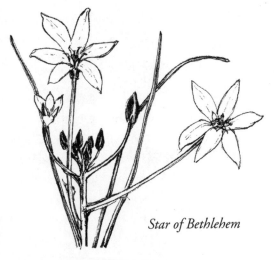

Star of Bethlehem

one stem, though this branches to form an 'umbel'—a flat-topped flowering head (hence *O. umbellatum*). Individual flowers are thus linked back to a common axis in the central stem: a miniature tree form. This structure is common to many plants, but with Star of Bethlehem the strength and clarity of the form is pronounced.

The Star of Bethlehem remedy is prepared by the boiling method (page 199). It is somewhat shocking to see these beautiful flowering stems collapse in the heat of boiling water. One might think this remedy should be made by the more gentle sun method. But it is not for a gentle condition. Fire transforms. It brings about a change in state. This can also be said of accidents, shock and trauma. They break up the pattern of the past and interrupt the established order of life experience.[5] At times this may be necessary to allow for new growth. When people experience the fire of change they may react with symptoms of grief and distress. Star of Bethlehem helps to reform a stable patterning in the emotional life. Dr Bach called it 'the comforter and soother of pains and sorrows'.[6]

Where Star of Bethlehem is needed to reassemble a pattern with clear lines of geometry and structure, White Chestnut dispels a repeating pattern of thoughts. These thoughts, said Bach, 'seem to circle round and round and cause mental torture'.[7] The link to Star of Bethlehem can be seen by imagining an accident and attendant shock. Star would bring comfort and ease the trauma. But suppose the sequence of events is played and replayed in the mind, like a tape recorder on an endless loop. That produces the White Chestnut state: 'thoughts which worry and will remain, or if for a time thrown out, will return'.[8]

White Chestnut

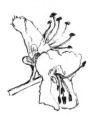

The flowers of White Chestnut, *Aesculus hippocastanum,* lack defined shape or design. Single flowers, thirty to forty of them, are held in a loose pyramid on a central stem. A complex spiral of small side branches hold sets of two, three or four flowers. The effect is made more irregular by the fact that on these smaller stalks the blooms open randomly through the weeks of early summer. Bursts of varying intensity pulse through the massed light of the flowering candles. Each single flower has five amorphous white petals, delicate and beautiful, but uneven in form. The

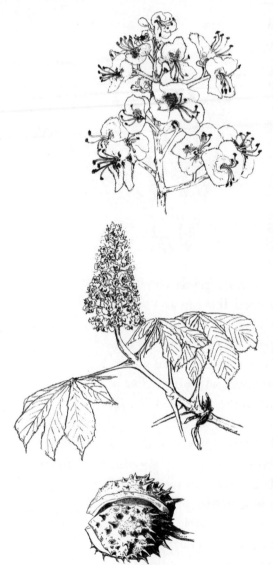

centre of each flower is splashed with yellow, which quickly turns to red on pollination. Fringed with hairs, the petals grow larger as the bud opens. The botanical form varies: some flowers are infertile—this limits the number of seeds once the first flowers are fertilized, setting a restraint on the future generation.* In a perfect White Chestnut flower there are five sepals, five petals, seven stamens, one pistil and a three-chambered ovary containing two rudimentary seeds. Another contrast with the clear form of Star. The seven stamens are very prominent, curving out like tongues from a mouth. Altogether the impression is one of change, movement and asymmetry. The flowers are not disorderly but do not conform to a clear pattern or geometry.

If few flowers set seed, fewer still develop as ripe fruits; maybe only two or three from each flowering head. These are the well-known conkers of the horse chestnut tree. They fall in October, the outer case splitting open when they hit the ground—indicative of the plant gesture, as the form is broken apart when it reaches earth. The prickle-studded seed case is designed both to cushion the fall and to ensure that the sphere breaks open. The spikes, like Gorse leaves (page 148) and the prickles of Wild Rose (page 269), stimulate action in order to break the mental pattern. This is vital if the seed of a new future is to be set free. As if to confirm the varying form of the White Chestnut flowers, no two of these 'conkers' are exactly alike. Gathered by schoolchildren for conker fights, they are involved in more hitting and breaking apart.[9] If not removed, a hundred small saplings may grow beneath a tree in springtime. But they will fail through lack of light and moisture.

---

* G. S. Boulger gives a concise description of the complex arrangement of the flowers: *Each 'thyrse', as they are technically termed, from the triumphal sceptre, or 'thyrsus', of*

The horse chestnut tree has a characteristic outline, with a forked trunk and radiating boughs. The branches have a curious habit of curving and drooping, rather like Larch. It is a weak form, lacking integrity and upright gesture. The roots spread over the surface of the ground and do not penetrate deeply into the earth. The wood splits easily and limbs will often break off in high winds. Mature trees rarely live more than 200 years, usually less. The bark starts out lithe and smooth but becomes fractured: rough squares peel away from the trunk like scales, uneven and unstructured. Only the leaves have a more powerful and 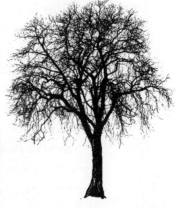 regular form. Five, six or seven leaflets form a palmate or compound leaf; the largest may be as much as thirty centimetres long. The single leaflet is strongly ribbed with a prominent skeleton, the edges jagged, the surface smooth and hairless. Here, at least, is an indication of determination and clarity, as with Impatiens.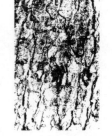

White Chestnut is prepared by the sun method—the only remedy of the Second Nineteen which is not a boiler. Puzzling perhaps? If all the other mother essences which Dr Bach made in 1935 used his new boiling method, why did he suddenly change for White Chestnut? It was not merely the convenience of sunshine in an otherwise cloudy summer (page 201). The most cogent argument is that Bach had already made a boiling remedy from this species: Chestnut Bud.[10] Though he used leaf buds and not open flowers for Chestnut Bud (page 207) the remedy comes from the whole tree and aspects of the whole tree inform the gesture. So Chestnut Bud must be closely related to White Chestnut. Indeed, this is so. Both speak of breaking up repeated patterns, but White Chestnut, because it uses the flowers and the sun method, is aimed more at a mental pattern, less at the life action. There is a difference in the level of consciousness involved.

Bacchus, is borne on a stout stalk, the branches of which are given off in a somewhat complex manner, forming a series of one of those spiral 'cymes' that puzzle the student of structural botany. The flowers nearest the stalk on the lower branchlets are the first to open, and receiving the full benefit of the nutriment prepared in the young and vigorous leaves, develop both stamens and pistils, so that they will be still represented amid the storms of the autumn equinox by the well-known globular fruits. The upper part of the thyrse bears flowers which are generally exclusively staminate, or male, and disappear after the discharge of their pollen; so that, eight, six or more commonly but two or three fruits will in autumn be the sole result of all the beauty of an entire pyramid of blossoms. (Boulger, G. S. *Familiar Trees*, Cassell & Co., 1906, Vol. 1, p. 12.)

This issue, concerning the level of consciousness involved, is complex but significant. Dr Bach's description for White Chestnut spoke of 'times when the interest of the moment is not strong enough to keep the mind full'.[11] This points to a problem of the mind, not an action of the will. The air element is predominant—that is why the leaves carry the strongest patterning (page 242). In this respect, there is a similarity to Clematis (page 47), which is in the same group as White Chestnut: *Not Sufficient Interest in Present Circumstances*.[12] What may appear to be a Clematis state can be White Chestnut; people have the same abstracted air. The overall gesture may be different, but there are elements in common: the white flowers, the rough bark, the smooth leaf and so on. In this same group for '*Not Sufficient Interest . . .*' is Chestnut Bud. Like Clematis and White Chestnut, Chestnut Bud lacks observation and involvement in life. But the boiling method, combined with the part of the plant used, brings out a different aspect in the remedy.

Red Chestnut

If a similarity in gesture notifies a similarity in emotional state then White Chestnut must be close to Red Chestnut—they are related species. Red Chestnut is like the white horse chestnut, but a slighter tree, of smaller build. The most obvious difference is in the flowers, which are rose-red, opening a week or two later than the white. Red Chestnut, *Aesculus carnea*, is the offspring of a cross between *A. hippocastanum*, White Chestnut, and *A. pavia*, the red buckeye of the southern United States. It dates from about 1818 so there is no possibility of some divine creation of this species at the beginning of time—it is a hybrid.[13] Nonetheless, *A. carnea*, Red Chestnut, does breed true and has become a species in its own right.

Bach described the Red Chestnut state as 'for those who find it difficult not to be anxious for other people'.[14] The story goes that he was doing some work in the garden at *Mount Vernon*, when he cut himself. According to Nora Weeks' account[15] he was chopping wood—though we might wonder what he was doing chopping wood at the end of May—when the axe slipped and he 'gashed his wrist'. He was in shock and given first aid*

---

* Nora Weeks in *The Bach Remedy News Letter* tells of 'first aid' being given in the June 1951 account and in December 1960, when the story was repeated. But in March 1970, when the item on Red Chestnut was published once again it speaks of Dr Bach being given Rescue Remedy (the Five Flower combination). Star of Bethlehem had only just been discovered in 1935 when the accident occurred. The question arises exactly when was the rescue combination actually formalized?

but, although 'pale and shaky and almost fainting from loss of blood',[16] it was the reaction of Nora and friends which claimed Bach's attention. He felt their fear and anxiety at his condition made matters worse. Nora noted that, at this time, so acute was his sensitivity that he experienced any worry, depression or fear in other people as an 'actual physical hurt'.[17] Feeling the worry of his friends, he declared that he had just experienced the emotional state for his next remedy: Red Chestnut's fear for the safety of others. A day or two later he found the flowers and made a mother tincture by the boiling method.

The story of Red Chestnut led Nora Weeks to conclude we are all susceptible to the influence of other people's thoughts, for good or ill. Negative thoughts, even if unexpressed, have a powerful impact. Thoughts for safety, health and success,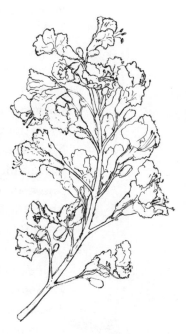
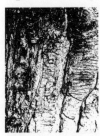 likewise. So the connection between Red and White Chestnut is here in the process of thinking: how to break or change the pattern of thought. Not surprisingly, the gesture of the two types of tree is similar. They have the same structure of trunk and branches, the same flaky bark, similar buds, similar leaves. But there are distinct differences. In all respects a Red Chestnut tree is less robust, more liable to disease and damage. The seeds are much smaller, the casing smooth and often empty—no valuable conkers here! The strength of the remedy comes more from the power in the colour of the flowers.

Being a hybrid, Red Chestnut often shows variations between one tree and another. Some flowers are deep orange or vermilion, others more pink and touched with a mauve-red. There is a yellowy centre which darkens after pollination. So there is both change and variety in flower colouring. None of the other Bach flowers is so strongly coloured.* Bach said of people who need Red Chestnut, 'often they have ceased to worry about themselves . . .'.[18] It is as if the red flowers voice an outward concern, not a fear for the self—red is coming towards you, an active,

---

* Red Chestnut, Gentian, Heather, Elm, Larch, Pine and Honeysuckle are all red in colour and each of these remedies, in the positive state, speaks of contentment and confidence in the present circumstances. That relates to the needs of a Red Chestnut fear.

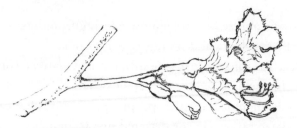

stimulating colour, projecting energy. This contrasts with White Chestnut and Clematis, which internalize. Red Chestnut fear for others is also in contrast to the Chicory 'over-care for the welfare of others'[19] which, with the recessive blue flowers is really an internal concern for self.

Whence comes the Red Chestnut state? Dr Bach noted a concern for others, 'especially those dear to us'.[20] It is as if, in the past, something did indeed happen to someone loved: Red Chestnut is a renewed response to that traumatic life event. These people's fear is partly based upon such a memory and, as with Honeysuckle (page 264), the red flowers call into the present, saying 'stop!' to the pattern of the past. Another look at Nora's concern for Dr Bach's wood-cutting accident indicates that this was not the first time Nora saw Edward in pain and needing help.[21] Any person in a Red Chestnut state resonates with accidents and mishaps which they remember, projecting that image upon a child or loved one:

> *If they return late, there is the thought that some accident must have happened; if they go for a holiday, the dread that some calamity will befall them. Some illnesses become* [grave concerns, as if] *very serious complaints, and there is a great anxiety even for those who are not dangerously ill. Always fearing the worst and always anticipating misfortune for them.*[22]

Red Chestnut is like maternal concern for a daughter. That does not exclude fathers and sons, rather it addresses the mother in us all: protecting and caring for the vulnerable. Red Chestnut is a weak tree, in contrast with Oak or Elm; it needs protection. With stooping branches, tumbling like tresses of hair, Red Chestnut has a feminine appearance. Yet the red flowers are powerful. This gesture speaks of empathy and an understanding which appreciates how others feel; of sensitivity and openness which does not overwhelm; of strength and the determination to give emotional support.

Bearing in mind that Bach was being thrust (Nora called it 'passing through') from one emotional state to another, we might consider what really was happening at this time. Back in 1928 (page 31) he left behind the physical laboratory, with its petri dishes, flasks and retort stands, and travelled out from London with the only laboratory he now needed: he was conducting experiments upon himself. By 1935, he must have been both fascinated and appalled by what those experiments had revealed. The experience of successive emotional states and the process of searching for a remedy must have been almost familiar by now. Yet so many questions remained. How did he come upon each successive experience? Were they merely accidental? If planned, then planned by whom? If some other agency was guiding this process of discovery or forcing Bach along a particular path, then who or what was it? Was Bach following the instructions of his teachers? If so, who were they, and how did they communicate? If the process of discovery originated only with Bach himself (his higher self or soul being the instructing voice) then how did he distinguish that voice? In chapter four of *Free Thyself* he wrote:

> *Our soul (the still small voice, God's own voice) speaks to us through our intuition, our instincts, through our desires, ideals, our ordinary likes and dislikes; in whichever way it is easiest for us individually to hear. How else can He speak to us? Our true instincts, desires, likes or dislikes are given us so that we can interpret the spiritual commands of our soul by means of our limited physical perceptions, for it is not possible for many of us yet to be in direct communion with our Higher Self.*[23]

Clear enough, apparently. But the discovery of each new remedy also brought him into a state where he was acutely suffering the very problems of separation from higher self.

Of Dr Bach's writings and letters little or nothing comes from this period, the summer of 1935. He wrote notes for an essay on pain[24] and a short *cri de cœur* explaining, perhaps, his view of what was happening to him:

> *No man would be a leader amongst others for any length of time unless he were more expert in his special branch of knowledge than his followers: whether it be army, statesmanship or whatever it may be. It therefore follows, to be a leader against trouble, difficulties, disease, persecution and so forth, the leader must still have a greater knowledge, a more intimate experience than, pray God, his followers need ever suffer.*[25]

But the most eloquent account of how he felt and what he was experiencing came from the remedies he found and the indication for their use.

Pine

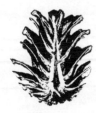

So, by the end of May, he felt a failure. Despite his hard work and the constant attempt to make progress he was discontented and blaming himself for a lack of success. Dr Bach a failure? Who would believe it? Ridiculous! No, not ridiculous; he felt a failure, not *was* a failure. His description for Pine reads as a clear statement of his circumstances. He is saying: 'I blame myself. Even though I have been successful, I know that I could have done better. I work hard but I make errors and I am dissatisfied with what I achieve.' What is the origin of this state of mind? Putting it baldly, it derives from severity of the father. If Red Chestnut concerns apprehension in the mother then Pine concerns stricture from the father.

Many people have written books about Dr Bach's remedies. Often these are based upon an author's case notes, describing the remedies according to practical experience in diagnosis and therapeutic use. Taking three such authorities it is interesting to compare their descriptions for Pine. Chancellor, who compiled his book using material from Nora Weeks,[26] focused upon the self-condemnation associated with Pine, contrasting Pine and Rockwater. Rockwater people feel good about themselves and are proud of their harsh values, Pine people feel bad about themselves and are discontented with their efforts. But Chancellor does not tell us why. Mechtild Scheffer, who says she based her book upon fourteen years' experience in Germany,[27] goes more deeply. She pivots the action of the remedy on the Old Testament/New Testament values of God's severity and forgiveness. The Pine state, she says, comes from 'dogmatic, excessively moral concepts and powerful commandments'.[28] Using keywords she makes reference to the Protestant work ethic, guilt about sex, an all-seeing God, suffering and penitence, moral severity, the expectation of punishment. There is, for her, a clear link to Christian salvation, Jesus Christ and the sins of the world.[29] For a third authority, there is the description provided by Richard Katz and Patricia Kaminski in their American *Flower Essence Repertory*. The Pine person, they write, feels a disproportionate guilt. 'These feelings may arise from childhood, when the person learned to internalize blame for dysfunction in the family system, or they may stem from a religious background which emphasizes sin and error more than salvation and grace'.[30] They go on to point out the context of giving in for-giving. That is, of not withholding love from the self, of releasing energy that is blocked and not holding on to past patterning.

All these help to describe Pine; they are based upon experiences of various people which trace their roots back to the remedy state. Scheffer's description narrows to a Christian view of guilt and forgiveness, while Katz and Kaminski make a more open appeal to 'Father and Fathering Forgiveness'. Katz and Kaminski also make a significant cross-reference to 'time relationship', their subject heading for remedies which have a connection to the past. This will be borne out by observation of the life history of the tree.

A few observations about Edward Bach and his possible relationship with father and family help to complete the background. He was 'a delicate boy'[31] and while Weeks recalled his boyhood determination to be a doctor he actually began work, aged sixteen, in his father's brass foundry. As the oldest son, perhaps he was expected to enter the family business. He worked there, unhappily, for three years before telling his father he wanted to be a doctor—clearly he took a long time to approach the conversation. According to Weeks he felt that he could not ask his family for money. In chapter five of *Heal Thyself* Bach stated and restated his view that parents must not interfere with the will of their child: 'independence, individuality and freedom should be taught from the beginning and the child should be encouraged as early as possible in life to think and act for himself. All parental control should be relinquished step by step . . .'.[32] He repeated this in *Free Thyself*: 'so many suppress their real desires and become square pegs in round holes: through the wishes of a parent . . .'[33] and on the next page 'some from childhood have the knowledge of what they are meant to do, and keep to it throughout their lives: and some know in childhood, but are deterred by contra-suggestions and circumstances, and the discouragement of others'.[34] Why make such an issue of this unless he had felt himself to be constrained by the expectations of his father? The potential for family difficulty was clearly there. And it is a part of the quality of Dr Bach's discoveries that they were not merely theoretical but grounded in the reality of his (and everyone's) life experience.

So Pine is an emotional state Bach understood; it spoke with the voice of his past:

> *For those who blame themselves. Even when successful they think that they could have done better, and are never content with their efforts or the results. They are hard-working and suffer much from the faults they attach to themselves.*

Sometimes if there is any mistake it is due to another, but they will claim responsibility even for that.[35]

For Bach it may have been a straightforward case of amplifying this emotional state and finding the flower which resonated in response: by now he must have become practised at this procedure. Observation of the Pine tree's gesture is almost separate and independent of the remedy description; there is little obvious correlation. However, in the life cycle of the tree we can begin to see how this remedy manifests itself in the form of the Scots Pine, *Pinus sylvestris*.

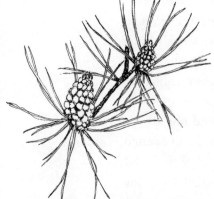

Pine is a conifer, one of a group of trees which share characteristics such as narrow, needle-like leaves, resinous sap and a fruit in the form of a woody cone. They are called gymnosperms because the seeds are 'naked' (page 212)—'their ovules, which later become seeds, are born exposed on the scale of the immature cones or female flowers'.[36] The only other gymnosperm in the Bach range is Larch. In evolutionary terms gymnosperms are older than other flowering plants; they formed the major component of vegetation which was compressed to make coal and so relate to the fire element formed within the earth. This immediately links Pine to the past and deep processes of change.

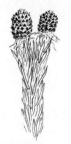

Male Pine flowers

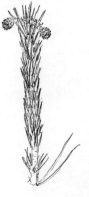

Female Pine flowers and immature cones

Pine is an emotional condition which develops over time. Like a mole it burrows out of sight, reappearing unexpectedly. Or, as with certain traumatic events, it remains buried in memory, to surface years later. This delay can be seen in the process of pollination and growth of the seed. While the flowers of Red and White Chestnut change colour almost immediately, to signal fertilization, Pine has a prolonged period of incubation during which seed embryos develop. The process is complex. It takes nearly a year for the male pollen grain and the female ovule to mature fully inside a cone and for fertilization to occur.[37] During this time cones remain outwardly unchanged; in January or February they are still small brown knobs, as seen last summer, bending over at the end of shoots. When spring arrives a new shoot will grow upwards and produce flowers. Meanwhile the cone, now sitting under the branch, swells and begins to form seeds internally. These will not be ready until the following spring, when the cone is nearly two years old. So three stages of cone growth can be seen on a branch: the female flower, last year's immature cone and the ripe cone of the year before. A picture of successive generations: grandparent, parent and child.

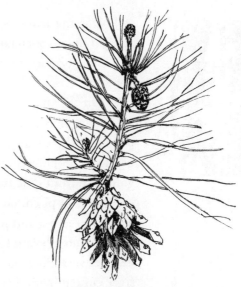

When the seeds are ripe the cone will open and release them. Here too the Pine tree behaves in a most remarkable way: the cone opens and closes according to the conditions. When it is wet the woody bracts close up, sealing the seeds in their compartments. Only when the air is dry and warm will they open. It is protective behaviour yet controlling of the future. Take a dry cone and run water over it and you will see all this happen; it takes a few minutes. The seeds have a small wing and are carried away from the parent tree, anything up to 750 metres.[38] This

Three generations together

slow drifting down to earth is paralleled in other remedy plants whose seeds are carried on the wind: Clematis, Wild Oat, Aspen, Hornbeam, Larch. Each of them shares a quality of detachment, of not being directly engaged in life at the present moment. For people in a Pine state, this debility is in the need to escape from memories of parental control; their inner child still feels something has been done which is wrong. They are held in the past.

Germination among Pine seeds is very good: in the positive remedy condition there is a strong drive to take up life opportunity. Johns quotes a nice passage by Sir T. D. Lauder in his *British Trees*:

> *It is curious to observe how the work of renovation goes on in a Pine forest. The young seedlings come up as thick as they do in the nurseryman's seed-beds; and in the same relative degree of thickness do they continue to grow till they are old enough to be cut down. The competition which takes place between the adjacent individual plants creates a rivalry that increases their upward growth, whilst the exclusion of air [and light] prevents the formation of lateral branches, or destroys them after they are formed.[39]*

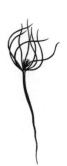

Does competition among siblings also play a part in the remedy? The trees grow up straight and tall, strong 'I' forms, independent and individually powerful. They are able to withstand exposure, cold winds and snow, because the fine leaves and bare trunk offer less resistance than other trees.

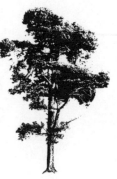

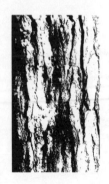

Just as the trunk is straight, so too the root; where possible it goes straight down. Such taproots show a connection to the past and to family (see Chicory, page 102). The bark is rough, broken and peeling, with the appearance of half-healed wounds which weep, oozing resin from the tree. On the upper trunk the bark becomes papery and scabrous with a blotchy, amber colour breaking out through the skin like eczema or psoriasis. There is a strange kind of secret in this, as though the tree would like to hide the very thing which reveals itself—that is in the nature of guilt. Sap from Pine trees was used to make turpentine for paints. It also is a source of pitch, tar and a range of gums and resins which are used as weatherproofing and preservatives. Pine oil is distilled from the leaves: it is used as an inhalant for coughs and bronchitis and as a disinfectant. The link between Pine and household cleansers is both amusing and serious since contamination is associated with guilt.

Scots Pines are the natural forest trees of Scotland. As in Beech woods, Pines exclude light from the understorey: nothing else can grow. Old Pine needles also form a slow-rotting and acidic blanket at the foot of the tree which deters other species—a picture of intolerance. But, while Beech is intolerant of others (page 223), Pine is intolerant of self. In England Pines are planted rather than self-sown; on hilltops and other prominent positions they show boundaries and paths. Richard Mabey in *Flora Britannica*[40] confirms what was observed by Alfred Watkins in *The Old Straight Track*,[41] that Pines marked drove-roads across the Welsh borders. On the old Trewyn estate, not far from Abergavenny, clumps of Pines are said to have been planted at the edge of the property so that the

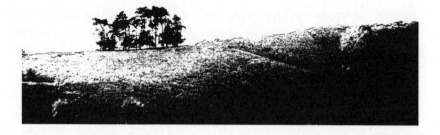

Edwardian owner could stand on his terrace and point out to his guests the extent of his family's land. Because they are used as signals or markers, such trees have a solitary air. It is not quite loneliness but the sense of standing apart. We speak of wind sighing in the Pines: it is a lament of sadness, a memory of regret.

Clearly Pine is a complex remedy state. It involves more than guilt and self-blame. It contains a personal life story for the individual, parts of which may be hidden or suppressed. Pine helps to establish way-markers in the biography or life journey, like the hilltop clumps of trees which are prominent in a landscape. Acting within the detail of a person's feelings, Pine also helps to straighten out tangled and confused emotions—just as Pine's needle-leaves are narrow and straight. The leaves are similar to those of Larch and they offer the same thought of needing to clarify and reassess self-worth. But Pine, being an evergreen, keeps its leaves through the winter, hanging on to the past. Each year some new leaves appear with the new shoots which also bear flowers—the older leaves fall after three or four years. The dark red female flowers, so strong and upright at first, bend around through ninety degrees during the summer. They continue to turn and face downwards as the cone develops. It is an expression of turning again to look at the past, the experience of your life on earth.

The Pine remedy can take us on a journey to reassess the past so we can be more accurate about present circumstances. Just as Pine involves this time relationship, so too does Honeysuckle. Nora quoted Dr Bach as saying of Honeysuckle:

Honeysuckle

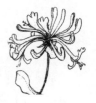

> *This is the remedy to remove from the mind the regrets and sorrows of the past, to counteract all influences, all wishes and desires of the past and to bring us back to the present . . . .*[42]

It is rather as if Pine had pushed Bach back towards his childhood to re-evaluate family involvements and, mentally, he had become stuck there—and so needed Honeysuckle to get back to the present.

Honeysuckle also links to Clematis. Clematis looks to the future, dreaming of better times to come; Honeysuckle dreams of the past and does not expect such happiness again. The two remedies are like the two faces of the god Janus—one looking forward to the New Year, the other looking to the old—after whom January is named. Significantly, *Lonicera caprifolium,* which is Bach's Honeysuckle, begins to break into leaf in December-January, when the sun is in the constellation of Capricorn. True, *caprifolium* is derived from the Latin *capri,* 'of goats', and this is followed in French by 'Chèvre-feuille', the German 'Geißblatt' and in Italian 'Capri-foglio'.[43] But apart from goats having an appetite for young leaves at any time of year, *caper* the goat takes us nowhere. However, the astrological sign Capricorn, ruled by Saturn, slow planet of memories

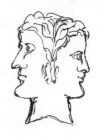

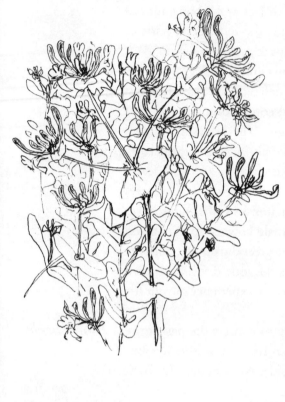

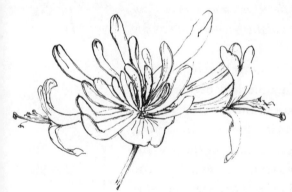

and old age, does have a mythology and symbolism which speaks of Honeysuckle's link to the past. But after all, *caprifolium* is only a name.

The gesture of the plant confirms Bach's observations. Honeysuckle is a shrubby climber with multiple trailing stems, very much like Clematis (pages 47–8). It threads through branches of other supporting hedgerow trees. In old age the bark becomes fibrous, although the younger shoots are notably smooth. Like Clematis, it has a simple, glabrous leaf. The flowers are also constructed in a similar way, with multiple individual blooms on a single head—what is called a terminal whorl. There are many features which distinguish the two plants, but similarities illustrate their kinship as remedies. The contrast is seen in the detail of taxonomy, colour and structure of the flower, the seed and means of reproduction, the terrain in which the two plants grow, in the life span and seasonal cycle.

Externally, the Honeysuckle flowers are strikingly red. Like Red Chestnut, their energy is moving forward (page 255). The buds have a sealed end: crimson tubes formed by five petals fused together along their length. These swell until, curling backwards, the bell of the flower is revealed, shaped like a small trumpet, as if sounding a clarion call, a reveille. The stamens pop out, spreading like fingers. This happens in the evening around seven pm, taking two or three minutes for a flower to open. For all its bright colouring, Honeysuckle is primarily a flower of the night. And at night the sweet scent draws in the insects required for pollination.

Sir Ferdinand von Mueller (1825-96), a German botanist who emigrated to Australia at the age of thirty-two, studied *Lonicera caprifolium* and found six different species of hawkmoth which visited the plant. The significance of this was noted by Sir John Lubbock (1843-1913). A keen follower of Darwin, Lubbock pointed out[44] that only the Hawkmoth, with its exceptionally long proboscis, was able to extract all the nectar in the long, slender tube of the flower.[45] Hawkmoths hover like hawks and as they do so they must brush against the flowers' sexual organs. The pollen has 'needle-like prickles, so that it sticks to the soft fluff of the moth's body'[46] and is then carried on to an adjacent style for pollination. Pollination occurs on the night the flower opens. The bright white interior of the flower, which acted as a beacon to the moths, turns dusky yellow by the second day. As with White Chestnut the signal is immediate. The intimacy of this adaptation between flower and moth appears to confirm Darwin's theories of natural selection, but it also illustrates the gesture of the Honeysuckle flower which ignores daytime insects and proffers nectar for nocturnal moths. Dreaming is a nocturnal process. In the Honeysuckle state memories are projected on the dark screen of sleep; either a literal sleep or the symbolic sleep of people without *interest in present circumstances*. Thinking of the past puts one to sleep in the present. The sweet scent of Honeysuckle makes the same point: nothing can transport the imagination so quickly to the past as a smell—scent is the gatekeeper of memory.

The leaves of *L. caprifolium* are capable of independent movement: the stalk turns the leaf to receive the most light.[47] Olive leaves have the same property (page 179). But those leaves growing towards the end of a shoot, beneath the flowering head, have no stalks and are perfoliate (or connate): two join together around a stem, forming one disk-shaped leaf. This perfoliate leaf is specific to Bach's Honeysuckle and is not found on others, such as *L. periclymenum*. These leaves form stages or platforms. It has been suggested that they represent a link between Honeysuckle and reincarnation. Certainly they do suggest a process of passing time, just as the flowers do with their red buds, the white interior of those freshly opened, then the third stage, yellowed after pollination—a three-day picture of yesterday, today, tomorrow.

Honeysuckle forms red berries. These cluster at the end of the stalk, piled on the small plate of a rounded leaf. They are eaten by birds which may evacuate the seeds in another hedgerow. But unlike Holly (page 237) the seedlings can only grow where there is sufficient light; Honeysuckle wants to come into the bright light of day. The shrub extends outwards and upwards. Propagation also occurs by means of adventitious roots. These grow from any stems which fall back to touch the earth—a form of growth characteristic of the common Blackberry, *Rubus fructicosus,* which, while not a Bach flower, shares many gestural characteristics with Honeysuckle. Of the Bach flowers, Willow and Mimulus also form adventitious roots (pages 54 and 220). The positive statement in each case includes a willingness to come into the present and take up life opportunities as they occur. Putting it to the negative, with Mimulus one is held back by fear of the future; with Willow resentment holds a person back because of difficult experiences; with Honeysuckle a desire for dreams and memories leads to living in the past. As the stems travel over the ground a new plant, separating from the parent, can take root and grow upwards.

Lonicera caprifolium is not a British native. Of those authorities who list it, most say that it is a denizen of the Mediterranean and rare or very rare in Britain. (The common honeysuckle, *L. periclymenum,* is found throughout Britain and northwest Europe). So how and when did Bach come upon Honeysuckle; where did he first find it and make the mother essence? Henslowe, in *British Wild Flowers,* said that it had been found in woods in Oxfordshire[48] though a recent *Flora of Oxfordshire*[49] lists it as 'rare', found only at Goring and Mapledurham. It is known that Dr Bach planted some slips of Honeysuckle in the front garden at *Mount Vernon,* where it still grows today. It is wishful thinking to suppose that there is some virtue in this individual plant not found in others. It is the gesture of the plant which is important, not the fact that Dr B. had his hand upon it. In *The Twelve Healers & Other Remedies* he gave the following description for Honeysuckle:

> *Those who live much in the past, perhaps a time of great happiness, or memories of a lost friend, or ambitions which have not come true. They do not expect further happiness such as they have had.*[50]

Perhaps he felt the little Oxfordshire cottage needed it.

18 · Apathy, Depression and Despair

*L*ITTLE BRIAR ROSE IS A STORY told by the Brothers Grimm.[1] It was popularized by Walt Disney as the cartoon *Sleeping Beauty*. The story is well known: everybody remembers the princess who is cursed to prick her finger on a spindle, how the king ordered every spindle in the land to be burned, then the fateful day when the princess climbs a tower and sees an old woman busy spinning flax. Curious to try to spin herself, the princess no sooner touches the spindle than the magic decree of the thirteenth wise woman (in some versions a fairy, in others a wicked witch) is fulfilled and everyone in the palace falls into a deep sleep which lasts one hundred years. Around the castle a thick hedge of thorns grows up. The story of the sleeping princess 'Briar Rose' encourages many princes to attempt rescue but they die, impaled on the thorns. At last, one prince comes to the hedge and finding it in flower he succeeds in passing through. And when he kisses Briar Rose, of course, all reawaken; the couple marry and live happily ever after.

Wild Rose

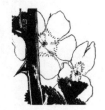

The story can be read in different ways and its symbolism disputed. Going up into a tower may indicate a higher level of consciousness. The act of spinning could symbolize thinking or mental awareness, but more especially making those connections which are the threads of meaning in life. A pricked finger might suggest menarche or intercourse to some, a loss of innocence, or an action which wounds, linked to the will—to be pricked by a spindle means this wilful action somehow breaks the thread of life. Falling asleep means gliding through life, taking it as it is, without any effort to improve things (Bach's indication for Wild Rose). The coming of the princes, impaled upon thorns, may show the repeated attempts to achieve reunification of the soul or self through the union of male and female. This is done over many lifetimes during the hundred years. The kiss which awakens Briar Rose leads to a deeper joy in life and rebirth in the lost kingdom of nature. All depends upon how the tale is interpreted. But there is a link here to the symbolism and gesture of the Wild Rose, which Dr Bach chose as remedy for those who become apathetic and allow their will to fall asleep.

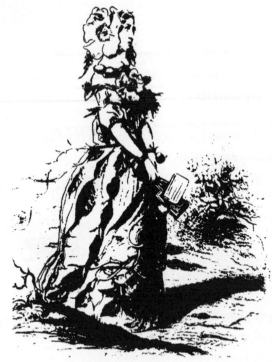

Eglantina

This association between Briar Rose and spinning is reinforced in a curious way by an engraving dating from 1847 by the French caricaturist J. J. Grandville (1803-1847). He illustrated a book, *Les Fleurs Animées,* with flowers in human form. The brief story accompanying the illustrations explains how flowers have tired of their settled life in nature and beg the Flower Fairy to allow them to experience human qualities. For thousands of years, say the flowers, we have supplied mankind with their themes of comparison, metaphors and language of poetry. In return 'men lend to us their virtues and their vices, their good and bad qualities, and it is time we had some experience of what these are'.[2] Eglantina, Wild Rose, will become a literary lady. But Grandville's illustration shows her in a moody pose, carrying carding combs, her wrists bound by entwined stems, so that she either cannot, or does not wish to use them. Carding wool is a preliminary to spinning; both were undertaken as a matter of routine by women in traditional communities who would spin as they walked. So carding combs are symbolic of being occupied with productive work; spinning with the hands or spinning with the mind. 'Nothing is made without carding and spinning,' Eglantina seems to say, 'and I am tired of doing it. I can no longer be bothered!' She is a perfect picture of arrested process which characterizes the Wild Rose state:

> *Those who without apparently sufficient reason become resigned to all that happens, and just glide through life, take it as it is, without any effort to improve things and find some joy. They have surrendered to the struggle of life without complaint.*[3]

Remember that this emotional state, as with others of the Second Nineteen, is the result of some life trauma or changed circumstances. The key words are resignation and surrender.

Wild Rose, *Rosa canina,* can be either white or rose pink: shades of both Clematis and Honeysuckle. And the same gesture is there in the stems which, although they start off energetically, thrusting up vertically,

when free of support curve over and turn back towards the
earth (Clematis pages 47–8, Honeysuckle page 264). Roses
put out new growth in August and September, at the end of
the summer, and so leave it late in the year (like Gentian, page
128). These gracefully arching stems, fresh green and flexible,
are an echo of spring. The thorns, which are a bright, flesh-
pink when young, act as hooks, helping the plant to gain
stability. This is important, because the long stems would
otherwise be blown about by the wind, damaging the plant.
When a person becomes 'resigned to all that happens' they are
indeed blown as the wind wills, without structure or direction
of their own. Hiding in the hedge, Wild Rose usually gains
support from others.

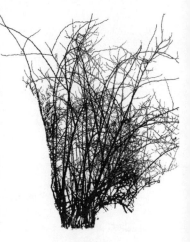

Wild Rose

The hooks or thorns are fiercely prominent and extremely
sharp. Approach Wild Rose and you will never escape without
a scratch; blood will be drawn. Here we see again the image
of forceful stimulus found in Gorse (pages 146–7) which will
jab at apathy and weak will. The thorns are curved downwards, shaped like a canine tooth (hence *Rosa canina)* and
they share the tooth's ripping and tearing disposition. In the
converse of the Wild Rose state a person takes hold and will
not let go; with terrier-like determination they keep working
at a problem until it is solved. *Rosa canina* is also known as
Dog Rose though it is also supposed that Dog derives from
dague, Old French for dagger.[4] The sharpness of the prickles
is followed by the jagged edge of the leaves. The surface of
the leaf is smooth, without hairs to indicate sensitivity to the
environment around.

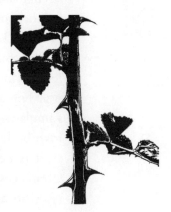

The simple five-petalled flowers are the largest in the Bach
range: up to fifty millimetres across. The central part of the
flower is filled with golden-yellow stamens, a star burst of
strength. The petals open as a flattened dish, as if to absorb
all possible light, like a satellite receiver searching for signals
and stimulus. While Rock Rose opens in a similar way, lying
back to face the sun, Wild Rose faces out in all directions.
The remedy is more concerned with activities of life on earth
and human participation (or the lack of it). Compare the
floral gesture of Wild Rose with that of Oak (page 154). Oak

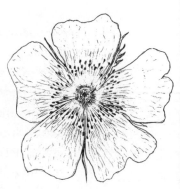

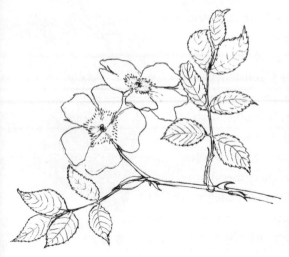

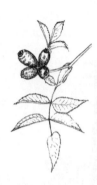

is powerfully-structured, with very small, hidden flowers; the emotional state is determined and represents a fully-engaged, even over-active will force. The same idea is expressed in the small flowers of Vervain. By contrast, the large, flamboyant rose with its loose plant structure illustrates lack of will and lack of clear determination. Dr Bach pointed towards this as he grouped Cerato, Clematis and Scleranthus opposite Honeysuckle and Wild Rose (page 280); all have the same unstructured form and a similar confused mentality.

Red rosehips contain high concentrations of vitamin c, important for strength and health. Those who suffer the Wild Rose lassitude and mental fatigue would find physical stimulus and refreshment from rosehip tea or syrup. Little hairs cushion the seeds within the hip and these provided playful children with itching powder[5] in the days before television eroded interest in the natural world. The irritant effect of these hairs echoes the prickling of the thorns. Like the stinging nettle (*Urtica urens*), Wild Rose stimulates a physical response. Indeed, there is a link between nettle and rose; both are markers of human settlement. In Scotland, where many crofters were dispossessed of their land and homes during the Highland Clearances, tumble-down ruins can still be found where people lived 150 years ago. They are marked by Wild Rose and nettles. Nettles grow wherever urine has fouled the ground and Wild Rose where human endeavour has been defeated by time and troubles (like Gorse).

Roses are said to be long-lived. At Hildesheim, near Hanover in Germany, there was and may still be a Wild Rose more than a thousand years old.[6] Time certainly plays a part in the nature of the plant: we can see this in germination. *Rosa canina* seeds have a low viability, often below thirty per cent, even in nursery conditions. There is little inclination to take up the opportunity of life. Tests have shown[7] a noticeable delay in germination until the second year, indicating a slow response, a lack of effort, delayed reaction. Two other plants in the Bach range share this feature of delayed germination: Hornbeam[8] and Mustard. Hornbeam, like Wild Rose, waits until the second spring before the seed breaks open and develops; both display a similar apathy and weariness. Mustard seeds can wait, buried in the earth, for many years before they germinate. The Mustard emotional state develops through lack of interest in life and a will-less emptiness.

The key to understanding Mustard, as a Bach flower remedy, is given in an observation by Johns in his *Flowers of the Field*: 'a common weed in cornfields, sometimes springing up in profusion from recently disturbed ground, though previously unknown there'.[9] It is not uncommon for wild plants to appear suddenly but Mustard can swamp a field of corn with yellow flowers among the green stalks, like the red poppies which used to be seen in ripening wheat or barley—an unexpected invasion. It is like the sudden and unexplained onset of depression or despair which Bach described for this remedy:

Mustard

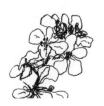

> *Those who are liable to times of gloom, or even despair, as though a cold dark cloud overshadowed them and hid the light and the joy of life. It may not be possible to give any reason or explanation for such attacks.*[10]

The farmer ploughs a field, plants seeds and, as they germinate and grow, weeds appear among the crop. These days such weeds are quickly eradicated, sprayed with chemicals as soon as they appear, but in the 1930s they were a common sight. Charlock, or wild Mustard as it is also known, was a real nuisance—'probably the most troublesome of all annual weeds of arable land'.[11] It competes for light and air by overgrowing other plants, more or less smothering them; harvests may be reduced by as much as fifty per cent.[12] It also takes nutrients from the soil and harbours pests like turnip fly and gall weevil.[13] No wonder farmers wanted to be rid of it.

Bach first saw Mustard growing in the Sotwell area in the early summer. He sent some of the flowers to The Royal Botanic Gardens, Kew, asking for identification (his letter dated May 12th 1935). They replied that the specimens were probably *Brassica (sinapis) arvensis* a flower which reaches full flowering in early June. ('June is the month in which ordinarily it is most abundant').[14] So his first sight was of weeds growing among the corn (like biblical tares) but not yet fully in flower. Perhaps he even had a conversation with the farmer and so learned about the unusual life cycle of *Sinapis arvensis*. Writing in 1852 about *The Weeds of Agriculture*, George Sinclair, gardener to the Duke of Bedford, commented:

> *It is well known that the seeds of charlock, poppy and camomile, lie for ages in the bowels of the earth uninjured; and it is only when brought near the surface, that they can be made to vegetate, and then only under peculiar circumstances of the surface soil in which they lie. It has*

long been observed, that the prevalence of charlock and poppies occur
periodically. In one year every field will have an abundant share of one
or both these weeds: and it sometimes happens, that for ten years at a
stretch, neither will appear in injurious quantity. Hence the old saying,
'it is a charlock year'....[15]

What actually controls the appearance of *Sinapis arvensis* has more to do
with the depth of ploughing. If the blade of the plough should pull deep,

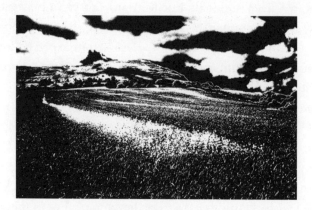

soil carrying old Mustard seeds will be brought to the surface. Evidence of
this may sometimes be seen when panels of Charlock appear in a field, as
the set of the plough has changed. A single plant may carry 4,000 seeds,
so that millions may lie buried, a seed bank waiting for an opportunity
to surface.[16]

As an emotional state, Mustard is a kind of depression which waits,
unseen, for an opportunity to surface. Its origins will have been in the
past, buried deeply, even beyond memory. By looking at the natural
history of the plant, two things can be seen. One, the darkness which
clouds the 'light and joy of life' comes from within the earth; it is born
of past experiences (karma if you will) which the individual carries as
unresolved material, ungerminated seeds. To use another analogy, it is
like the psychological baggage many carry, filled with who knows what.
The second point: Mustard plants only develop when a field is left empty,
the soil bare. The Mustard state follows disturbance of the settled pattern
of life (ploughing) and only takes root in the mind because there is some
inactivity in the will (an empty field). That is why Mustard is alongside
Honeysuckle and Wild Rose in the sequence of discovery—Nora Weeks
put Mustard there[17] and so did Bach, in the group for *Not Sufficient*
Interest in Present Circumstances.

So Mustard is an opportunist pattern of interference, a form of possession, which takes up residence only because of the weakness of the host. This idea is hinted at by some writers who speak of dark forces overshadowing the soul, of separation and a fall from grace.[18] The image of an empty, ploughed field (or even upturned earth) invites such thoughts. There is something unnatural about land devoid of all plants. Today, when farmers spray fields with weed-killer, before planting and ploughing, there is cause to wonder about the effect on the psyche of the planet. Eradicate all plants from a field and what will enter? The psyche of the planet may be too abstruse a concept, but the complex relationships of plant to earth, of biodiversity and subtlety in thought are the very things forced under by the bulldozer of materialism. The farmer increases his yield at harvest by removing unwanted competition from weeds: charlock hardly grows in arable land today. But does its extinction as a species leave us less protected from the 'cold, dark clouds' of depression?

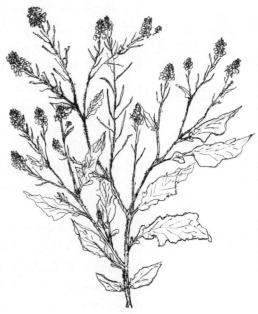

Mustard can germinate after autumn ploughing, although it may not survive the winter; more usually it appears with spring. When it grew in cornfields (European cereal crops, not American sweet corn) it was just slightly taller than wheat or barley, about seventy-five centimetres, taking shelter from other plants. These days it is more commonly seen on roadside verges and embankments where repairs and earthworks have disturbed the ground. Leaves and stems are rough, bristling with stiff hairs (hispid)—like the stinging nettle, but without the irritant poison. The seeds though, when eaten, are stimulating, hot and tangy: *sinapis* is derived from the Greek word for mustard. The leaves are irregularly lobed; these plants lack symmetry and balance. The flowers however, are cruciform: four brilliant yellow petals on short stalks cluster near the top of the stem. The intense yellow of the massed flowers makes for a clear brightness which

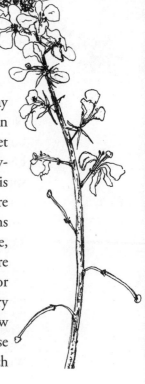

dispels gloom, like sun breaking through clouds, enlivening the earth. This is the action of the remedy; it dispels gloom. But it does so by helping the person to understand and come to terms with the problem. Katz and Kaminski make the point that in the Mustard state 'the consciousness finds it difficult to penetrate to the cause or meaning of such depression'[19]—the yellow flowers link to clear mental energy, which can help this understanding.

When afflicted by the Mustard state 'it is almost impossible to appear happy or cheerful', said Bach.[20] So Mustard can be used whenever a person appears depressed but for no clear reason: hence the oft-quoted Gentian for known cause and Mustard for unknown. True enough, but the Mustard depression derives from a clear source when we can find it. Something is there which actively invades or attacks the consciousness of the person. Bach spoke of a lack of 'explanation for such attacks . . .'.[21] Like Aspen (page 195), Mustard depression is based upon the action of unseen forces which manipulate the psyche of an individual.

Sweet
Chestnut

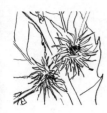

Each of the previous emotional states has its difficulty; each represents a particular pain or problem to overcome. Combine the worst of all of them, amplifying the feeling to a great intensity, and we arrive at the last of the Thirty-eight Bach flower remedies: Sweet Chestnut. There can be no doubt Edward Bach himself felt great anguish. Nobody could describe it so succinctly without knowing the experience:

> *. . . when the anguish is so great as to seem to be unbearable. When the mind or body feels as if it had borne to the uttermost limit of its endurance, and that now it must give way.*[22]

Nora Weeks mentioned that Bach suffered from a 'virulent rash which burned and irritated incessantly'[23] throughout June and July (page 229) but that was a small, outward, physical symptom of the mental and spiritual distress with which he was struggling. The Sweet Chestnut state, he wrote, is for 'when it seems there is nothing but destruction and annihilation left to face'.[24] The very light of life has been extinguished: it has been called the dark night of the soul.*

---

* Saint John of the Cross, born in Spain 1542, wrote *Noche obscura del alma*, (*The Dark Night of the Soul*), an account of progress towards union with God which entailed passing the threshold of desolation. One part of the narrative makes a comparison between Divine Light, its action upon the soul and the action of fire upon wood in both purging it of impurities and transforming it to light. *The Dark Night of the Soul*, Watkins 1905, pp. 167-174.

Many of the remedy plants have been described in terms of light (all plant life works to mediate light on earth), and the theme of darkness and light most strongly characterizes this remedy. There is something subterranean about the Sweet Chestnut state, a depth of feeling like the oppression of mines where sunlight never enters. Yet, even in the darkest labyrinth a luminous thread of meaning still guides the soul;[25] here that thread is lost. The point has been made that overcoming difficulties leads to the evolution of soul qualities (page 202) and that remedies of the Second Nineteen are concerned with this process of turning suffering into learning. Also that the boiling method, using fire from within the earth, speaks of this transformation. So here, with the last of the boiling remedies, there is a final darkening of the light as soul-flame certainties are extinguished by materiality and suffocation of the spirit. Bach wrote that 'it is one for that terrible, that appalling mental despair when it seems the very soul itself is suffering destruction'.[26] This calls for the most powerful expression of light and regeneration in the plant kingdom, to pull consciousness up from the darkness of this underworld.

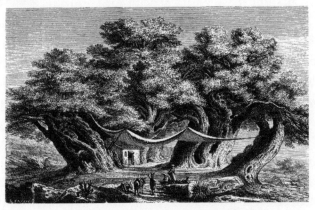

Chestnut of One Hundred Horses

The Sweet Chestnut tree, *Castanea sativa*, is among the mightiest of species. In winter the tree is a picture of huge, spiralling forces, upthrust energy in trunk and bough. A single tree can be eight metres in girth, like the one beside the river Grwyne Fawr, above Glangrwyney, between Abergavenny and Crickhowell. Five or six people are needed to link hands and encircle such a trunk. Others are recorded as being far bigger: *Castagno del Cento Cavalli* (Chestnut of One Hundred Horses) on the west side of Mount Etna, in Italy, was said to be more than fifty metres

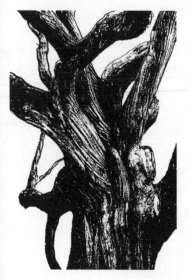

in circumference, although quite hollow.[27] An estimate of its age? 3,000 or 3,500 years old! British Chestnuts rarely live beyond 500 years, although the ancient giant at Tortworth in Gloucestershire is estimated to be 1,100.[28] Sweet Chestnut is a native of the Mediterranean and once formed great forests: a remnant can be seen on the western slopes of Mount Ochi, on the Greek island of Evia. It survives such dry conditions with a massive and deeply penetrating root structure. Johns remarked that the tree loves volcanic soil, which reinforces the idea that subterranean fire is resonant with the Sweet Chestnut condition.[29]

The bark is characteristically furrowed, deeply etched with force lines running parallel to each other like ribbons, which seem to draw strength upwards from the earth. These begin to open out and spiral around the tree when it is about 100 years old. Younger branches have a smooth, grey skin, like young Olive trees (page 175). Like Olive, the Sweet Chestnut has a great capacity for regrowth 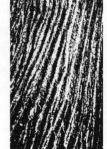 from the ground up, so that a coppiced tree will send up many young shoots. This may have accounted for the massive girth of *Castagno del Cento Cavallo* since trunks can fuse together if they make contact. The single bole of a tree is rarely more than twenty-five metres high but it stands powerfully, like a pillar. Branches often grow out horizontally and are liable to be torn from the trunk by the wind, weighted against the foliage. Old trees stand shattered and broken.

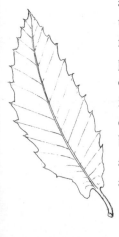

The leaves are large, simple and deeply notched, rather like Impatiens (page 43); the energy clear and directed. Smooth and glossy, they have a strong skeletal form which holds them stiffly in a rosette at the end of the branches. They are never attacked by insects. The male flowers grow from the axil of the leaf, pushing out away from the dark foliage, as long plumes, creamy white with pollen. The scent is variously said to be sickly or unmistakeably smelling of semen.[30] The catkins, unusually, are erect, in contrast to the downward drooping Aspens (page 196) which point to earth. Sweet Chestnut flowers are an explosion of fire, like rocket trails bursting into space. The surge of energy from the root, up the trunk, out along the branches into the leaves and flowers is a blast of power, lifting against gravity, shooting towards the stars.

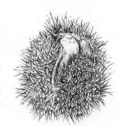

Female flowers are sited at the base of the male catkins; they are small, green and spiky. After pollination they swell to produce nuts enclosed in a bristly case which falls from the tree in autumn. The sharp spines, as with Gorse leaves, are more a sign of stimulus than any kind of protection for the tree or its fruit. Since flowering never begins before July, the growth of these nuts must be very rapid if they are to be viable seeds in Britain. Further south they flower earlier, grow fatter and the edible nuts are gathered for food. In all cases they germinate easily. Along with the faculty to regrow from the root up after coppicing, this is a sign of the vitality of the tree.

Making the mother essence, by the boiling method, is an extraordinary experience. The tree, so vast, is covered in flowers, from top to bottom. Only where a lowered branch reaches towards earth can they be picked. Then, pluck one of these creamy-headed creatures from the branch, with its spray of leaves and catkins, and the saucepan is already full and overflowing. Nora Weeks says, sweetly, 'gather about six inches of the twig with leaves, male and female flowers from as many trees as possible',[31] but this may not be practicable. . . . It is not a problem, however, it just illustrates again the immense vitality and exuberance of this remedy flower. When the essence has been made it is dark, reddish-brown, like mahogany—the taste sharp and stimulating, awakening. But the feeling it produces is gentle, a golden glow in the heart. Dr Bach said 'the cry for help is heard . . .'.[32] After the dark night, the sun rising.

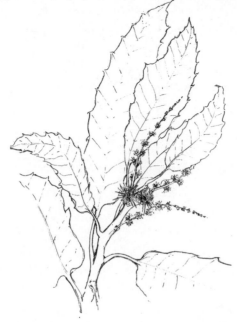

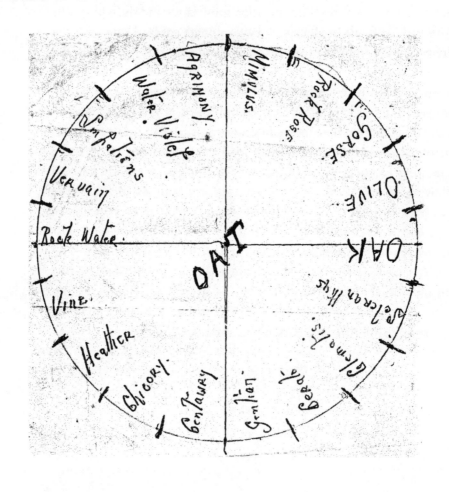

19 · The Pattern in Practice

WITH THE DISCOVERY OF SWEET CHESTNUT Bach's work was almost done: the sequence of Thirty-eight remedies was complete. Nothing remained but finalizing the descriptions and reprinting *The Twelve Healers*. Bach had begun to use the new remedies immediately, of course, and exchanged letters with colleagues who also reported their findings. 'What a splendid case of Aspen', he wrote in a letter to 'Dear Brother Doctor Wheeler', dated September 1935.[1] He continued: 'the more we use these remedies, both the new nineteen and the old nineteen, the more wonderful the results . . .'. Bach also began to explore the possibilities for organizing the remedies into some formal scheme. 'I have not yet quite thought out the table you sent, but hoping to let you have a reply about this quite shortly', he added as a postscript.[2] What table? What was he referring to?

In 1934 Bach had drawn a diagram with Oat at the centre of a circle, eighteeen of the other remedies around the circumference. Done at the time when there were just nineteen remedies, it was designed to explore relationships. Wild Oat is in the central position as if to ask the question—which direction should be taken? Was it a diagram used for dowsing? It is interesting to study such schemes but they are inevitably sterile unless the pattern works in practice. To place Mimulus opposite Centaury or Chicory next to Heather does little to assist diagnosis.

Later, when the full Thirty-eight remedies had been discovered, Bach set them out as if cohorts in a battle plan. Oat was opposite Walnut, Olive leading to Gorse and Oak. He was attempting to fit the remedies together, the Seven Helpers with the Twelve Healers, the Second Nineteen with the First. In a letter, written July 1st 1935, Bach wrote:

> *The prescription of these new remedies is going to be much more simple than at first appeared, because each of them corresponds to one of the Twelve Healers or the Seven Helpers.*
>
> *For example: supposing a case is definitely Clematis and does fairly well but not a complete cure, give the corresponding new remedy further to help the cure.*[3]

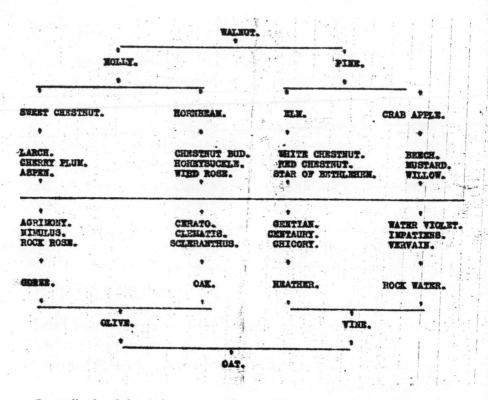

Crucially, he did not leave us with the full information as to how and why the new remedies corresponded with the old. 'Enclosed a list of those already worked out,' he wrote in the same letter, 'the rest we shall receive in due time.' In some cases the connection is obvious, as with Honeysuckle and Clematis. Cherry Plum links to Rock Rose, Aspen to Mimulus. But it is not equally clear which of the boiling remedies follows on from Water Violet or Impatiens. Arguments could be put forward but they lack clarity and falter. If the scheme had been useful it would have been written about before now.

In the end Bach settled for seven groups, allocating each of the Thirty-eight to one of them. Mimulus, Rock Rose, Aspen, Red Chestnut and Cherry Plum all worked with fear, so the first group was *For Fear*. Impatiens, Water Violet and Heather each concerned loneliness: so another group was *For Loneliness*. And so on for all of the Thirty-eight. The 'Seven Headings', as Bach called them, were written into the 1936 edition of *The Twelve Healers & Other Remedies* and have been used ever since. The only problem is that they too fail to work in practice. The seven headings look good on paper but do not lend themselves to practical application of the remedies. The idea behind the seven headings, undoubtedly, was to make it easier for people to understand the remedies. It was too complex to consider thirty-eight different states without some structure and order. An alphabetic listing from Agrimony to Willow was arbitrary and did nothing to guide the user. The problem still applies to someone coming new to the subject today, reading a book or leaflet. All the remedies are given equal weight and no differentiation. At least the seven groups offered a starting point. They are:

> For fear
> For uncertainty
> For insufficient interest in present circumstances
> For loneliness
> For those oversensitive to influences and ideas
> For despondency and despair
> For over-care for the welfare of others

But how can a person be sure of the difference between uncertainty and lack of interest in present circumstances? Those who know Bach remedies well can point the distinction but it is one made by the remedies themselves and not by a clear meaning of the headings. A Mimulus person could be described as oversensitive (nervous, shy, reactive); someone in a Gorse state (depressed and hopeless) might be seen as despondent and in despair, yet they are not placed in those groups. A lack of interest in present circumstances sounds like a good phrase to describe someone with the Hornbeam feeling though Bach put Hornbeam in the group for uncertainty. It can be confusing.

It seems likely that Bach based his seven headings on the seven chakras or energy centres of the body.[4] These would correspond with the 'seven principles' or archetypes he had written about in *Some Fundamental Considerations . . .*[5] in 1930 (page 89). In this scheme, by way of example, the loneliness remedies (Impatiens, Water Violet and Heather) correspond to the crown chakra (located by the pineal gland at the crown of the head) and the seventh principle, Spiritual Perfection. This type, he said, worked with the characteristics of the enthusiast, the puritan and the monk. All very well, but too intellectual for everyday use.

There is a similar problem with astrology. In the first edition of *The Twelve Healers* Dr Bach began finding correspondences between the twelve remedies and the twelve astrological signs:

> *These types of personality are indicated to us by the moon according to which sign of the Zodiac she is in at birth . . . . The secret of life is to be*

true to our personality, not to suffer interference from outside influences.
Our personality we learn from the position of the moon at birth; our
dangers of interference from the planets.[6]

But later he wrote 'I am being cautious as regards astrology and that is
why one left out the signs and the months in the first Twelve Healers'.[7]
Although he examined 'the exact placing of signs and planets and bodily
systems', it lacked certainty.[8] Furthermore, however useful astrology may
be to an astrologer, it complicated the simplicity of the remedies.[9] Bach
wanted to 'give general principles whereby people like you who have a
more detailed knowledge, may discover a great truth'.[10] The remedies
themselves must be open to serve all interests and not become narrowed
by arcane or esoteric specialism.

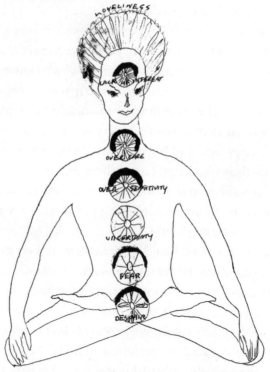

The seven chakras and seven groups

Clearly there was a tension here between what Bach knew about
astrology, chakras, and the spiritual path and what he could reasonably
expect others to know and understand. Having already alienated his
medical colleagues with metaphysics (page 79), he tried to avoid further
complications. Shortly before he died Bach rewrote the introduction to
The Twelve Healers & Other Remedies, eschewing all unnecessary science,

theories or knowledge 'apart from the simple methods described herein'.[11] He concluded 'there is little more to say, for the understanding mind will know all this . . .'. In other words—make of it what you can.

Yet there is a way in which the Thirty-eight Bach remedies can be presented straightforwardly so that anybody may make sense of them and appreciate the different qualities. It is the schema used for this book—the schema used by Bach himself in the unfolding story of their discovery. It is the system of 12:7:19, the Twelve Healers, the Seven Helpers and the Second Nineteen. The Twelve Healers are the twelve soul types, the type remedies; the particular nature with which we are born (pages 139–142). The Seven Helpers are chronic conditions, emotional states which have developed over time, which have become habitual and which may mask the true type. The Second Nineteen are reactive emotional and mental conditions which can occur as a response to life traumas. They may be long-lasting and deep-acting but can be traced back to a particular event which triggered the reaction. An understanding of these kinds of remedy is supported by an understanding of the difference between the two methods of preparation: the sun method and the boiling method.

Because the First Twelve remedies are closer to the beginning of this life they are not always apparent at first glance. They may be overlaid by complexity and the distortions of experience: the Seven Helpers and the Second Nineteen. Those who are closer to their origins, the more innocent, may more readily show their type as one of the First Twelve—children, animals, souls who have resolved or never encountered life problems. Those who have travelled further from home may have disguised their true feelings. For this reason the image is sometimes used of peeling back the layers of an onion, revealing progressive levels of emotional experience. A good image and one which probably came from Bach. The power of the idea can be properly appreciated if the onion's layers are 12:7:19.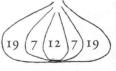

The core of a personality, therefore, is the type remedy. Dr Bach was an Impatiens, Nora Weeks probably a Water Violet. It shows the motivation for the life. In the Seven Helpers are seven ways in which an individual may mediate with life. These remedies are not invariably appropriate but one of the seven often shows the habitual approach: Vine is controlling, Wild Oat diffused, Oak full of endeavour. The outer layer shows the remedy states closest to the surface, the visible trauma of Star, the anger of Holly, the apathy of Wild Rose, the resentment of Willow. Take drops of a remedy from the Second Nineteen and the underlying chronic condition may be revealed. That in turn can lead to the type remedy. Where there is immediate trauma and obvious distress it is no good speaking of soul lessons: first repair the car and then see about completing the journey.

This suggests the Second Nineteen are easier to recognize than the soul types. They are likely to be the presenting emotional states, those nearest to the surface. They are the remedies which are used most widely—those which sell most.[12] Most popular is Walnut, then Larch, White Chestnut, Crab Apple and Star of Bethlehem. Mimulus and Impatiens top the chart of the Twelve Healers; Olive is the most popular of the Seven Helpers. Vine, Rock Water and Heather are the least used remedies: indicative of a need to better understand the Seven Helpers.

These seven remedies—Olive, Gorse, Oak, Vine, Heather, Rock Water, and Wild Oat—could be considered independently for the purposes of diagnosis, before turning attention to the type remedy. Bach made the distinction of whether 'the patient is pale' or 'high coloured', but gave no explanation.[13] Better to look at the person overall and assess the state of vitality and their use of energy. Remember this is the chronic condition, a key pointer to the state of health.

The Twelve Healers can most easily be recognized when a person is unwell: we revert to type (pages 293–4). Or the soul lesson may be recognized by looking back to moments of crisis and trauma. Bach said, look at the virtues you admire or dislike in other people.[14] It is equally possible to look at a formative event and consider the reaction to it. This may be something specific and personal or a more general event from childhood. In any case it is the characteristic behaviour of the individual which is significant. Often people say they react differently at different stages in their life. But there is no contradiction in this. Water Violets are not likely to develop into Centaury types or Vervain into Cerato. If a Scleranthus type develops the character of Gentian, then Gentian has become the passing mood and should be treated as such. Bach wrote:

> If in doubt between one or two, give both; they can be put into the same bottle. This also applies if the patient has two definite states present at the same time, such as fear and impatience.
>
> During an illness more than one state may be present, or one may follow another, then each stage should be treated as it occurs. In severe illness, there may be despair or fear; on recovery, indifference or discouragement;

*during convalescence, impatience or weakness; and so on. In such cases
each stage can be dealt with until it disappears and perfect health is
regained.*[15]

It is part of the beauty of the Bach remedies, however, that no one way
of working is right for all people. There is no need to be prescriptive about
how to use them. There is a wonderful opportunity to explore new ways
of working through a self-developmental approach to learning. But it
comes back to Dr Bach's aphorism in chapter ten of *Free Thyself*, 'to gain
freedom give freedom'.[16] It is important to remember that this freedom
is there only so long as it is not used to inhibit the freedom of others.
The Bach flower remedies were given to the world and there need be no
controls to limit their use.

People sometimes ask why it is that Edward Bach died at the relatively
young age of fifty. If he invented these wonderful remedies, so the
thought goes, could he not have healed himself and lived to be ninety
and a wise old man? Matters of life and death are rarely in our hands,
but in any event we can reply that Dr Bach died at the completion of
his life work. The first of the remedies he found, Impatiens, was his own
type remedy. Subsequently, he experienced the intensity of lifetimes in
a deep-diving immersion in the gamut of human emotion and mental
conditions. From loneliness to selfish passion, from hatred to despair, his
journey moved through the stations of human soul life; he ended with the
desolate anguish of Sweet Chestnut. At the same time he was physically
far from strong and suffered debilitating illness throughout his life. It is no
wonder that he died at fifty. However, the question implies some judgement upon Bach by supposing that illness and death represent failure on
his part. But that is to misunderstand an essential message of Dr Bach's
remedies: opportunities afforded by life should be welcomed, no matter
how difficult they may appear, no matter what the consequences.

There is an extension of this thought: there is more to be gained in
overcoming difficulties than in never having faced a problem. There
are those souls who appear to fall through life without friction, never
meeting resistance. But what do they learn? Such a charmed existence
does nothing for the evolution of consciousness; those who overcome
achieve greatness. Each one who masters a soul lesson contributes to
the building of a new world, 'exerting a continual pressure towards
perfection'.[17] Changing the habitual patterning of one of the Seven helps
'to realize the mightiness of our Destiny'.[18] Overcoming the adversity of

those states described by the Second Nineteen leads from darkness into light. But experience is brought from that darkness 'into the glorious sunshine of the knowledge of your Divinity'.[19] So it was knowledge and experience which Bach gained from his short life. It was gained through the discovery of the Thirty-eight flower remedies. With that knowledge and experience he was able to make a map of the metaphysical world. It is a map which can be used by anyone, whatever his soul journey, whatever stage in life has been reached.

At the end, just weeks before he died, Bach wrote to his friends—'dear lovely people'—asking them to carry on the work he had started, 'a Work that can rob disease of its powers, the Work which can set men free'.[20] In recent years this has appeared as just extravagance or, perhaps, the confusion of a man close to death. But suppose it was true. Was he claiming great powers for the remedies he had discovered? In part, yes. He believed they were capable of helping people make great changes, such that they might loosen the stranglehold of disease. The real secret, however, was that transforming the life transformed the power of disease: it was this which 'can set men free'.

Today disease and death control us ever more strongly with a litany of viruses, cancers and heart disorders. The causes may be vaccinations, environmental poisons, despoliation of food, or pollution of the elements—earth, water and air. For Bach the cause was clear and it is clear today:

> It is only because we have forsaken Nature's way for man's way that we have suffered, and we have only to return to be released from our trials. In the presence of the way of Nature disease has no power; all fear, all depression, all hopelessness can be set aside. There is no disease of itself which is incurable.[21]

It is a trumpet call to life.

Appendix I

The Story of the Travellers

Once upon a time nineteen travellers set out upon a journey . . . . That is the opening of the story which Bach told. To be accurate, he had sixteen travellers (he had only completed *The Twelve Healers & Four Helpers*) but that hardly matters.* In his tale, when they were lost deep in the forest at night, each of the travellers behaves according to type. Agrimony worries, Mimulus becomes afraid, Gorse gives up and thinks he will lie down and wait for death. Later, when they have safely found the path, they all show the positive strengths of their type: Mimulus knows no fear, Gorse tells of the sunrise in the morning. They go on to guide other travellers and are an example to those who have not made the journey before.

Although the story is conceived in the imagery of a fairy tale Bach did not develop the symbolism. All he wished to do was to show the remedy types relating to each other as a group and to illustrate the different ways in which each reacts to a common experience. It points towards a most useful tool for diagnosis. It is easy to see the different emotional reactions when we allow each person to tell their part in a story. In practical terms, this can be related to almost any mundane event. It might be going to town to get a haircut, to buy a new pair of shoes, or to complain about something, or what happens when we decide to go on holiday. How each of us deals with the situation will show how we take decisions, deal with a new experience or resolve difficulties. The remedies can help us with our life problems.

To tell the story of the travellers today, the nineteen remedies could be placed in a new situation, no longer walking through the forest but still on a journey—they are in a minibus, going as a group for a visit. Vervain is the organizer and has done a good job keeping everybody informed of the arrangements by email but now Clematis has overslept. Impatiens does not think they should wait any longer; ten o'clock means ten

---

* *Collected Writings of Edward Bach,* Ashgrove Press, pp. 75–6.

o'clock, he says. He has threatened to go on ahead in his own car; tense and irritable, he wants to get started. But who is going to drive the bus? Oak will do it, let the others sit back and relax, enjoy the trip. Relax? How can anybody relax? Mimulus is worrying about the traffic on the motorway and the speed they will be driving at, he gets so frightened. Chicory is feeling sick and has a headache and wants everybody to wait while Centaury is instructed to go to the shop to get some more tablets. Olive sits patiently in the bus, pale and exhausted. Scleranthus sits first at the front, then at the back and then at the front again. Water Violet watches the performance with disdainful amusement having chosen the only single seat available. At last Clematis arrives and after a telling off from Vine gets on board, takes out a CD player, dons headphones and listens to music.

'Where are we going?' Wild Oat wants to know. 'Who cares,' says Agrimony with a laugh, 'so long as there's a pub.' Rock Water looks disapproving and goes back to reading *The Twelve Principles of Perfection*. 'We are scheduled to visit a beautiful garden,' Gentian explains, 'though we probably won't make it,' he adds gloomily. Just at that moment there is a bang, smoke pours from the engine and the bus grinds to a halt. Gentian shakes his head. 'Typical,' he says to himself, 'just my luck.' Wide-eyed with fear, Rock Rose begins to panic. But Vine is already on his feet shouting for everybody to stay calm. Gorse, slumped in his seat, does not seem to have noticed what has happened. What will they do now, asks Cerato?

Vervain soon has things organized with the breakdown service and mentally has written the first of several strongly-worded letters to the hire company. While the engine is repaired the group must stay the night in a nearby hotel and this unexpected event seems to bring out the worst in everybody; only Heather seems happy and spends the time telling his life story to the receptionist. The rest of the party are arguing or in tears. Water Violet has gone up to his room and left them to it. It looks as though things cannot get any worse.

The next day Gentian wants to give up and go home, there seems little point in persevering. Gorse agrees. But little Rock Rose, taking courage in both hands says that they really must try to keep going and get to the garden; if everybody made a big effort to be positive then they can still manage it. Chicory is about to say that he has been making an effort all along but a look from Vine silences him. But, even if they are willing to try, how will they find the garden? Cerato wants to know. Should they just go around asking? At this point Water Violet steps forward, he can show them the way, since he has been there before.

So they set out again, trying to encourage each other all the while. Vine works hard to help the group and plans gently to tell Centaury that he does not need to be carrying everybody's cases: but Centaury is deep in conversation with Mimulus and just quietly smiles at Vine. Rock Rose has confidently asked Vervain for the roadmap and is asking Water Violet about the route while Vervain listens to them attentively. Gentian feels sure that they will make good time now. Chicory has stopped worrying about himself and is caring for Olive. Gorse looks out brightly at the passing fields and is making plans, Oak has let Scleranthus drive and is sitting with his feet up playing cards with Rock Water (who has forgotten to criticize). Wild Oat is happily writing a story about what has happened. Clematis has lent his music to Impatiens who is relaxing now, while Clematis looks around enjoying the present moment. Agrimony and Heather are sitting in silence, holding hands. And Cerato goes to sit next to Water Violet. They discuss the changed mood which has come about.

The road they have taken leads them at last to a car park beside a river. One at a time they walk across the nearby bridge. Impatiens is the first to cross, of course, and finds himself on the riverbank surrounded by tall balsams with pale mauve flowers which are visited by hundreds of bees. Impatiens feels drawn to the flowers. Breathing deeply, he begins to relax for the first time in months. Not far away he sees Mimulus stepping out into the stream on some rocks, laughing and singing quietly to himself as he admires some beautiful yellow flowers hanging over the water. And Clematis too is nearby looking up into the trees and gazing with rapt attention at some small white blossoms shining like stars against the dark green of the leaves. As the others cross the bridge they stop to talk with Impatiens, Mimulus and Clematis and look at their flowers. How alike they are one to the other. Then they wander away each in his own direction, looking to see if they too have a special place in the garden. And, of course, each one looks for their flower and finds it growing happily in perfect circumstances.

Rock Rose and Gentian have a little further to walk because they have to climb to the downland, further away from the river. Wild Oat wanders everywhere, all through the garden and finds that his particular grass is growing on the side of every path. There are olive trees and vines, gorse bushes and oaks. Poor Heather has a long solitary walk to the top of the furthest hill but he does not mind at all. Water Violet finds a beautiful pool of still water, not far from a spring, which splashes cold and clear on to the rocks. There is a perfect place for everyone.

Later in the day they drift back in groups of two or three towards the bridge. Here they meet someone who appears to be the gardener. As they talk and ask questions he tells them many things about themselves and their individual plants. Cerato wants to know why his flowers are blue; Mimulus asks why his live so close to the water. Oak asks about roots, leaves and flowers and what they mean. Every part of the plant, the gardener tells them, has a significance and represents a quality of being. Where and how a plant grows describes aspects of these qualities. Just as Clematis and Impatiens behave differently as people, so their plants behave differently. However, some plants or trees have qualities in common, they have deep roots or hairy leaves or a particularly upright gesture and those characteristics are shared by both the person and the plant. Within the garden there are many different beings, each with an individuality or soul. It is the soul quality which informs the way the plant grows.

While they are talking, Wild Oat is looking around. Pointing to another part of the garden, beyond where the olive trees are growing, he asks, hesitantly, who might those others be? Where he is pointing the land is disturbed and in places the ground ploughed; there are fields and hedges and great boulders grouped together in the centre of one field. Many of the trees there are flowering, covered in blossoms, and they make a great show of strength and purpose. Those, says the gardener, are the people who have suffered in life, they are learning how to transform their experience. The group of friends look puzzled but want to go over and say hallo. When they get there they meet Aspen, Elm, Red Chestnut, Willow, Wild Rose and all the others: there were nineteen of them as well.

With so many people talking together it is natural that they begin to move into groups. Red Chestnut begins to tell them how worried he had been when Mimulus was perched on the stones in the middle of the river. Cherry Plum, imagining how frightened he would have been, begins taking deep breaths to calm himself down. Aspen stands beside them, his leaves a-tremble. Wild Oat, Scleranthus and Cerato are soon talking to Gentian and Gorse. They have all met before, of course, but now Hornbeam comes to join them. Heather, Impatiens and Water Violet form a little group on their own. As they talk and learn about their individual life stories, they realize that they can help each other, and work together to help everyone.

Just how this story will end is not clear, for it is still going on.

Appendix II

Twelve Ways of Being Unwell

In illness, each of the twelve types reacts in a different way:

Impatiens is quickly ill and quickly well again, impatient to be up and doing. There may be pain and tension but the character of the person is sure to be irritable. The child lies ill and Mum comes to offer sympathy and kindness. But nothing is right and nothing is accepted.

'Would you like some nice hot milk, darling?'

'No! Just go away and leave me alone.'

When the doctor comes they want an instant cure.

Clematis people like being ill: all that time with nothing to do but dream. They sleep easily and if awake will want television or novels to distract themselves. If they have a fever the hallucinations add interest to a dull day. The whole metabolism will slow as they drift away from the world.

Mimulus, being the remedy for fear, carries an anxiety that the problem is more serious.

'I'm worried that I've got polyitis, it's what John's cousin had.'

'You'll be alright, don't worry,' says Dad, holding the child's limp hand. Large round eyes look up in a silent appeal.

The *Agrimony* patient though seriously ill makes light of the matter, talking to keep his visitors by the bedside. With the doctor he jokes about the problem.

'Have you heard the one about the man who thought he had a phantom limb? Well his wife…'.

'Please hold still Mr Jones, I've got to a tricky stage and this might hurt a bit.'

Chicory people like to be ill; it gives them an opportunity to get things organized around them.

'You can read me another story now, Daddy, then Lucy can come up after tea and play a game and then Mummy . . .'.

'I'm sorry, but I've got to go. Oh come on, don't start crying again my darling.'

Vervains know what is best for them and will not take advice, even from the doctor.
'I know you don't think you are ill, but I would still recommend a few days in bed.'
'Don't be ridiculous I can't afford the time and besides I have my multi-pack pills, here you should try some.'

Centaury, too, cannot be ill—who would wash and scrub and tend to the others? If, finally they succumb, the illness is characterized by weakness and debility.

Cerato says: 'Am I ill, do you think? I am not sure. Somebody said yesterday that I looked awful but I haven't the spots that Mary had. Perhaps we should see what the other doctor says when he gets here.'

With *Scleranthus* the symptoms come and go, they move about, the temperature is up and down. In the morning they want to stay in bed, by eleven they are up and dressed, then turn around and they are back in bed again. They cannot make up their minds if they are ill.

Water Violet people are even more withdrawn than usual. They are knowledgeable and calm, speaking to the doctor as an equal. They do not like to be fussed over.
'Just leave the tray on the chair, my dear, I will get it when I want it.'

Gentian gets depressed and, as Bach observed, is discouraged by any set-back in recovery. Then they see the perverse fate that led to their illness. 'It's just my luck to get flu again this week when I was planning that trip.'

Rock Rose's behaviour is not so obvious. They are mute, remember. They run a high temperature and struggle to keep their hold on life. Those around soon share the apprehension.

Appendix III

Which Plants Come From Where?

Plants have been on the move since the beginning. They colonize an area when it is suitable, only to abandon it when circumstances change. While some plants extend territory through their roots, others employ a winged seed to assist dispersal; birds and animals can be pressed into service as carriers. Whether by accident or design, mankind has assisted in the dispersal of plants. Whatever the mechanism, it is clear that plants can be taken to the four corners of the earth and, provided conditions are suitable, they thrive. *Impatiens glandulifera* is a clear case in point. It was imported from Kashmir by plant collectors and greedily consumed territory along the waterways once it had arrived in England.

The Roman armies took the Sweet Chestnut with them from the Mediterranean as they conquered north west Europe and brought vines to Britain (although they were not necessarily the first). Mimulus was introduced to the UK from the west coast of North America and as a reciprocal gesture, Scleranthus probably was taken to California—at the time of the gold rush in 1849, carried in animal feed. The English Elm was brought, not as seed but as sapling from France or Spain, to be used for hedging and as a landscape tree. Gorse was planted as cover for game birds. White Chestnut was introduced in the early seventeenth century from Macedonia. Star of Bethlehem may have been brought to England by the Crusaders. [See Maggie Campbell-Culver, *The Origin of Plants*, Headline, 2001]. Plants hunters like Earnest Wilson, 'Chinese Wilson' as he was called, made expeditions to send back specimens both for research and cultivation. Wilson was responsible for sending Cerato to the West.

All this points to the fact that plants do not know national boundaries. Even though certain geographical regions develop a unique flora, any plant may escape or be taken out from one region and introduced to another. Climate change alone forces the migration of plants: there are few species which could survive the cold in Britain during the last Ice Age, they had to travel south or perish. Equally, as the glaciers retreated, virgin soil was open for colonization by pioneers returning north. As with people, it is difficult to say who might be a true native. Consequently it is hard to see how Bach flower remedies can be claimed as English, rather than Irish, French or European—apart that is from the fact that Bach himself was English. Even Europe is too small a geographical enclosure if the origin of plants is properly considered.

```
HOLLY . . . . . Britian:  Europe.

CRAB APPLE . . Britian: Europe:  Western Asia:
               Himalayas.

ELM . . . . . Britian,  not native.

HORNBEAM. . . Wales:  Central and Southern England.

BEECH . . . . Temperate Europe.

OAK . . . . . Britian.  Europe:  Asia.

WILLOW. . . . Europe:  Temperate Asia.

ASPEN . . . . Britian:  North Europe:  Northern Asia.

PINE  . . . . Scotland:  North & Central Europe:
              North Asia.

RED CHESTNUT.  North America.

WALNUT . . . . Persia:  Himalayas:  Western Asia.

SWEET CHESTNUT. Southern Europe:  North Africa.

LARCH . . . . . Central Europe.

IMPATIENS . . . Himalayas.

CERATO . . . . Thibet.

CHERRY PLUM. . Caucasus.

MIMULUS. . . . North America.

WHITE CHESTNUT. Caucasus:  Balkans:  North India.
```

Dr Bach recognized all this, we may be sure. He typed a list of eighteen of the remedy plants and trees, indicating the region from whence they came. In *The Twelve Healers & Other Remedies* he noted that: 'All the remedies can be found growing naturally in the British Isles except Vine, Olive, Cerato, although some are true natives of other countries along middle and southern Europe to northern India and Tibet'. More significant than geography is the identification of the correct species—that is why Bach always provided the Latin name—for it is the plant which is important, not the country in which it grows.

It follows from this that anyone may make a Bach remedy, wherever they live, provided that the true species has been identified. There may be constraints upon the quality of the mother tincture, but territory is not one of them. How foolish, then, to suggest that Bach remedies can only be made at one location in England. Certainly neither Weeks, nor Bach before her, suggested that a location in the Thames Valley was in any way preferable to one in any other county or country. In the very first *Bach Remedy News Letter*, March 1950, Nora reported that a list of the plant names had been sent to Royal Botanic Gardens, Kew, so that Latin names might be verified. *Centaurium erythaea*, for instance, had been changed to *C. umbellatum*, *Impatiens roylei* to *I. Glandulifera*, Crab Apple was *Malus pumilia*, rather than *Pyrus malus*. Then came the note that 'friends in Australia' had found Centaury growing profusely in fields near Sydney. 'We should be interested to know which of the remedy plants grow wild in Africa, New Zealand, Switzerland, America'. [*Newsletter*, No. 1, March 1950, page 2]. In this first newsletter, as in every succeeding one, she provided full details of how to find and identify one of the Bach remedy flowers, so that people might prepare their own essences.

By *Newsletter* No. 3, in September 1950, Nora Weeks was already dealing with one of the most controversial questions concerning Bach remedies. Was it really true that anybody could make them? Surely only essences made by Dr Bach have a true potency. Or perhaps, only essences made by trained helpers at *Mount Vernon* could really be effective. Nora's reply?

> *Although it is a privilege to have stocks from Dr Bach's own preparations, any made by yourselves will be found to be just as potent. Many people have already made Tinctures both by the sun method and by the boiling method, and the medicines prepared from them have brought the same excellent results.*

Purists might argue that the best remedy should be made where the plant originated. After all, Bach made Olive and Vine in the Mediterranean. But then we would have to journey to China to prepare Cerato—an interesting prospect—as Wilson listed the Min river valley as the only place where he found it.

There is evidence that plants adapt and take a different form when growing in different localities. This is true of Agrimony, depending upon whether it is found in moist clay or dry chalk-downland. And it may well be that adaptation of form, brought on by differing environmental influences, leads to both species variation and the development of a new species. The *Ray Society* published monographs which noted the variation in species such as Campion (*Silene*) and Knapweed (*Centaurea*). Variant forms of Red Chestnut (*Aesculus carnea*) have already been noted. The tendency of *Mimulus guttatus* to hybridize with *M. luteus* has been used to advantage by nurserymen for many years. Mention should be made of Luther Burbank (1849-1926) who did pioneering work in California adapting plant forms so that he even grew a spineless cactus.

Nature is constantly in experiment—that was Darwin's thesis—and the 'sport' which throws up an unusual pattern may become the species of tomorrow. When making flower essences it is important to be aware of this potential for variation and instability. These in turn are influenced by the provenance of an individual plant and its location.

Appendix IV

Homœopathy, Dilutions and a Numbers Game

When Dr Bach discovered his new remedies he made them available through the leading homœopathic pharmacies in London: Keane & Ashwell, Epps and Nelsons. Just as he had developed the Bach nosodes and made them available to a wider public, so too his flower remedies. He had not thought of patenting a new medicine but made his discoveries immediately and widely known to those who might make use of them: doctors. The chemists (he listed them in *The Twelve Healers*) had 'very kindly undertaken the distribution of these remedies at a moderate price'. In 1936, a single remedy cost 8d, postage 2d. By today's prices, with postage at 27p, the single remedy would cost £1.08. A full set of twelve remedies were to cost five shillings: moderate indeed.

By working through the homœopathic pharmacies, Bach employed the best means available—there were no health food stores in 1930. Homœopathic remedies represented the only alternative to conventional medicine. But just because he availed himself of this service we should not be drawn to the conclusion that the Bach flower remedies were homeopathic medicines, either then or subsequently. This was a convenience, no more. In his writings Bach made it clear that the flower remedies were not homœopathic. At first, the Bach Centre supported this view. In the *Bach Remedy News Letter* (September 1951), Frances Wheeler wrote 'these remedies are not homœopathic, nor are they prepared by homœopathic methods'. Even after the death of Nora Weeks there was an announcement, in June 1978, when John Ramsell wrote:

> . . . *we sometimes label our packages 'Homœopathic Tinctures'. This reference must not be taken literally. . . . The homœopathic methods of succession and tituration do not apply. This means there can be no such determined levels of potency as 6x, 12x, or 30x etc., in relation to the Bach Remedies.*

We can agree on that. But if Bach remedies are not homœopathic why label them as such?

The deceit of calling them homœopathic remedies was confirmed in 1980 when an announcement was placed in the American Homœopathic Journal which effectively gave homœopathic status to Bach remedies in the USA. Significantly, Richard Katz and Patricia Kaminski of the North American Flower Essence Society resisted this move. In a monograph entitled *Flower Essences & Homœopathy*, 1983, they conducted a forensic analysis of the issues. They concluded that homœopathy and flower essence therapy were related but essentially different.

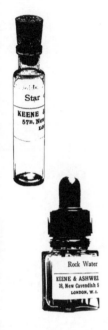

The very earliest labels carried simply the name of the remedy: Star of Bethlehem, Rock Water, without any indication of potency. An advertisement, dated June 1933, in *Heal Thyself* (the magazine produced by J. Ellis Barker, which had previously used the title *The Homœopathic World*), offered *The Twelve Bach Remedies* in 'disc' form. Presumably this was some kind of pill. The advertisement was placed by Nelson's Pharmacy of 73, Duke Street, London. The remedies were offered for sale at twelve shillings, post extra, more than double the price Bach had announced.

It is unclear just when the Bach Centre began bottling and selling direct to the public. While the newsletter offered various books for sale it never directly promoted the remedies, preferring to encourage people to prepare their own. But at a certain point John Ainsworth, the Chief Pharmacist at Nelsons, advised Nora Weeks that Bach remedies would be better protected if the authorities regarded them as homœopathic. To provide a notional homœopathic dilution the labels then indicated: 'active ingredients: 1-240 per cent of an aqueous infusion of the flowers of . . .'. In March 1963 the *Bach Remedy News Letter* carried a short piece on labelling. Here Nora Weeks wrote 'we have decided to conform to these [pharmaceutical] regulations and state on the stock bottle labels the quantities and percentages of the flowers contained in them'.* The quantity 1:240 per cent is meaningless, however. It is possible to have 1: 240; one percent is possible (i.e. 1:100), but not 1:240 per cent. It was a pseudo-homœopathic dilution, apparently, designed to represent the quantity of the original flowers present in the bottle. In the sun method this quantity would have been zero, in every case. In the boiling method

---

* 'We had a big quantity of the Rescue Remedy labels printed and can supply them to those practitioners who also sell the Rescue Remedy, if they will write and let us know how many they need.' Nora was referring to the current practice of people preparing their own rescue remedy from the five stock bottles: Cherry Plum, Clematis, Impatiens, Rock Rose, Star of Bethlehem. It was then a formula and not a branded product.

a dry ash test could have established a figure but it would have had no real meaning since the Bach remedies were and are based upon a quality and not a quantity. The label of Rock Water, incidentally, read 'active ingredients: 1-240 per cent of solarized Aqua Petra'.

In Weeks and Bullen's *Bach Flower Remedies Illustration & Preparation* (1964), we can read that the actual dilution used at this time was two drops of mother tincture in one ounce of brandy (30 ml). The exact levels of dilution had varied. In 1933 Bach had recommended that one drop of mother tincture potentized eight ounces of water (250 ml), 'from which doses may be taken by the teaspoonful as required' (*Collected Writings*, p. 81). Later in the same year he called mother tincture 'stock' (*Collected Writings*, p. 67), and under 'method of dosage' he spoke of four drops added to a four ounce bottle (125 ml). He said 'bottles of the remedy supplied by the chemist are stock and are to be used for medicating four-ounce bottles as described here'. The same formula was repeated in 1934 (*Collected Writings*, p. 57). Does this mean that Keane & Ashwell, Nelsons and Epps were all handing over mother tincture to customers?

By 1936 Bach wrote in *The Twelve Healers & Other Remedies* that two drops should be taken from stock bottles and added to a 'small bottle nearly filled with water; if this is required to keep for some time a little brandy may be added as a preservative' (*Collected Writings*, p. 46). So he is now down to two drops in a small bottle. This might be taken directly by mouth or diluted again 'in a little water, milk or any way convenient'.

In the *Bach Remedy News Letter* of June 1950 Weeks gave a clear account of how the remedies were prepared. This was repeated in *Bach Flower Remedies Illustration & Preparation*. Here at least there was no confusion. There are three stages:

  I.   The preparation of the mother essence
  II.   The making of the stock bottle (two drops in 30 ml)
  III. The medicine bottle for dosage.

It seems unlikely that Nora was acting contrary to Bach's instructions. The earlier contradictions have the appearance of being experimental. The labelling and declared 'potency' is another matter.

Two drops of mother tincture in 30 ml of brandy, for preparing stock, sounds easy. But as soon as the production volumes begin to rise it must have been necessary to make up larger quantities of stock before pouring into the small bottles. (In 1981 the Bach Centre offered stock bottles for sale in the following sizes: 5 ml, 8 ml, 10 ml, 30 ml, 35 ml.) If two drops in 30 ml is correct it follows that sixty-six drops are required for one litre. But what actual dilution is that? Drops and millilitres are not equivalent measures. A drop is a variable quantity depending upon the size of the dropper (or lip) and the specific gravity of the liquid. This point was noted by Hahnemann who conducted experiments to establish that 100 drops of alcohol (52.6 per cent) = 2.7 ml, 100 drops of water = 6.28 ml (P. Bartel, *Hahnemann's Legacy*). Similar experiments have established that 100 drops of brandy at 40 per cent alcohol = 2.91 ml. A 30 ml bottle of brandy, therefore, contains some 1,000 drops. This gives a dilution of two drops per 1,000 or 1:500. Mother essence is brandy and water (20 per cent alcohol) and 100 drops = 3.80 ml, giving a dilution of 1:395. It must be stated that this is calculated on the basis of the pipette which gives the largest drop; dilutions as low as 1:800 would be produced by smaller drops, from different pipettes.

These figures bear no relation to the 1:240 per cent discussed above. John Ainsworth left no explanation and it is doubtful whether Nora Weeks understood the calculation. It was probably based upon the old measures of a drachm, a drop and a minim. Because the volume of drops varied, pharmacists had long ago adopted a standard measure:

60 drops or minims = 1 drachm = 1/8 fluid ounce.

A fluid ounce contained 480 such 'standard' drops. A notional dilution of 1:240 for Bach remedies follows. But this is not 1:240 per cent.

When Nelsons Pharmacy was sold, John Ainsworth set up Ainsworth Pharmacy, at the premises of Keane & Ashwell in New Cavendish Street. Some years later Nelsons bought the business of Bach Flower Remedies Ltd. In their attempt to register Bach remedies as homœopathic they revived the old 1:240 per cent dilution, explaining it like this:

> *1:240 per cent is an outdated scale of measurement. Bach Flower Remedies are akin to homœopathic remedies, therefore the same labelling conventions are used and the dilution is expressed using the decimal or x scale. The 5x dilution is calculated as follows:*
>
> *Step One – the basic mother tincture produces a dry residue of 1% i.e. 1 in 100.*
>
> *Step Two – This is mixed with an equal quantity of brandy, 1 in 2.*
>
> *Step Three – There are 1,000 drops of grape alcohol (brandy) 27% in 30 ml. Two drops of Mother Tincture are added to this 2 in 1,000 or 1 in 500.*

5x is calculated as follows:

1/100 x ½ x 1/500 = 1/1000,000 or 10⁵ = 5x

This is ingenious but it has little bearing on the truth. There is no dry residue of 1%; 27% grape alcohol cannot be called brandy.

The same booklet went on to claim that Bach remedies function homœopathically because:

1. They are potentized.
2. The stock is diluted, without a traceable active ingredient.
3. They do not contain the physical plant but the pattern of energy.
4. The sun and boiling methods are recognized by the British Homœopathic Pharmacopoeia.

To reply to the points in order:

1. There is no serial dilution, succession or other homœopathic process involved in preparing Bach remedies.
2. No traceable active ingredient is found in the mother tincture before dilution—not so in homœopathy where the mother tincture is prepared from the physical material.
3. See 2; there is no change in polarity (page 57) as in classical homœopathy.
4. The British Homœopathic Pharmacopoeia included Bach remedies only at the insistence of Nelsons, who employed two of the five members of the Scientific Committee (1993).

In July 2000 Nelsons abandoned their attempt to register Bach remedies as homœopathic in the UK. In other countries they continue to promote them as homœopathic medicines.

This whole subject of dilution can be understood easily once it is accepted that Bach remedies are qualitative and not quantitative. Again this is a clear contrast with homœopathy which employs multiple high potencies to different effects. The surprise in homœopathy comes when we realize that the serial dilution leaves no measurable quantity of the original material in the remedy. With Bach's flower essences there never was a measurable quantity. From the beginning the mother tincture and the remedy were only qualities: a pattern which cannot be measured, at least not by physical means. This quality is a means of recognition, the character which makes the remedy what it is. A quality is recognized as a signature or gesture: like a phrase of music, it is not made more by virtue of volume. The signature written into the spring water of a mother essence is like a signature which proves identity, it is not clearer for being written larger.

Dilution therefore is managed not by quantity but quality. When Bach was experimenting in the 1930s he varied the measures. By the time he died he had settled on a formula which worked. There is no need to imagine that the remedy has greater strength at stock or even mother tincture level, provided the pattern is properly there and its integrity has been maintained. In the same way there is no need to increase the dose in order to gain greater benefit. It is repetition of the pattern which determines dosage, not the size of the physical body or the intensity of the difficulty.

Appendix V

Chronology from 1886 to 2002

1886   24 September, Edward Bach born, Moseley, near Birmingham.

1903-6   Worked at his father's brass foundry.

1906-12   Medical School, Birmingham and London.

1912   Graduated MRCS, LRCP; postgraduate training.

1913   14 January, married Gwendoline Caiger.
       University College Hospital, London.

1915-19   Bacteriological research.

1916   Daughter born to Edward Bach and Kitty Light.

1917   5 April, Gwendoline Bach died of diphtheria at Golders Green, London.

       2 May, Edward Bach marries Kitty Light of Islington, London.

       July, Bach collapsed at work, received surgery for cancer.

1918   Influenza epidemic.

1919   March, appointed to London Homœopathic Hospital; research at Nottingham Place laboratories, London W1.

1920   April, read paper *Vaccine Therapy* . . . to London Homœopathic Society.

       Research with F. H. Teale.

1922   Began Harley Street practice, London and moved to laboratories at Park Crescent.

       Development of the seven Bach nosodes.

       Separated from Kitty.

1924   Read paper *Intestinal Toxaemia* . . . at British Homœopathic Congress, London.

1925   Wrote *Chronic Disease a Working Hypothesis* with Dr Charles E. Wheeler.

1927   Read paper *Chronic Disease…* at International Homœopathic Congress, London.

1928   September, discovered *Impatiens, Mimulus and Clematis* at Crickhowell.

November, read paper *Rediscovery of Psora* at British Homœopathic Society.

1929   Gave up nosode therapy.

1930   January, published *Preparing Vaccines* ...

February, published *Some New remedies & New Uses.*

May, closed medical practice and left London.

Bettws-y-Coed, Wales, developed type theory.

Abersoch, Wales, developed sun method; wrote *Heal Thyself.*

July, Pwllheli, Wales.

August/September, Cromer, Norfolk, found *Agrimony, Chicory, Vervain Centaury, Cerato, Scleranthus.*

Some Fundamental Considerations . . . listed eleven new remedies, including Cotyledon and Arvensis.

1931   February, *Heal Thyself* published,

Ye Suffer From Yourselves, talk at Southport, Cheshire.

March, left for Wales.

May, staying near Abergavenny.

June, at Lewes in Sussex, *Water Violet.*

July, in Thames Valley, found *Gentian.*

September, Westerham in Kent, made *Gentian.*

Winter in Cromer.

1932   Spring, in London, consulting rooms in Wimpole Street.

Wrote *Free Thyself* in Regents Park, published privately it listed twelve remedies, including *Rock Rose,* made at Westerham in June.

Autumn, returned to Cromer, *The Twelve Healers.*

November/December, advertised remedies, correspondence with General Medical Council.

1933   April, Marlow, Buckinghamshire, *Gorse.*

May, Cromer, *Oak.*

August, Abergavenny, Wales, *Rock Water, Heather.*

Autumn, Cromer, *The Twelve Healers & Four Helpers.*

1934   March, left Cromer.

1934	April, Sotwell, Oxfordshire, at *Wellsprings* and *Mount Vernon*.
(*cont.*)	June, *Olive, Vine, Wild Oat, The Twelve Healers & Seven Helpers*.
1935	Discovery of Second Nineteen, and the boiling method.
1936	September, *The Twelve Healers & Other Remedie* published.
	24 September, *Healing by Herbs…* a lecture at Wallingford.
	October, *Masonic Lecture*.
	27 November, Bach died at Ladygrove Nursing Home, Didcot. Causes of death listed as cardiac failure and sarcoma. Nora Weeks was sole beneficiary under his will. Death certificate for E. Bach, medical practitioner of *Wellsprings*, Sotwell,
1937	New edition of *The Twelve Healers & Other Remedies*.
1938	*To Thine Own Self Be True,* by Mary Tabor.
1940	*Medical Discoveries* … Nora Weeks' biography of Bach.
1950	March, *The Bach Remedy News Letter*, first issue.
	June newsletter described in detail the 'sun method of potentizing'.
	December newsletter described how to prepare Rescue Remedy putting two drops of each the five remedies into a dosage bottle.
1951	September newsletter stated categorically that the remedies are not homœopathic.
1955	A fund created to purchase Mount Vernon.
1958	Formation of *The Dr Bach Healing Trust*. It had three objectives: to purchase property (Mt Vernon) for 'the work of flower healing', to pay for its maintenance, and to 'promote and expand the work' as the Trustees think fit. The first trustees were Nora Weeks, Victor Bullen and Frances Thomas.
1964	*Bach Flower Remedies Illustration & Preparation,* Nora Weeks and Victor Bullen.
1971	Chancellor's *Handbook* published.
	Nickie Murray and John Ramsell joined the Bach Centre.
1973	Ramsell and Murray became trustees of *The Dr Bach Healing Trust*.
1974	Weeks and Bullen began trading as Dr Edward Bach's Team.
1975	May, Victor Bullen died, leaving everything to Nora Weeks.
1976	April, Weeks, Murray and Ramsell trade as Dr Edward Bach's Centre.

1978   January, Nora Weeks died, leaving her residual estate to the trustees of *The Dr Edward Bach Trust* 'to be used in their absolute discretion in the furtherance of their work . . . the receipt of the Treasurer or other proper officer of the Trust shall be a good and sufficient discharge . . . '.

1979   February, Ramsell registered trademark 'Bach Flower Remedies', UK.

Bach's description of 'methods of preparation' removed from *The Twelve Healers & Other Remedies*.

September newsletter announced that the Weeks & Bullen book *Bach Flower Remedies Illustration & Preparation* will not be reprinted.

1983   Ramsell and Murray formed company Bach Flower Remedies Ltd, transferring all assets of Dr Edward Bach Centre to the company.

1984   28 February, further registration of 'Bach Flower Remedies' as trademark in UK by Bach Flower Remedies Ltd.

1985   Ramsell's daughter, Judy Howard joined the Bach Centre.

1986   Bach's writings out of copyright. Publication of *Collected Writings of Edward Bach*.

Murray left Bach Centre, retiring to Crete and then California.

1987   Murray sold shares in Bach Flower Remedies Ltd to BFR (Mount Vernon) Ltd, owned by Ramsell.

Bach Flower Remedies Ltd dissolved.

1988   Publication of *Healing Herbs of Edward Bach—a practical guide to making the remedies*.

1989   Four further trademarks using the name 'Bach' registered in UK by BFR (Mount Vernon) Ltd.

Healing Herbs began production of Bach flower remedies.

1991   January, BFR (Mount Vernon) Ltd made exclusive agreement with A. Nelson Ltd for packaging and marketing of remedies.

Two further trademarks using the name 'Bach' registered in UK by BFR (Mount Vernon) Ltd.

1993   Nelsons buy BFR (Mount Vernon) Ltd for 4.3 million pounds, reforming the company as Bach Flower Remedies Ltd (No 2).

British Homœopathic Pharmacopoeia carried monographs on Bach flower remedies, listing dilutions as 5x, using ethanol 22%.

1997   26 February, Healing Herbs applied to High Court for revocation of trademarks containing the word 'Bach'.

1998   April, High Court, London (Mr Justice Neuberger) decided that 'Bach' is generic and cannot be used as a registered trademark.

1999   October, Court of Appeal, London, upheld High Court decision.

2000   House of Lords rejected further appeal on trademark decision.

Endnotes

INTRODUCTION

1. These court hearings were the result of an application by the author to remove the marks 'Bach' and 'Bach Flower Remedies' from the list of registered trademarks in Britain. The first hearing took place in April 1998, the appeal in October 1999. The House of Lords later rejected an application to rehear the case and refer it to the European Court. The text of the first two judgements can be read online at www.healing-herbs.co.uk, under 'Legal Debate'.

2. *Collected Writings of Edward Bach,* Bach Educational Programme, 1987. p. 13.

3. Ibid.

4. Ibid., p. 126.

5. Eliade, Mircea, *The Sacred & the Profane,* Harcourt, Brace & World, 1959, pp. 52, 149-150.

6. *Collected Writings,* op. cit., pp. 12-13.

7. A randomized double-blind study at Exeter University used Bach remedies to alleviate exam stress. The sample was too small, only 45 people. Nevertheless, 'participants taking the verum reported lower anxiety than those taking placebo on day three of the study. However, this result needs to be interpreted with great caution as we had no *a priori* expectation of this finding...'. In other words, we did not expect the remedy to show a result on day three and so ignored the finding. Not very scientific. The authors nonetheless felt confident to report: Bach remedies ineffective in relieving exam stress. [N. C. Armstrong, E. Ernst, *A Randomized, double-blind, placebo-controlled trial of a Bach Flower Remedy,* Prefus, November 1999.]

8. Bose, Sir Jagadis Chunder, *Plant Autographs and their Revelations,* Longman, Green and Co., 1927.

9. Watson, Lyall, *Supernature,* Hodder & Stoughton, 1973, pp. 247-248. Tompkins, Peter, & Bird, Christopher, *The Secret Life of Plants,* Allen Lane, 1973, pp. 17-26.

10. Zimmer, Carl, *Evolution, The Triumph of an Idea,* Heinemann, 2002.

11. Rose, Hilary and Stephen, *Alas Poor Darwin,* Jonathan Cape, 2000, p. 4.

12. Darwin, Charles, *The Movements and Habits of Climbing Plants,* John Murray, 1937, p. 183.

CHAPTER 1. A GROWING SENSITIVITY

1. *Collected Writings of Edward Bach,* Bach Educational Programme, 1987, pp. 183-4.
2. Ibid., p. 217.
3. Ibid., p. 224.
4. Weeks, Nora, *The Medical Discoveries of Edward Bach Physician,* C. W. Daniel Co., 1973, p. 23.
5. A digest of the book appears in *Collected Writings of Edward Bach,* in the chapter 'Intestinal Toxaemia in its Relation to Cancer', reprinted from *The British Homœopathic Journal,* October 1924.
6. *Collected Writings,* op. cit., p.194
7. Bach, Edward and Wheeler, Charles E. *Chronic Disease, a working hypothesis,* H. K. Lewis, 1925, pp. 9-14.
8. *Collected Writings,* op. cit., p. 208.
9. Ibid., op. cit., p. 221.
10. Ibid., p. 211.
11. Ibid., p. 125-126.
12. Ibid., p. 216.
13. Ibid., p. 183 ff.
14. *Organon of the Medical Art,* Dr Samuel Hahnemann, edited by Wenda Brewster O'Reilly, transl. Steven Decker, Birdcage Books, Washington U.S.A., 1996.
15. *Collected Writings,* op. cit., p. 192.
16. Ibid., p. 60.
17. Ibid., p. 215.
18. Ibid., p. 115.
19. Ibid., p. 100.
20. Ibid., p. 52.
21. *Luke* 4, 23.
22. *Organon,* op. cit., p. 150.
23. Ibid., pp. 232-243.
24. Ibid., p. 277.
25. *Collected Writings,* op. cit., p. 193.
26. Ibid., p. 177 ff.
27. Ibid., p. 150.
28. *Medical Discoveries,* op. cit., pp. 39-40.

CHAPTER 2. DOWN BY THE RIVERSIDE

1. Weeks, Nora, *The Medical Discoveries of Edward Bach Physician,* C. W. Daniel, 1940, p. 41.
2. Ibid., p. 39-40.
3. Ibid., pp. 25, 30, 39, 41.
4. Ibid., p. 25.
5. Ibid., pp. 134-41.
6. Ibid., p. 136.

7. Ibid., p. 48.

8. Ibid., pp. 138-139.

9. Royle's book *Illustrations of the Botany of the Himalayan Mountains*, 1839, was probably the first to list *Impatiens*.

10. Inaccurately quoted by Mehta, Ashrin in *100 Himalayan Flowers*, 1991 from F. S. Smythe *The Valley of the Flowers*, Hodder & Stoughton, 1938, p. 68.

11. Mabey, Richard, *Flora Britannica*, Sinclair Stephenson, 1996, p. 275.

12. Bach's own comments on what intuition is and how to use it can be read in *Collected Writings—Free Thyself*, chapter 4, pp. 93-4 and in *Heal Thyself*, chapter 7, pp. 146-7.

13. Isaac Asimov makes this bold definition for us in *Forward the Foundation*, 1993, p. 62. Equally the O.E.D. will serve for definitions. Asimov is interesting in that he attempts some kind of analysis of the processes of intuition but it does not go very far.

14. Published in *The Bach Remedy Newsletter*, March 1971.

15. *The Original Writings of Edward Bach*, C. W. Daniel, 1990, p. 92.

16. *Collected Writings of Edward Bach*, Bach Educational Programme, 1987, p. 174.

17. Loc. cit.

18. Loc. cit.

19. *Original Writings*, op. cit., p. 181.

20. *Collected Writings*, op. cit., pp. 26-7.

21. *Original Writings*, op. cit., p. 181.

22. *Collected Writings*, op. cit., p. 21.

23. Ibid., p. 174.

24. Ibid., p. 54.

25. *Collected Writings*, op. cit.

26. Ibid., p. 174.

27. I am grateful to Hugh G. Baily of London for the etymology.

28. *Collected Writings*, op. cit., p. 175.

29. Ibid., p. 175.

30. Ibid., p. 151.

31. Ibid., p. 106.

32. Ibid., p. 176.

33. Wingate, Peter, *The Penguin Medical Encyclopaedia*, Penguin Books, 1972, p. 157.

34. *Collected Writings*, op. cit., p. 166.

35. Ibid., p. 106.

36. Ibid., p. 175.

37. Ibid., p. 166.

38. Ibid., p. 64.

39. Mrs Grieve says of *Clematis vitalba* 'this variety is also said to contain clematine' which she calls a violent poison. Grieve, Mrs M., *A Modern Herbal*, Jonathan Cape, 1977, p. 206. Also it is noted by Professor Henslowe in *British Wild Flowers*, S.P.C.K., 1910, p. 1: 'it is very narcotic in its properties . . .'

40. *Collected Writings*, op. cit., p. 166.

41. Ibid., p. 174.

42. *Organon of the Medical Art,* Dr Samuel Hahnemann, edited by Wenda Brewster O'Reilly, transl. Steven Decker, Birdcage Books, Washington U.S.A., 1996. Glossary, pp. 235-243.
43. *Collected Writings,* op. cit., p. 173.
44. Loc. cit.
45. *Original Writings,* op. cit., pp. 98, 99.
46. *Collected Writings,* op. cit., p. 81.
47. Ibid., p. 87.
48. Ibid., p. 174.
49. Ibid., p. 63.
50. Turner, W. J., in *Nature in Britain,* Collins, 1946, p. 86.
51. Allen, Mea, *Darwin and his Flowers,* Faber, 1977, pp. 250-3.
52. Ridley, H. N., *Dispersal of Plants Throughout the World,* L. Reeve & Co., n.d. p. 187.
53. *Collected Writings,* op. cit., p. 81.
54. Ibid., p. 105.
55. Ibid., p. 175.
56. Gimbel, Theo, *The Colour Therapy Workbook,* Element Books, 1993, p. 16.
57. Ibid., p. 79.
58. Ibid., p. 176.
59. *Organon,* op. cit., Glossary, p. 340.
60. *Collected Writings,* op. cit., pp. 183-194.
61. Ibid., pp. 193-4.
62. Loc. cit.

CHAPTER 3. THE SUN METHOD

1. *Collected Writings of Edward Bach,* Bach Educational Programme, 1987, p. 171.
2. Ibid., p. 109.
3. Ibid., p. 88.
4. Ibid., p. 170.
5. Weeks, Nora, *The Medical Discoveries of Edward Bach Physician,* C. W. Daniel, 1940, p. 49.
6. This information comes from Richard Katz and Patricia Kaminski of *The Flower Essence Society,* California, U.S.A.
7. *Medical Discoveries,* op. cit., p. 44.
8. I am indebted to Rachel Carter for tracing this connection.
9. *Mrs Beeton's Household Management.* Ward Lock & Co. New Edition, *circa* 1920, p. 1401, *illust.* opposite p. 1392.
10. *Medical Discoveries,* op. cit., p. 39.
11. *Collected Writings,* op. cit., p. 171.
12. Ibid., p. 109.
13. Ibid., p. 174.
14. *The Original Writings of Edward Bach,* C. W. Daniel Co., 1990, pp. 97-8.
15. *Collected Writings,* op. cit., p. 47.

16. Dr Jacques Benveniste, *Understanding Digital Biology*, writing at www.homeopathyhome.com as at March 2001.
17. *Medical Discoveries*, op. cit., pp. 50-51.
18. *Collected Writings*, op. cit., p. 167.
19. Ibid., p. 169.
20. Ibid., p. 117.
21. *Medical Discoveries*, op. cit.. p. 67.
22. *Collected Writings*, op. cit.. p. 174.
23. *Medical Discoveries*, op. cit., p. 67.

CHAPTER 4. HEAL THYSELF—FREE THYSELF

1. *Collected Writings of Edward Bach*, Bach Educational Programme, 1987, p. 192.
2. Ibid., p. 100.
3. Ibid., p. 160.
4. Ibid., pp. 157-172.
5. Weeks, Nora, *The Medical Discoveries of Edward Bach Physician*, C. W. Daniel, 1940, p. 134.
6. *Collected Writings*, op. cit., p. 157.
7. Ibid., pp. 157–8.
8. Ibid., p. 158.
9. Loc. cit.
10. Ibid., p. 159.
11. Ibid., p. 142.
12. Ibid., p. 127.
13. Ibid., p. 148.
14. Ibid., p. 30.
15. Ibid., p. 112.
16. Ibid., p. 130.
17. Ibid., p. 115.
18. Ibid., p. 102.
19. Ibid., p. 131.
20. Loc. cit.
21. Ibid., p. 78.
22. Ibid., p. 160.
23. Loc. cit.
24. Loc. cit.
25. Ibid., p. 92.
26. Ibid., p. 111.
27. Ibid., p. 114.
28. Ibid., p. 115.
29. There are two contemporary novels that grapple with this idea: *Soul Flame* by Barbara Wood and *The Physician* by Noah Gordon.
30. *Collected Writings*, op. cit., p. 119.
31. *The Bach Remedy Newsletter*, March 1956, p. 3.
32. *Collected Writings*, op. cit., pp. 23, 24, 28.

33. Ibid., p. 29.
34. Ibid., p. 104.
35. Loc. cit.
36. Ibid., p. 83.
37. Ibid., p. 30.
38. Ibid., pp. 32-33.

CHAPTER 5. NOT THE RIGHT REMEDY

1   *Collected Writings of Edward Bach,* Bach Educational Programme, 1987, p. 160.
2. Loc. cit.
3. Ibid., p. 99.
4. Ibid., p. 161.
5. Loc. cit.
6. Mrs Grieve, M., *A Modern Herbal,* Jonathan Cape, 1931.
    Potter's New Cyclopaedia of Botanical drugs and preparations, Potter & Clarke
    Ltd, 1975.
7. *Potter's New Cyclopaedia of botanical drugs and preparations,* C.W. Daniel, 1988,
    pp. 265-266.
8. *Collected Writing,* op. cit., p. 176.
9. Ibid., p. 166.
10. Ibid., p. 167.
11. Loc. cit.
12. Ibid., p. 161.
13. Ibid., p. 169.
14. Loc. cit.

CHAPTER 6. CROMER

1. *The Original Writings of Edward Bach,* C. W. Daniel Co., 1990, p. 190.
2. Weeks, Nora, *The Medical Discoveries of Edward Bach Physician,* C. W. Daniel
    Co., 1940, p. 64.
3. *The Teachings of Don Juan, 1968, A Separate Reality, 1971, Journey to Ixtlan, 1972,
    Tales of Power, 1974,* all available as Penguin Books.
4. Quoted by Nancy Price in *Where the Skies Unfold,* George Ronald, 1947, p. 5.
5. *Medical Discoveries,* op. cit., p. 64ff.
6. *Philippians* 4, 7.
7. *Collected Writings of Edward Bach,* Bach Educational Programme, 1987,
    pp. 116-117.
8. Ibid., pp. 75-76.
9. Ibid., p. 105.
10. Grieve, Mrs M., *A Modern Herbal,* Jonathan Cape, 1977, p. 13.
11. *Collected Writings,* op. cit., p. 41.

12. Ibid., p. 79.
13. Mrs Grieve, op. cit., p. 14.
14. Weeks and Bullen, *Bach Flower Remedies Illustration & Preparation*, C. W. Daniel Co., 1964, p. 24.
15. *Collected Writings*, op. cit., p. 105.
16. Ibid., p. 63.
17. Ibid., p. 45.
18. Ibid., p. 165.
19. Ibid., p. 166.
20. Ibid., p. 104.
21. Ibid., p. 84.
22. Professor Henslowe, *British Wild Flowers*, Society for Promoting Christian Knowledge, London, 1910, p. 174.
23. Johns, Rev. C A. *Flowers of the Field*, Society for Promoting Christian Knowledge, London, 1899, p. 416.
24. Mrs Grieve, op. cit., p. 197.
    Blunt, Wilfred, *The Compleat Naturalist, A Life of Linnaeus*, Collins, 1971, p. 198.
25. Johns, op. cit., p. 361.
26. Mabey, Richard, *Flora Britannica*, Sinclair-Stevenson, 1996, p. 360.
27. *Collected Writings*, op. cit., p. 104.
28. Chancellor, Philip M., *Handbook of the Bach Flower Remedies*, C. W. Daniel, 1973, p. 72.
    Scheffer, Mechtild, *Bach Flower Therapy*, Thorsons, 1986, pp. 67-69.
29. Henslowe, op. cit.. p. 173.
30. Long, H.C. *Weeds of Arable Land*, Ministry of Agriculture and Fisheries, H.M.S.O., 1929, p. 92.
31. Loc. cit.
32. *Collected Writings*, op. cit., p. 166.
33. Ibid., p. 47.
34. Ibid., p. 169.
35. Ibid., p. 107.
36. Loc. cit.
37. Loc. cit.
38. Loc. cit.
39. Loc. cit.
40. Ibid., p. 79.
41. Loc. cit.
42. Ibid., p. 45.
43. Loc. cit.
44. Loc. cit.
45. Ibid., p. 69.
46. Ibid., p. 106.
47. Loc. cit.
48. Ibid., p. 84.
49. Ibid., p. 79.
50. Henslowe, op. cit., p. 198.

51. John Milton, Sonnet 16, *On His Blindness.*
52. *Collected Writings,* op. cit., p. 42.
53. Ibid., p. 106.
54. Ibid., p. 165.
55. Ibid., p. 54.
56. Brickell, Christopher and Sharman, Fay, *The Vanishing Garden,* John Murray, 1986, p. 4.
57. Ibid., p. 65.
58. Briggs, Roy W. *A Life of Ernest H. Wilson,* HMSO, 1993, p. 120.
59. Lauener, L. A., *The Introduction of Chinese Plants into Europe,* SPB Academic Publishing, 1996, p. 40.
60. *Collected Writing,* op. cit., p. 87.
61. Ibid., p. 79.
62. Loc. cit.
63. Ibid., p. 168.
64. Ibid., p. 38.
65. *Weeds of Arable Land,* op. cit..
66. *Collected Writings,* op. cit., p. 68.
67. Druce, G. C., *The Flora of Berkshire,* Clarendon Press, 1897, p. 417.
68. Bowen, H. J. M., *The Flora of Berkshire,* Holywell Press, Oxford, 1968, p. 166.
69. Roe, Captain R. G. B., *The Flora of Somerset,* 1981, p. 66.
70. *Collected Writings,* op. cit., p. 168.
71. Ibid., pp. 93 and 147.
72. Ibid., p. 168.
73. Loc. cit.
74. Ibid., p. 106.

CHAPTER 7. THE LAST OF THE FIRST TWELVE

1. Burrell, W. B., *British Plant Life,* Collins New Naturalist, 3rd edition 1962, p. 94.
2. Proctor, M., Yeo, P., and Lack, A., *The Natural History of Pollination,* Collins New Naturalist, 1996, pp. 325-328.
3. *Collected Writings of Edward Bach,* Bach Educational Programme, 1987, p. 66.
4. Tillyard, E. M. W., *The Elizabethan World Picture,* Chatto and Windus, 1943, p. 25.
5. *Collected Writing,* op. cit., p. 171.
6. Shakespeare, *Antony & Cleopatra,* V, ii, 88.
7. *Collected Writing,* op. cit., p. 108.
8. Ibid., p. 40-41.
9. Ibid., p. 109.
10. Ibid., pp. 66-67.
11. Ibid., p. 109.
12. Ibid., p. 67.
13. Ibid., p. 109.

14. Loc. cit.
15. Loc. cit.
16. Allan, Mea, *Darwin and his Flowers*, Faber and Faber, 1977, pp. 264-276.
17. Ridley, H. N., *Dispersal of Plants Throughout the World*, L. Reeve & Co., n.d. pp. 187, 189.
18. *Collected Writings*, op. cit., p. 138.
19. Grigson, Geoffrey, in *Nature in Britain*, Collins, 1946, p. 103-4.
20. *Collected Writings*, op. cit., p. 169.
21. Loc. cit.
22. Ibid., p. 107.
23. Loc. cit.
24. Ibid., p. 80.
25. Lousley, J.E. *Wild Flowers of Chalk and Limestone*, Collins New Naturalist, 1969, p. 31.
26. *Collected Writings*, op. cit., p. 107.
27. Ibid., p. 80.
28. Weeks, Nora, *The Medical Discoveries of Edward Bach Physician*, C. W. Daniel Co., 1940, p. 84.
29. Loc. cit.
30. *Collected Writings*, op. cit., p. 108.
31. Ibid., p. 77.
32. Ibid., pp. 36, 63.
33. Clarke Nuttall, G., *Wild Flowers as They Grow*, Waverley Book Company, n.d., vol. 4, pp. 184-185.
34. *Natural History of Pollination*, op. cit., p. 338.
35. Ridley, H.N. *Dispersal of Plants Throughout the World*, L. Reeve & Co., n.d. pp. 523.
36. Salisbury, Sir Edward, *Downs and Dunes their plant life and its environment*, G. Bell & Sons, 1952, p. 50, 67-68.

CHAPTER 8. THE ARCHITECTURE OF THE TWELVE HEALERS

1. *Collected Writings of Edward Bach*, Bach Educational Programme, 1987, pp. 95-98, 119, 157.
2. Ibid., p. 100.
3. Ibid., p. 80.
4. Weeks, Nora, *The Medical Discoveries of Edward Bach Physician*, C.W. Daniel Co., 1940, p. 44.
5. Thompson, D'arcy, *On Growth and Form*, Cambridge University Press, 1961 edition, p. 326.
6. *Collected Writings*, op. cit., pp. 77, 78, 80.
7. Ibid., p. 97.
8. Ibid., p. 96.
9. Loc. cit.
10. *Matthew* 10, *Luke* 12.

11. *Collected Writings,* op. cit., p. 97.
12. Ibid., p. 103.
13. Ibid., p. 104.
14. Ibid., pp. 97-98.

CHAPTER 9. THE FOUR HELPERS

1. Weeks, Nora, *The Medical Discoveries of Edward Bach Physician,* C.W. Daniel Co., 1940, p. 86.
2. *Collected Writings of Edward Bach,* Bach Educational Programme, 1987, pp. 84-6
3. Ibid., p. 68.
4. Ibid., p. 84.
5. Ibid., p. 83.
6. Loc. cit.
7. Loc. cit.
8. Ibid., p. 78.
9. Ibid., pp. 69-70.
10. Ibid., p. 70.
11. Loc. cit.
12. Loc. cit.
13. Loc. cit.
14. Loc. cit.
15. Loc. cit.
16. Mabey, Richard, *Flora Britannica,* Sinclair-Stevenson, 1996, p. 233.
17. *Collected Writings,* op. cit., p. 71.
18. Fritsch, F.E. & Salisbury, E.J., *Plant Form and Function,* G.Bell & Sons , 1938, pp. 149, 507-509.
    Huxley, Anthony, *Plant and Planet,* Allen Lane, 1974, pp. 229, 279.
    Professor Henslowe, *British Wild Flowers,* Society for Promoting Christian Knowledge, London, 1910, p. 70.
19. *Flora Britannica,* op. cit., pp. 230- 233.
    Henslowe, op. cit., p. 69-70.
20. *Collected Writings,* op. cit., p. 71.
21. Loc. cit.
22. Loc. cit.
23. Mitchell, Alan, *Trees of Britain,* Collins, 1996.
    Paterson, J.M., *Tree Wisdom,* Thorsons, 1996.
24. Edmund Spenser, *The Ruines of Rome,* Stanza 28, quoted by William Gilpin in *Remarks on Forest Scenery & Other Woodland Views, Edinburgh,* 1834, p. 68. Spenser compares ancient Rome and her past glories to a fallen oak, loved and honoured but almost dead.
25. Brimble, L.J.F., *Trees in Britain,* Macmillan, 1946, p. 263.
26. *Collected Writings,* op. cit., p. 44.
27. Tansley, A.G., *Oaks and Oakwoods,* Methuen, 1952.
28. *Collected Writings,* op. cit., p. 71.

29. Ibid., p. 72.
30. Ibid., p. 44.
31. Shakespeare, *Measure for Measure,* II, ii, 116.
32. *Collected Writings,* op. cit., p. 44.
33. Ibid., p. 73.
34. Ibid., p. 72.
35. Ibid., p. 56.
36. Ibid., p. 41.
37. *The Bach Remedy Newsletter,* June 1956, Vol. 2 No. 2, pp. 12-13.
38. *Collected Writings,* op. cit., p. 70.
39. *The Original Writings of Edward Bach,* C.W. Daniel Co., 1990, p. 92.
40. Barnard, J. & M., *The Healing Herbs of Edward Bach,* Ashgrove Press, new edition, 1995, pp. 25-26.
41. *Collected Writings,* op. cit., p. 74.
42. Ibid., pp. 60, 47.
43. Ibid., p. 74.
44. Weeks, N. and Bullen, V., *Bach Flower Remedies Illustrations and Preparation,* C.W.Daniel, 1964, p. 52.
45. *Collected Writings,* op. cit., p. 73.
46. Ibid., p. 56.
47. Ibid., pp. 73, 108.
48. Steve Johnson of Alaskan Flower Essence Project was among the first to use this term to designate essences made more by time and place than from any plant species growing in a locality.
49. Baring, Anne, & Cashford, Jules, *The Myth of the Goddess,* Viking Arkana, 1991, pp. 15-18.
50. Jones, Frances, *The Holy Wells of Wales,* Cardiff University Press, 1992 (1st published Aberystwyth, 1954), p. 1.
51. Ibid., p. 22.
52. *Collected Writings,* op. cit., p. 46.
53. Ibid., p. 73.
54. Ibid., p. 45.
55. Watkins, Alfred, *The Old Straight Track, its Mounds Beacons, Moats, Sites and Mark Stones,* Methuen, 1925, p. 59, *passim.*
56. Underwood, Guy, *The Pattern of the Past,* Museum Press, 1968.
57. Leather, Ella Mary, *The Folk-lore of Herefordshire,* Sidgwick & Jackson, 1912, pp. 10-14.
58. Sant, Jonathon, *Healing Wells of Herefordshire,* Moondial, 1994.
59. *Holy Wells of Wales,* op. cit., pp. 96-107.
60. *Folk-lore of Herefordshire,* op. cit., p. 13.
61. *Collected Writings,* op. cit., p. 73.
62. *Holy Wells of Wales,* op. cit., p. 195.
63. Bradney, Joseph, Alfred, *A History of Monmouthshire, The Hundred of Abergavenny,* Mitchell Hughes and Clarke, 1906, Academy Books, 1991. Volume 1, part 2a, pp. 158-159.
64. *Collected Writings,* op. cit., p. 73.
65. Loc. cit.

CHAPTER 10. THE SEVEN HELPERS

1. *Collected Writings of Edward Bach,* Bach Educational Programme, 1987, p. 61.
2. Weeks, Nora, *The Medical Discoveries of Edward Bach Physician,* C. W. Daniel Co., 1940, p. 101.
3. Ibid., p. 102.
4. *Collected Writings,* op. cit., p. 55.
5. Loc. cit.
6. Ibid., p. 56.
7. Darwin, Charles, *The Movements and Habits of Climbing Plants,* John Murray, Cheap edition, 1937, p. 137.
8. *Collected Writings,* op. cit., p. 55.
9. Ibid., p. 45.
10. Ibid., p. 56.
11. Loc. cit.
12. *Luke,* 6, 44.
13. *Collected Writings,* op. cit., p. 141.
14. Ibid., p. 55.
15. Ibid., p. 55.
16. Hepper, F. Nigel, *Illustrated Encyclopaedia of Bible Plants,* Inter Varsity Press, 1992.
17. *Book of Job,* 14, 7-9.
18. *Psalms* 128, 3-4.
19. Hepper, *Bible Plants,* op. cit., p. 114.
20. *Matthew,* 26, 36ff.
21. *Luke,* 24, 50.
22. Bauussen, Olivier and Chibois, Jacques, *Olive Oil,* Flammarion, 2000, p. 11.
23. *Collected Writings,* op. cit., p. 39.
24. Ibid., p. 56.
25. Loc. cit.
26. Ibid., p. 55.
27. *Medical Discoveries,* op. cit., p. 113.
28. Plues, Margaret, *British Grasses,* L. Reeve, 1867, p. 223.
29. Ibid., p. 224.
30. Parnell, Richard, *The Grasses of Britain,* William Blackwood, 1845.
31. *Collected Writings,* op. cit., p. 56.
32. Ibid., p. 39.
33. Loc. cit.
34. Chancellor, Philip, *Handbook of the Bach Flower Remedies,* C. W. Daniel Co., 1971, p. 217.
35. *Medical Discoveries,* op. cit., pp. 101-102.
36. *Collected Writings,* op. cit., p. 99.

CHAPTER 11. THE FIRST OF THE SECOND NINETEEN

1. Weeks, Nora, *The Medical Discoveries of Edward Bach Physician*, C.W. Daniel Co., 1940, p. 111 ff.
2. Ibid., p. 113.
3. Ibid., p. 114.
4. *Collected Writings of Edward Bach*, Bach Educational Programme, 1987, p. 37.
5. Ibid., p. 8.
6. Loc. cit.
7. Hadfield, Miles, *British Trees, a guide for everyman*, J. M. Dent, 1957, p. 328.
8. *Collected Writing*, op. cit., p. 117.
9. Ibid. p. 43.
10. Loc. cit.
11. Druce, G. C., *The Flora of Berkshire*, Clarendon Press, 1897, p. 441.
12. Holbrook, A.W., *Dictionary of British Wayside Trees*, Country Life, 1936, p. 49.
13. Clouston, Brian & Stansfield, Kathy, *After the Elm . . .*, Heinemann, 1979, p. 10.
14. Hadfield, *British Trees*, op. cit., p. 227.
15. *After the Elm . . .* op. cit., p. 66.
16. By Monsieur Gérard Wolf of Paris.
17. Ball, Stefan, *Flower Remedies*, Blitz, 1996, p. 55.
18. Gilpin, William, *Remarks on Forest Scenery and Other Woodland Views*, new edition, Edinburgh, 1834, Vol. 1, p. 90.
19. *Medical Discoveries*, op. cit., p. 114.
20. *Collected Writing*, op. cit., p. 37.
21. Loc. cit.
22. Chancellor, Philip M., *Handbook of the Bach Flower Remedies*, C. W. Daniel, 1973, p. 43.
23. Gilpin, *Remarks on Forest Scenery . . .* op. cit., p. 68.
24. Johns, Rev. C. A., *British Trees and Shrubs*, George Routledge, n.d., p. 99.
25. Folkard, Richard, *Plant Lore, Legends and Lyrics*, Sampson Low, 1884, passim.
26. Step, Edward, *Wayside and Woodland Trees*, Frederick Warne, n.d., p. 58.
27. Johns, op. cit., p. 100.
28. *Collected Writing*, op. cit., p. 37.

CHAPTER 12. THE BOILING METHOD

1. *Collected Writings of Edward Bach*, Bach Educational Programme, 1987, pp. 47-48.
2. Weeks, Nora, *The Medical Discoveries of Edward Bach Physician*, C.W. Daniel Co., 1940, p. 115.
3. *Collected Writings*, op. cit., p. 48.
4. Ibid., p. 23.
5. *Medical Discoveries*, op. cit., p. 114.
6. *Collected Writings*, op. cit., p. 112.

CHAPTER 13. HOLDING BACK FROM INVOLVEMENT IN LIFE

1. *Collected Writings of Edward Bach,* Bach Educational Programme, 1987, p. 40.
2. Ibid., p. 128.
3. Ibid., pp. 121-2.
4. Ibid., p. 129.
5. Weeks, Nora, *The Medical Discoveries of Edward Bach Physician,* C.W. Daniel Co., 1940, p. 21-22.
6. Subtitle of *Heal Thyself.*
7. *Collected Writings,* op. cit., p. 128.
8. Loc. cit.
9. Ibid., p. 40.
10. Ibid., p. 42.
11. Loc. cit.
12. Loc. cit.
13. Evelyn, Sir John, *Silva, or A discourse of Forest Trees and the Propagation of Timber in His Majesty's Dominions,* with notes by A. Hunter (second Hunter edition) 1786, Vol: 1, p. 280.
14. Boulger, G. S. *Familiar Trees,* Cassel & Co., n.d., vol. 3, p. 137.
15. Hadfield, Miles, B*ritish Trees,* J .M. Dent, p. 49.
16. Wordsworth, William in *Description of Scenery of the Lakes,* quoted by Rev. C. A. Johns, *British Trees,* George Routledge, n.d., p. 229.
17. Russ Collins, www.beyond.fr/flora/larch.html
18. Johns, Rev. C. A., *British Trees and Shrubs,* George Routledge, n.d., p. 231.
19. *Collected Writings,* op. cit., p. 38.
20. Loc. cit.
21. Clarke Nuttall, G., *Trees and How they Grow,* Waverley Book Company, n.d., p. 49.
22. Quoted by Johns, *British Trees and Shrubs,* George Routledge, n.d., p. 137.
23. Wilks, J. H., *Trees of the British Isles in History and Legend,* Frederick Muller, 1972.
    Patterson, Jacqueline M., *Tree Wisdom,* Thorsons, 1996.
    Neither book even mentions Hornbeam by name.
24. Buxton, Edward North, *Epping Forest,* Stanford, 1911, p. 115.
25. Ridley, E. N., *Dispersal of Plants Throughout the World,* L.Reeve, n.d., pp. 72, 96.
26. *Collected Writings,* op. cit., p. 38.

CHAPTER 14. FINDING FAULT WITH THE WORLD AROUND US

1. Weeks, Nora, *The Medical Discoveries of Edward Bach Physician,* C.W. Daniel Co., 1940, p. 114.
2. *Collected Writings of Edward Bach,* Bach Educational Programme, 1987, p. 43.
3. *Medical Discoveries,* p. 114.
4. *Collected Writings,* op. cit., p. 43.
5. Loc. cit.

6. Fuller, quoted by Archie Miles, *Silva, The Tree in Britain*, Ebury Press, 1999, p. 191.
7. *Ezekiel*, 17, 5-6.
8. Johns, Rev. C. A., *British Trees and Shrubs*, George Routledge, n.d., p. 172.
9. Porter, Roy, *The Greatest Benefit of Mankind*, Harper Collins, 1997, p. 270.
10. Chancellor, Philip, *Handbook of the Bach Flower Remedies*, C. W. Daniel, 1971, p. 228.
11. *Collected Writings*, op. cit., p. 45.
12. Loc. cit.
13. Katz, Richard and Kaminski, Patricia, *Flower Essence Repertory, A comprehensive guide to North American and English Flower Essences for emotional and spiritual well-being*, 1994, p. 299.
14. *Medical Discoveries*, p. 12.
15. *Collected Writings*, op. cit., p. 45.
16. Step, Edward, *Wayside and Woodland Trees*, Frederick Warne & Co., n.d., p. 24.
17. Boulger, G. S. *Familiar Trees*, Cassel & Co., n.d., vol. 3, p. 111.
18. Ibid., p. 110.
19. Mitchell, Alan, *Trees of Britain*, Collins, 1996, p. 229.

CHAPTER 15. WHAT HAS GOT INTO YOU?

1. *Collected Writings*, op. cit., p. 44.
2. Loc. cit.
3. Wingate, Peter, *The Penguin Medical Encyclopaedia*, Penguin Books, 1972, p. 404.
4. *Collected Writings*, op. cit., p. 44.
5. Loc. cit.
6. Ibid., pp. 151, 205ff.
7. Ibid., p. 192.
8. Ibid., p. 161.
9. Ibid., p. 2.
10. Ibid., p. 44.
11. *Medical Discoveries*, op. cit., pp. 115-117.
12. *Medical Discoveries*, op. cit., p. 116.
13. *Collected Writings*, op. cit., p. 42.
14. Loc. cit.
15. Ibid., p. 43.
16. Quoted by Mrs Grieve *A Modern Herbal*, Jonathan Cape, 1977, p. 844.
17. Quoted by Boulger, *Familiar Trees*, Vol. 1, p. 88.
18. Mrs Grieve, op. cit., p. 842.
19. Miles, Archie, *Silva, The Tree in Britain*, Ebury Press, 1999, p. 265.
20. Baring, Anne, & Cashford, Jules, *The Myth of the Goddess*, Viking Arkana, 1991, p. 321.
21. Ibid., p. 326.
22. Johns, *British Trees*, op. cit., p. 146.

23. Evelyn, Sir John, *Silva, or A discourse of Forest Trees and the Propagation of Timber in His Majesty's Dominions,* with notes by A. Hunter (second Hunter edition) 1786, Vol: 1, p. 169. Evelyn quotes Virgil and Catullus, Latin poets who refer to this custom.

24. Moldenke, H. N. & A. L., *Plants of the Bible,* Chronica Botanica, 1952, p. 119.

25. Weeks, Nora and Bullen, Victor, *Bach Flower Remedies Illustration & Preparation,* C. W. Daniel, 1964, p. 72.

26. Chancellor, op. cit., p. 201.

27. Clarke Nuttall, G., *Trees and How they Grow,* Waverley Book Company, n.d., p. 90.

28. Ridley, H.N. *Dispersal of Plants Throughout the World,* L. Reeve & Co., n.d. p. 379.

29. Chancellor, op. cit., p. 201.

30. Loc. cit.

31. Mrs Grieve, op. cit., p. 844.

32. Parkinson, John, *Paridisi in Sole Paradisus in Terrestris,* reprinted from the edition of 1629, Methuren & Co., 1904, p. 594.

33. Howard, A. L., in *Nature in Britain,* Collins, 1946, p. 39.

34. Evelyn's, *Silva,* op. cit., Vol: 1, p. 168.

35. *Collected Writings,* op. cit., pp. 41-42.

36. Ibid., p. 42.

37. Loc. cit.

38. Chancellor, op. cit., p. 107.

39. Loc. cit.

40. Damasio, Antonio, *The Feeling of What Happens,* Heinemann, 1999, p. 51.

41. Ibid., p. 54.

42. Ibid., p. 56.

43. Johns, *British Trees,* op. cit., p. 116.

44. Briggs, D. & Walters, S. M., *Plant Variation and Evolution,* Cambridge University Press, Second edition 1984, p. 39.

45. Professor Henslowe, quoted by Mrs Grieve, op. cit., p. 406.

46. Darwin, Charles, *The Movements & Habits of Climbing Plants,* John Murray, 1937, p. 183ff.

47. Mabey, Richard, *Flora Britannica,* Sinclair Stephenson, 1996, p. 251.

48. Ibid., p. 248.

49. Williamson, John, *The Oak King, The Holly King and the Unicorn,* Harper Row, 1986, p. 58ff.

50. Graves, Robert, *The White Goddess,* Faber, 1961, 180.

51. See Folkard, Richard, *Plant Lore, Legends and Lyrics,* Sampson Low, 1884, p. 40 ff. *et passim.*

52. Chancellor, op. cit., p. 47.

53. Vickery, Roy, *Oxford Dictionary of Plant Lore,* Oxford University Press, 1995, p. 139.

54. Weeks and Bullen, op. cit. p. 76.

55. Chancellor, op. cit., p. 107.

CHAPTER 16. THE COMING OF THE LIGHT

1. *Collected Writings of Edward Bach*, Bach Educational Programme, 1987, p. 171.
2. Ibid., p. 156.
3. Ibid., pp. 96ff., 161ff.

CHAPTER 17. MAKING THE PATTERN, BREAKING THE PATTERN

1. Emboden, William A., *Leonardo da Vinci on Plants and Gardens*, Christopher Helm, 1987, p. 77.
2. *Collected Writings of Edward Bach*, Bach Educational Programme, 1987, p. 43.
3. Loc. cit.
4. Parkinson, John, *Paridisi in Sole Paradisus in Terrestris*, reprinted from the edition of 1629, Methuren & Co., 1904, p. 136.
5. See *Patterns of Life Force*, Julian Barnard, Bach Educational Programme, 1986, p. 43 *et passim*.
6. *The Bach Remedy Newsletter*, December 1958, p. 93.
7. *Collected Writings*, op. cit., p. 40.
8. Loc. cit.
9. For a full description of conkers and conker fights see: Mabey, Richard, *Flora Britannica*, Sinclair Stephenson, 1996, pp. 260-64.
10. Monsieur Gérard Wolf of Paris was the first person to make this observation to me.
11. *Collected Writings*, op. cit., p. 40.
12. Ibid., pp. 39-40.
13. Hadfield, Miles, *British Trees, a guide for everyman*, J. M. Dent, 1957, p. 396.
14. *Collected Writings*, op. cit., p. 37.
15. *The Bach Remedy Newsletter*, June 1951, Vol. 1, No. 6, p. 37.
16. Loc. cit.
17. Loc. cit.
18. *Collected Writings*, op. cit., p. 37.
19. Ibid., p. 45.
20. Ibid., p. 8.
21. Weeks, Nora, *The Medical Discoveries of Edward Bach Physician*, C. W. Daniel Co., 1973, pp. 114-116.
22. *Collected Writings*, op. cit., p. 9.
23. Ibid., p. 93.
24. Ibid., pp. 26-27.
25. Ibid., p. 21
26. Chancellor, Philip M., *Handbook of the Bach Flower Remedies*, C. W. Daniel, 1973, Preface.
27. Scheffer, Mechtild, *Bach Flower Therapy*, Thorsons, 1986, Introduction.
28. Ibid., p. 135.
29. Ibid., p. 136.

30. Katz, Richard and Kaminski, Patricia, *Flower Essence Repertory, A comprehensive guide to North American and English Flower Essences for emotional and spiritual well-being,* 1994, p. 353.
31. *Medical Discoveries* op. cit., p. 9.
32. *Collected Writings,* op. cit., p. 139.
33. Ibid., p. 97.
34. Ibid., p. 98.
35. Ibid., pp. 42-3.
36. Mitchell, Alan, F. *Conifers,* Forestry Commission Booklet No. 15, H.M.S.O., p. 4.
37. Brimble, L.J.F., *Trees in Britain,* Macmillan, 1946, pp. 40, 63.
    Proctor, M., Yeo, P., and Lack, A., *The Natural History of Pollination,* Collins New Naturalist, 1996, pp. 273-4.
38. Hadfield, Miles, *British Trees, a guide for everyman,* J. M. Dent, 1957, p. 68.
    Ridley, E. N., *Dispersal of Plants Throughout the World,* L. Reeve, n.d., p. 72.
39. Johns, Rev. C. A., *British Trees and Shrubs,* George Routledge, n.d., p. 210.
40. Mabey, Richard, *Flora Britannica,* Sinclair Stephenson, 1996, p. 23.
41. Watkins, Alfred, *The Old Straight Track, its Mounds Beacons, Moats, Sites and Mark Stones,* Methuen, 1925, p. 62, *passim.*
42. Chancellor, op. cit., p. 111.
    The Bach Remedy Newsletter, June 1954, No. 18, pp. 133-135.
43. Grieve, Mrs M., *A Modern Herbal,* Jonathan Cape, 1977, p. 409.
44. Lubbock, Sir John, *British Wild Flowers considered in relation to insects,* Macmillan & Co. 1893, p. 118.
45. The same point is made by J. E. Taylor in *Flowers their origin, shapes, perfumes and colours,* W. H. Allen, n.d., p. 220.
46. Clarke Nuttall, G., *Wild Flowers as They Grow,* Waverley Book Company, n.d. vol. 3, p. 38.
47. Ibid., p. 40.
48. Professor Henslowe, *British Wild Flowers,* Society for Promoting Christian Knowledge, London, 1910, p. 128.
49. Killick, Perry & Woodell, *The Flora of Oxfordshire,* Pisces Publications, 1998.
50. *Collected Writings,* op. cit., p. 39.

CHAPTER 18. APATHY, DEPRESSION AND DESPAIR

1. There are very many versions of Grimms' Fairy Tales, I have worked from *Household Tales by the Brothers Grimm,* Eyre & Spottiswoode, 1946, p. 204-6.
2. *The Court of Flora, Les Fleurs Animées,* Introduction by Peter A. Wick, George Braziller, New York, 1981.
3. *Collected Writings of Edward Bach,* Bach Educational Programme, 1987, p. 39.
4. Lang, David C., *The Complete Book of British Berries,* Threshold Books, 1987, p. 60.
5. Mabey, Richard, *Flora Britannica,* Sinclair Stephenson, 1996, p. 193.
6. Genders, Roy, *The Scented Wildflowers of Britian,* Collins, 1971, p. 96.

7. Rowley, G. D. *Germination in Rosa Canina*, American Rose Annual 1956.

8. Evelyn, Sir John, *Silva, or A discourse of Forest Trees and the Propagation of Timber in His Majesty's Dominions*, with notes by A. Hunter (second Hunter edition) 1786, vol. 1, p. 49.

9. Johns, Rev. C A. *Flowers of the Field*, Society for Promoting Christian Knowledge, London, 1899, p. 65.

10. *Collected Writings*, op. cit., p. 40.

11. H. C. Long, *Weeds of Arable Land*, H.M.S.O., Ministry of Agriculture & Fisheries, 1929, p. 45.

12. Ibid., p. 14.

13. *Destruction of Yellow Charlock*, Ministry of Agriculture & Fisheries Advisory leaflet, 1946.

14. Hulme, F. E., *Familiar Wild Flowers*, vol. 3, Cassell & Co., 1910, p. 125.

15. Sinclair, George, *Hortus Gramineus Woburnensis*, 4th Edition with *The Weeds of Agriculture* added, Ridgways, 1852, p. 336.

16. *Weeds of Arable Land*, op. cit., p. 20.

17. Weeks and Bullen, *Bach Flower Remedies Illustration & Preparation*, C. W. Daniel Co., 1964, pp. 86-92.

18. Katz, Richard and Kaminski, Patricia, *Flower Essence Repertory, A comprehensive guide to North American and English Flower Essences for emotional and spiritual well-being*, 1994, p. 346.
    Scheffer, Mechtild, *Bach Flower Therapy*, Thorsons, 1986, p. 124.

19. Katz, Richard and Kaminski, Patricia, *Flower Essence Repertory*, 1994, p. 346.

20. *Collected Writings*, op. cit., p. 40.

21. Loc. cit.

22. Ibid., p. 43.

23. Weeks, Nora, *The Medical Discoveries of Edward Bach Physician*, C. W. Daniel Co., 1973, p. 116.

24. *Collected Writings*, op. cit., p. 43.

25. See George Macdonald's *Curdie and the Princess*

26. Chancellor, Philip M., *Handbook of the Bach Flower Remedies*, C. W. Daniel, 1973, p. 185.

27. Figuier, Louis, *The Vegetable World*, Chapman & Hall, 1867, p. 358.

28. Pakenham, Thomas, *Meetings with Remarkable Trees*, Weidenfeld & Nicolson, 1996, pp. 168-9.

29. Johns, Rev. C. A., *British Trees and Shrubs*, George Routledge, n.d., p. 105.

30. *Flora Britannica*, op. cit., p. 84.

31. Weeks and Bullen, *Bach Flower Remedies*, op. cit., p. 90.

32. Chancellor, op. cit., p. 186.

CHAPTER 19. THE PATTERN IN PRACTICE

1. *Collected Writings of Edward Bach*, Bach Educational Programme, 1987, p. 24.
2. Loc. cit.
3. *Collected Writings*, op. cit., p. 23.
4. In May 1987 Jean Addison sent me a picture combining seven chakras with seven groups and seven colours as she supposed Dr Bach had done. The colours, which derived from the poster produced by the Bach Centre, were those selected by Dr Bach for each of the groups.
   In 1998 Philip Salmon and Anna Jeoffroy published *Dr Bach's Remedies and the Chakras* which forms the basis of their teaching programme Energy Works.
5. *Collected Writings*, op. cit., p. 162.
6. Ibid., pp. 77-78.
7. Ibid., pp. 16-17.
8. Loc. cit.
9. See Lilly, Sue, *Healing with Astrology*, Capall Bann, 2002.
10. Ibid., p. 16.
11. Bach, Edward, *The Twelve Healers & Other Remedies*, C. W. Daniel Company Ltd, 1968.
12. Based upon the volume of remedies sold by Healing Herbs Ltd. There are interesting variations between different countries and between different years.
13. *Collected Writings*, op. cit., pp. 55-6.
14. Ibid., p. 104.
15. Ibid., p. 68.
16. Ibid., p. 102.
17. Ibid., p. 154.
18. Loc. cit.
19. Ibid., p. 156.
20. Ibid., p. 33.
21. Ibid., p. 61.

Index

[Page references in *italics* refer to illustrations,
and in **bold** to the major account of the subject.]